Breakthrough Leadership

ACHIEVING ORGANIZATIONAL ALIGNMENT THROUGH HOSHIN PLANNING

Mara Minerva Melum and Casey Collett

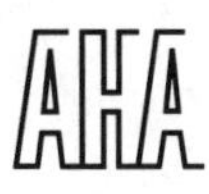

AHA books are published by American Hospital Publishing, Inc., an American Hospital Association company

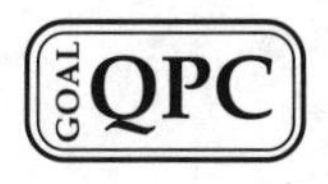

The views expressed in this publication are strictly those of the authors and do not necessarily represent official positions of the American Hospital Association or GOAL/QPC.

Library of Congress Cataloging-in-Publication Data

Melum, Mara Minerva.
Breakthrough leadership : achieving organizational alignment through hoshin planning / Mara Minerva Melum, Casey Collett.
p. cm.
Includes bibliographical references and index.
ISBN 1-55648-133-0
1. Medical care—Quality control. 2. Health facilities—Quality control. 3. Total quality management. I. Collett, Casey. II. Title. III. Title: Hoshin planning.
[DNLM: 1. Total Quality Management—methods. 2. Delivery of Health Care—organization & administration—United States. 3. Health Facilities—organization & administration—United States. 4. Organizational Innovation. 5. Health Planning—United States. W 84 AA1 M56b 1995]
RA399.A1M45 1995
362.1'068'5—dc20
DNLM/DLC
for Library of Congress

94-48029
CIP

AHA Catalog no. 169108
GOAL/QPC Catalog no. 4160P

Printed in the USA

AHA is a service mark of the American Hospital Association used under license by American Hospital Publishing, Inc.

Text set in Century Textbook
3M—04/95—0398

Audrey Kaufman, Senior Editor
Nancy Charpentier, Editor
Peggy DuMais, Production Coordinator
Cheryl Kusek, Cover Designer
Marcia Bottoms, Executive Editor
Brian Schenk, Books Division Director

We dedicate this book
to our families:

to our husbands, Eric and Dennis

to our children,
Daniel and Arielle
and
Aaron, Liese, Miriam, and Jordan

to our brothers and sister,
Frank, Ellen, and Gene

and to our parents,
Daniel and Phyllis Minerva
and
Edward and Pauline Teufert

We are thankful beyond words for you –
the most important focus in our lives.

Contents

List of Figures

About the Authors

Mara Melum is president of the Minerva Leadership Institute, Inc., a management consulting and applied research company based in St. Paul, Minnesota. The company specializes in leadership, quality management, and strategic planning.

Ms. Melum serves as coach to CEOs, senior executives, and boards of trustees, assisting them to focus and align the organization, continuously improve quality, and exceed customer expectations. She also assists communities in improving health outcomes and health status. Ms. Melum has been a pioneer in working to advance the state of the art of strategic planning, and to transfer industrial quality management approaches to service businesses.

Ms. Melum has extensive experience both in top organizational leadership positions and as a coach and consultant. She has served as special consultant to the 3M Corporation, senior vice-president of HealthOne Corporation, vice-president of Metropolitan Medical Center, vice-president of the Minnesota Hospital Association and Association of Homes for the Aging, and consultant and policy analyst at InterStudy.

Ms. Melum is an administrative board member for the Minnesota Quality Award. She has also served as lead senior examiner for the Minnesota Quality Award and chairperson of the Northeast Council for Quality. She is a member of the GOAL/QPC health care application research committee, is chairperson of the GOAL/QPC Task Force on the Integration of TQM and Outcomes Management, and is vice-chairperson of the Northeast Metro Technical College Advisory Board. Ms. Melum is coauthor of numerous books and articles, including the AHA books *Total Quality Management: The Health Care Pioneers* and *The Changing Role of the Hospital: Options for the Future.*

Mara Melum holds an MPA degree from the Maxwell School at Syracuse University and a BA degree, with honors, from the Woodrow Wilson School at Princeton University.

Casey Collett, PhD, is president of Collett & Associates, an international management and consulting firm specializing in quality systems and strategic planning. For six of her ten years at Hewlett-Packard Company, Dr. Collett developed, used, and taught hoshin planning. In her own practice and as an affiliate of GOAL/QPC, Dr. Collett consults and trains across a broad client base, which includes organizations in health care, education, government, and industry.

Casey Collett received her PhD, MS, and BS degrees from Purdue University and has taught courses in organizational behavior in the Department of Management at Oregon State University. She has coauthored several GOAL/QPC publications, including two texts on the topic of daily management, research reports on process management and TQM in higher education, and a facilitator's guide for implementing TQM in K–12 education. Her current research interests include practical ways to manage processes and the spiritual basis of quality management.

Contributors

Jon T. Beste is vice-president of planning, SSM-Ministry Corporation, and CEO, SSM-Diversified Health Services. SSM-Ministry Corporation, in Milwaukee, is a Wisconsin-based multihospital system and the parent corporation of SSM-Diversified Health Services, a shared services entity. In his role within SSM-MC, Mr. Beste is responsible for business planning and development activities that promote the establishment of regionally integrated health care delivery networks in Wisconsin. As CEO of SSM-DHS, he is responsible for all shared services initiatives, including group purchasing.

Lisa Boisvert is a member of the teaching/consulting faculty at GOAL/QPC and the director of the Instructional Services Division. She has previously held the positions of director of new product development and coordinator of TQM research for GOAL/QPC. Her previous experience includes directing community-based human service programs and designing and delivering adult basic education curricula. She is a contributing author to *Putting the "T" in Health Care TQM/A Model for Integrated TQM: Clinical Care and Operations,* published by GOAL/QPC (1992), coauthor of the *Coaches Guide to The Memory Jogger™ II,* published by GOAL/QPC (1995), and author of several articles related to the application of TQM to health care and other environments.

Sister M. Lois Bush, BSN, MSN, MBA, is president and CEO of Sisters of the Sorrowful Mother Ministry Corporation. Previously she was the Assistant Provincial of the Congregation and was responsible for the redesign of the Orders hospitals from independent facilities to a health care system. This was preceded by fourteen years in progressive nursing and nursing leadership positions within the Congregations hospitals.

Geoffrey Crabtree is director, strategic planning and market services, Southwest Texas Methodist Hospital, in San Antonio. He is on the advisors board of the Alliance for Healthcare Strategy and Marketing. He is also a member of the American Marketing Association, American Society for Hospital Marketing, and American Society for Health Care Marketing and Public Relations of the American Hospital Association. Mr. Crabtree is a presenter and speaker on customer-focused planning in health care (hoshin planning) regionally and nationally.

Lois Gold, MA, MEd, EdD, is vice-president Citibank, N.A, Citicorp. Previously she was Americas field operations quality manager, medical products group, Hewlett-Packard. She was responsible for implementing quality systems for America's (U.S., Canada, and Latin America) sales, services, marketing center, field support center, and health care information systems group. While working in corporate quality (Hewlett-Packard), she developed the internal paper: "Implementing Total Quality Control at Hewlett-Packard."

Brad Harrington, MA, is group quality manager, Hewlett-Packard Medical Products Group. Mr. Harrington has been with Hewlett-Packard since 1980 and has held numerous management positions in quality and human resources in the U.S. and in Europe. During this time, he has designed and delivered training in areas of career development, total quality management, and organizational change. Mr. Harrington is also an acting contributor to the Center for Quality Management (CQM) where he has served on the editorial board of the *CQM Journal*, been a member of the CQM steering committee, and has chaired the CQM networking committee.

Dona Hotopp, MA, is director, health care services, GOAL/QPC. She is also director, health care application research committee, whose 35 members from health care and consulting organizations develop leading-edge quality management methodologies in health care. Ms. Hotopp codeveloped and coteaches GOAL/QPC's introductory and advanced TQM in health care courses and has consulted and trained for five years in TQM for academic medical centers, hospitals, associations, and nursing homes. She is coauthor and coeditor of *Putting the "T" in TQM in Health Care* and GOAL/QPC's *Integrated Planning Research Report.* Since opening GOAL/QPC's Pittsburgh office in 1992, Ms. Hotopp has consulted with local manufacturing, education, and service organizations in total quality and strategic planning and has researched TQM methods in Japan. She formerly served as the executive director of a labor management committee in New York state.

Gerry Kaminski, DA, is vice-president of total quality management at Bethesda, Inc., Cincinnati, Ohio. Dr. Kaminski has provided leadership for the corporationwide implementation of total quality management at Bethesda since 1988. She has presented at national meetings on a variety of TQM-related topics such as overall implementation strategies, quality function deployment, and hoshin planning. Dr. Kaminski's previous work experience includes 18 years in higher education plus 5 years of health care experience as a medical technologist. She is a member of the American Society for Quality Control, the Association for Quality and Participation, and the GOAL/QPC health care application research committee.

Owen McNally, MBA, MSW, is director of total quality management at Our Lady of Lourdes Medical Center in Camden, New Jersey. His responsibilities include designing and implementing quality management initiatives. Mr. McNally has spoken at a number of quality conferences on the integration of strategic and hoshin planning. He previously served as the executive vice-president of a municipal engineering firm, a township manager, and the administrator of a social service organization. Mr. McNally is a member of the American Society for Quality Control, the Association for Quality and Participation, the GOAL/QPC health care application research committee, and the Advisory Board of PACE (Philadelphia Area Council on Excellence).

Louis E. Monteforte, Sr., MS, is transmission quality planning director for AT&T Network Systems in Morristown, New Jersey. Mr. Monteforte began his AT&T career in June 1979 at AT&T Bell Laboratories in Whippany, New Jersey, as a member of the technical staff. In July 1986, he became department chief of component engineering at North Carolina Works. In 1988, he returned to Whippany, where he was named supervisor of the SLC® Product Design Group.

Since November 1990, Mr. Monteforte has assumed the responsibility of developing quality strategies for AT&T's Transmission Systems Business Unit (TSBU). As the manager of transmission quality planning, he led the TSBU team that prepared the Malcolm Baldrige National Quality Award application and implemented a total quality management system in the TSBU. Mr. Monteforte earned a bachelor of science degree in mechanical engineering from Manhattan College in 1979 and a master of science degree in mechanical engineering from Rutgers University in 1981.

Foreword

From Gail L. Warden (CEO and president, Henry Ford Health System, Detroit, Michigan)

As leaders in health care, we are faced with particularly challenging times. We must balance the need for economic discipline with our commitment to continually improve the quality of the services we provide. Major changes in the health care environment – including reimbursement changes, managed care growth, and delivery system consolidation – require that, now more than ever, health care organizations plan a course of action that will ensure the survival of the organization and enable it to fulfill its mission. This book helps leaders plan and successfully implement such a course of action.

Strategic thinking is the essence of strategic planning. It is the type of thinking that determines the future direction of the organization. It enables the senior management team to define and clarify the organization's future strategic profile. Insights gained through strategic thinking are then translated into organizational reality with strategic planning. The process of strategic planning utilizes many tools and techniques, but it never replaces the need for strategic thinking and entrepreneurial risk taking. Hoshin planning, the subject of this book, builds on a strong foundation of strategic thinking – thinking about what is the most important focus for the organization to break through to new heights of success. As health care leaders, we must challenge ourselves to maximize the benefits of integrated health care systems and create internal environments empowered to move these systems forward to meet the health care needs of our nation.

The success of an integrated health care system depends on a number of factors, such as organizational structures, policy decisions, and managerial actions. It also depends on the development of a common whole. By adopting the concepts of total quality management (TQM), an organization can begin the cultural change needed for integration and internal strategic alignment. The fundamental principles of TQM are customer focus, process knowledge, use of data, and methods for designing and testing change. The organization that understands and applies these principles is able to move systematically and efficiently closer and closer to its vision. Strategic planning and quality planning are then united. The organization, as a whole, can focus on identifying the most critical goals and align all parts of the system toward achieving them. This is the essence of hoshin planning.

Leaders must remember that the hoshin planning process is a two-way street requiring a vision from the top and continuous dialogue with operations to understand the underlying processes and complexities of implementation. The vision must be translated into long- and short-term goals specifically related to the key processes. Knowledge of the linkage between customer requirements and the key processes is critical. Both development and implementation of the plan must include a broad cross section of employees. Communication in all directions is vital. The concepts of system and a system vision are not universally understood in an integrated health system, particularly at the level where care is provided to patients and their families. To bridge the gap, a collaborative planning process must link the vision to operations.

In this book, Mara Melum and Casey Collett communicate in a practical manner the value of hoshin planning and identify the valuable lessons learned by organizations that utilize this methodology. Strategic thinking and planning are critical in an era of change and reform. To survive and succeed, we must create and deploy a vision that aligns our future course with our customers' needs and expectations. It is a challenge and an opportunity vital to our future. Hoshin planning can help us to break through to new heights of success as we face this challenge–and build on the exciting opportunity to focus the power of our organizations and our people on what is most important.

From Robert King (executive director, GOAL/QPC, Methuen, Massachusetts)

It is a pleasure to have the opportunity to write a foreword to this book–both because the subject is so important to American industry today and because the book will help executives identify an important key to their success in the coming decade. In these few remarks, I will try to lend some credence to the importance of hoshin management [hoshin planning], speak of its place in the total quality scheme, and emphasize what we have learned to date about the keys to success.

Hoshin is truly a powerful tool. In 1988, when Ford Motor Company CEO Don Petersen and director of quality Jim Bakkan were retiring and the quality planning group was putting together a quality plan for the new leadership, I was called in to Ford headquarters to advise a benchmarking team headed to Japan. One of the questions I insisted they ask every company they visited was, "What do you know about *hoshin kanri*?"–a Japanese system used to focus improvement efforts. One of the team's visits was to Honda headquarters. For three hours they quizzed Honda vice-presidents on quality staffing and allocation of resources to achieve quality. As the time neared a close, they asked, "What do you know about *hoshin kanri?*" "Well, that is the most important thing we do!" came back the reply. In fact, Ford now also sees hoshin kanri as a key to its success in becoming the largest auto company in the United States by the end of the decade–with the best quality of any auto company in the world.

Ford is not the first auto company to choose hoshin to achieve a leadership position. In the early 1980s, Toyota was tied with Nissan for domestic auto business in Japan. Each had about 25 percent. Toyota decided to develop a superior cross-functional hoshin system and was able to achieve and maintain 40 percent domestic auto market share.

In the early 1990s in the United States, we have seen many other dramatic successes. In a tough computer market, one company used hoshin to move from number 3 to number 2 and to establish a leadership role in laser technology. A hospital in mid-America was struggling with costs related to declining bed utilization as the health care practice shifted from inpatient to day surgery. Problems developed as the hospital continued to spend its budget while falling short on income. A turn to hoshin not only brought staffing in line with costs, but soon made the hospital the dominant health care player in what had been a very competitive health care marketplace.

A U.S. consumer products company tried hoshin in one division and saved so much money the second year that the division was reluctant to tell top management. The division was afraid of criticism for how inefficient it must have been in the past!

Many U.S. companies keep their hoshin activity a closely guarded secret because they do not want their competition to catch on to their key to success. So it is particularly timely that this text will lay bare some of the "secrets" of hoshin for American executives in general and for health care executives in particular.

We cannot understand hoshin without knowing its place in total quality. We cannot succeed at hoshin without having its prerequisites in place. So we turn now to a brief look at hoshin's place in total quality management.

One of the problems total quality management has faced in the United States is a watering down by opportunists who, at best, have a superficial understanding of the concept. Dr. Naguchi, the executive director of the Japanese Union of Scientists and Engineers (JUSE), has given one of the best definitions of TQM. "Total quality", he says, "is all employees in all departments, every day, improving or maintaining quality, cost, yield, procedures, and systems to give customers products and services that are most economical and best qualified to meet customers' needs."

This total quality represents a fundamental departure from the Taylor model of management developed at the beginning of this century. In Taylor's view, not every supervisor was smart enough to figure out the best way to do a job. So for him the key to business success was to have an engineer design the job and then to get operations to carry out the job the way the engineer had set it up. This led to a departmentalized approach.

The transition from a Taylor-based organization to a TQM organization takes an average of five years once the groundwork has been laid. We refer to the transition plan as the *customer-driven master plan* to keep the focus that serving the customer better is one of the reasons for the change. The transition process builds from simple to complex. The first phase involves building the skill of all employees to make improvements in their particular area of work. This is called *daily management.* When each individual has mastered these skills and the whole organization has this skill level, then the whole organization can be mobilized to work on one or two organizationwide improvements. This is called *hoshin management.* When the organization can do one or two organizationwide improvements, then it can expand its organization improvements into more areas, such as quality, cost, and delivery. This is called *cross-functional management.*

As the understanding of these improvement systems has developed and grown, we developed a model to show the various parts. (See GOAL/QPC TQM Wheel.)

Each of the major phases of total quality–daily management, hoshin management, and cross-functional management–can be looked at in terms of:

1. What–the processes for change
2. Who–the human dimension
3. How–the tools

The items included in each area are not exclusive to that area but are basic to and representative of that area.

1. *Daily management:* In daily management, the key processes are continuous improvement and standardization. Every process is continuously improved in a plan-do-check-act (PDCA) cycle. Each gain that is made is captured or held

GOAL/QPC TQM Wheel

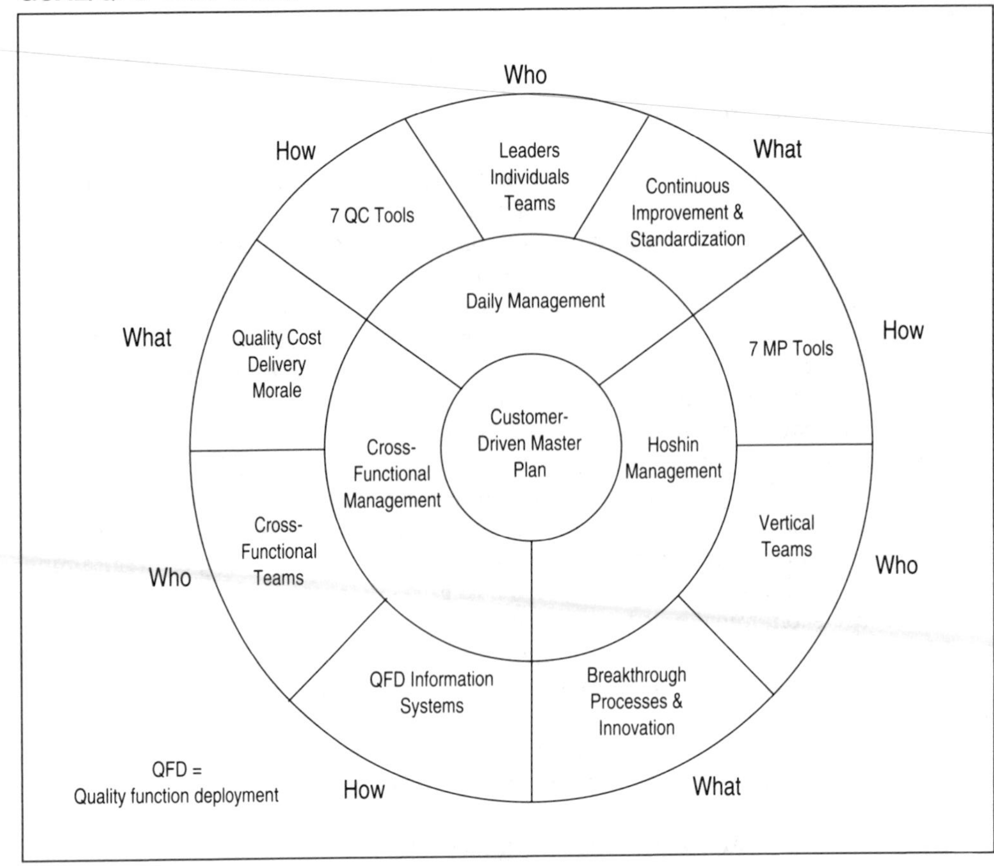

in a standardize-do-check-act (SDCA) cycle. The shift back and forth between continuous improvement and standardization should become as natural as breathing in and out.

The people involved are teams and individuals. Oftentimes not enough attention is paid to the human dimension of leading and facilitating teams. Also, not all improvement happens in teams. Each individual is personally responsible for holding the gain and for continuous improvement in his or her own area of responsibility.

The tools used are most often the basic tools called the *seven quality control (7QC) tools.* These are the check sheet, the run chart, the Pareto chart, the fishbone chart, the histogram, the control chart, and the scatter diagram. Other times people get involved in more sophisticated tools such as experimental design.

2. *Hoshin management:* In hoshin management, employees take the skills they have learned and apply them to an organizationwide problem. The key process is determining the most important organizational breakthrough that will move the whole organization forward.

   The people involved are initially top management and then eventually every employee. Top management needs to select the most important breakthrough area, and then each employee has to determine how he or she can contribute. A process called "catchball" ensures alignment of improvement activity vertically from the top to the bottom of the organization and horizontally across departments.

The seven management and planning (7MP) tools include the affinity chart, the relations diagram, the tree diagram, basic matrixes, decision matrixes, the process decision program chart, and the arrow or PERT diagram. These tools were originally grouped together in Japan in the early 1970s to help expand total quality into service and administration, but they have become even more popular in the United States as a basis for hoshin management.

3. *Cross-functional management:* In cross-functional management, organization-wide improvements are expanded. Quality, cost, delivery, and morale are improved on an organizational basis.

   These efforts are coordinated initially by the total quality steering committee and then eventually are coordinated by a single executive leading a team that is often a diagonal slice through the organization.

   Very few U.S. organizations are mature enough in total quality to do it from a cross-functional perspective. But many organizations have been quick to use the tools of quality function deployment (QFD). This group of tools–which includes matrixes, value and reliability engineering, and new concept selection–is helping organizations make major breakthroughs for customers.

How total quality is rolled out varies from organization to organization. The customer-driven master plan spells out the sequence in which the change effort will be introduced to the organization. System dynamics is a helpful tool to identify leverage points. A steering committee consisting of the key executives of the organization is responsible for drafting the master plan and modifying each year based on a review of successes and problems in the total quality implementation.

Finally, let me offer a few thoughts about what we have learned about successful hoshin implementation. First of all, an organization needs to be clear as to why it is doing total quality. Is the organization struggling under the weight of new kinds of competition and health care regulations? Then total quality may be used to chart a more successful competitive course for the organization and to streamline its paperwork system. Is the hospital's average length of stay too long for the industry or area? Then total quality can help chart a way to get significantly reduced length of stay while improving outcomes. Is the health care system a recent merger of many smaller units with vastly different cultures? Then total quality can help create a new, homogeneous culture focused on wellness of community and profitability. Total quality is a major undertaking, and the first step is to be clear as to why it is essential to a specific organization.

The second key to success in hoshin is to make the review process the top priority. It is only through thoroughly understanding past successes and failures that you can identify the most effective leverage points that hoshin can address. Many Japanese companies use the plan-do-check-act cycle to determine the organizational changes required to meet new visions. Nothing is more critical to successful hoshin management than a thorough review process.

A third important key to success is to identify the timetable for the hoshin process. It is important to know the months in which the organization will update the five-year plan, the three-year plan, and the one-year plan. This is important so that these tasks get done and also important so that people know when their particular issues will be dealt with.

A fourth key to success when beginning hoshin management is to keep the focus to one or two key breakthroughs. When I first taught a hoshin course for an information division of defense logistics at the Department of Defense, the division had at least a dozen priorities, all based on directives from the Pentagon. It was impossible at that time for those involved to deal with the thought that they had to select one or two priorities for special attention. And yet that is precisely the challenge that every organization wanting to do hoshin must tackle successfully.

A fifth key to success is not to rush into hoshin before employees are adept at daily management. Employees need to know how to identify problems, solve them, and hold the gain in their own department before they are asked to do that organizationwide. If the capability is not there on the department level, then failure is ensured on the organization level. Is there a faster way? Several organizations have started hoshin at the top level of the organization for the first couple of years and then dispersed it through the rest of the organization as each area mastered daily management.

I would like to thank Mara and Casey for inviting me to write this foreword and for their important contribution to the study of this powerful system. And success to you, the reader, in your investigation into hoshin and how it may bring your organization the dramatic results it has brought to others.

Preface

> All human progress has been a series of breakthroughs and many, perhaps most of these, have not been formally organized. Yet they happened. Why, then, do we talk of an organized approach?
>
> The answer is that an organized approach can greatly increase the probability that we will really get a breakthrough, and can drastically shorten the time for doing it.[1]

This book is our contribution to the leaders of organizations who are working hard to achieve breakthroughs. It is the culmination of two decades of work to discover which organized approaches to leadership really make a difference in long-term success.

Over the years, we have observed the tendency of executives – ourselves included – to work hard to stay up to date on the latest management approaches, to try them out with great intentions and much enthusiasm, only to leave them to wither away when initial grandiose expectations are not achieved. We have seen this cycle lead to employee skepticism about any change. It has also led to management skepticism about whether any organized approach to leadership can be creative, customized, and timely enough to work well in a unique company.

We believe that there must be a better way to build, support, and to lead successful organizations. We believe that we can learn from nature. The instinctive behaviors in a V-shaped formation of geese – choosing a leader, deciding on a destination, communicating directions, focusing on the destination as one cohesive unit – "all foster collective wisdom in the group." As AT&T leaders recognize, "When this behavior becomes instinctive, as it is in nature, the business will be in full flight and moving in a common direction."[2]

Hoshin planning, the subject of this book, helps organizations move in a common direction, in full flight. It brings together, in an organized yet flexible approach, the best of many of the planning and management approaches that we have worked with over the years. And hoshin planning has long-term staying power, because it provides the means to focus and align organizations, two things that will *always* be critical. We are writing this book because we believe that hoshin planning, done well, has the potential to help organizations breakthrough to new heights of success – and to find new joy in the flight.

How the Book Is Organized

This book is an executive guide to hoshin planning. Our purpose is to increase understanding and use of hoshin planning as a means to achieve breakthroughs and long-term success. We have tried to find a balance in this book among describing what hoshin planning is, discussing how to do it well, and sharing real-world experiences of organizations that are implementing hoshin planning. There are 16 chapters and 3 appendixes, presented as an increasingly detailed continuum of information. They are organized into three parts: I. Introduction to Hoshin Planning, II. How Hoshin Planning Works, and III. Case Studies of Hoshin Planning in Action.

Chapter 1: The Value of Hoshin Planning discusses needs that hoshin planning can help address, its major benefits, and some of the organizations using hoshin planning.

Chapter 2: Definition of Hoshin Planning provides an overview of what hoshin planning is and how it works. It defines hoshin planning and discusses the name. It describes the complementary relationship between hoshin planning and other management strategies – such as TQM, CQI, reengineering, benchmarking, and critical pathways – and the relationship of hoshin to strategic planning. Chapter 2 also includes an introduction to the four major steps of hoshin planning, which are described in more detail in chapters 5 through 9.

Chapter 3: Hoshin Planning Key Success Factors discusses six factors that contribute to successful hoshin planning. The chapter also describes the evolution of hoshin planning in an organization as the success factors grow stronger with time and experience.

In *Chapter 4: Organizing and Customizing Hoshin Planning* the tone of the book begins to shift from the concept and theory of hoshin planning to more emphasis on how to implement it. The purpose of chapter 4 is to assist leaders to organize and customize hoshin planning to the unique needs of the organization. It describes three categories of questions that need to be addressed up front by the CEO and top leadership team: (1) Why are we implementing hoshin planning? (2) When should we start to implement it? and (3) How will we implement it? Chapter 4 includes a leaders' hoshin planning implementation worksheet.

In *Part II: How Hoshin Planning Works,* chapter 5 introduces the process, while chapters 6 through 9 provide increasing detail on the four basic steps of hoshin planning. The chapter for each step clarifies the purpose and results, notes leadership issues, describes implementation tasks, offers lessons learned and helpful hints, and discusses roles and responsibilities. A health care example is woven throughout the chapters to illustrate the major tasks.

These chapters stress selected tasks and techniques that have been particularly useful to the early pioneers in hoshin planning. Additional, more detailed, and more comprehensive information on each step and on related tools and techniques appears in the case studies in part III, in the appendixes and resources in part IV.

In *Part III: Case Studies of Hoshin Planning in Action,* the direction of the book shifts to the experience of organizations that have implemented hoshin planning. Chapters 10 through 15 present case studies of four of the first health care organizations to embark on hoshin planning, along with case studies of two of the hoshin planning pioneers, AT&T and Hewlett-Packard. The case studies discuss benefits and results, problems encountered and how they were addressed, factors that contributed to success, how hoshin planning worked in the organization, roles of top leaders, and lessons learned. Finally, as an interesting aside, chapter 16 presents a brief case study of the Wright brothers, finding a metaphor for hoshin in their work.

Appropriate chapters include recommended actions for top leadership. Appendixes provide additional information on tools and techniques that can be used in hoshin planning, as well as sample hoshin plans.

Leaders may use this book in a number of ways. Top executives may be particularly interested in the overviews in chapters 1 through 4, and the recommended actions for top leadership. Executives, managers, and clinical leaders with additional hoshin planning implementation responsibilities may find the how-to detail included in chapters 5 through 9 and in the appendixes helpful. The case studies, with their diversity and depth, offer insights to everyone committed to improving organizational success.

We encourage readers to adapt hoshin planning to their unique organizations. As noted by Sister Lois Bush, president of SSM-Ministry Corporation:

> To do hoshin planning is not the goal – to use hoshin planning to create breakthroughs for the organization and the people it serves is the goal.[3]

Hoshin planning, like any substantial change effort, is not an easy, quick fix. But, as the organizations described throughout this book illustrate, the results are real and worth the effort. Hoshin planning provides a better way to work together. It weaves a *Golden Thread* throughout the fabric of the organization, so each person can clearly see how he or she is connected to the organization's most important goal, to its customers, and to one another. And when one *sees* things differently, one can then begin to *do* things differently.

References

1. Juran, J. *Managerial Breakthrough.* New York City: McGraw-Hill, 1964, p. 17.
2. AT&T Quality Steering Committee. Policy deployment: Setting the direction for change. Indianapolis: AT&T, 1992, inside cover page.
3. Sister M. Lois Bush, president and CEO, SSM-Ministry Corporation. Personal communication to Mara Melum, July 12, 1994.

Acknowledgments

We are indebted to many people for their contributions to this book. First, we thank our husbands – Eric and Dennis – and our children – Daniel, Arielle, Aaron, Liese, Miriam, and Jordan – for their encouragement, patience, and support in helping us make this vision become a reality.

It has been a pleasure to work with our publishers – American Hospital Publishing, Inc., and GOAL/QPC. Thanks to Audrey Kaufman at AHPI for originally championing the need for this book and for wise counsel and perspective throughout its development. We recognize and appreciate the commitment and hard work of Nancy Charpentier, our editor at AHPI. Thank you to Dona Hotopp at GOAL/QPC for guidance to ensure that the book adds value to the field – and for personal contributions based on leadership of the GOAL/QPC health care application research committee and her own work in hoshin planning and total quality management.

We are indebted to the case study authors for enriching this book and for giving of their time to share their hoshin planning experience with others. Thank you to Jon Beste, Lisa Boisvert, Sister Lois Bush, Geoffrey Crabtree, Lois Gold, Brad Harrington, Dona Hotopp, Gerry Kaminski, Owen McNally, and Lou Monteforte – and to your colleagues at AT&T Transmission Systems Business Unit, Bethesda, Inc., Hewlett-Packard, Our Lady of Lourdes Medical Center, SSM-Ministry Corporation, and Southwest Texas Methodist Hospital – for serving as leaders and role models in the quest to focus and align organizations to achieve a vision.

We appreciate the insights and wise counsel that Gail Warden and Bob King have contributed in writing the forewords that place this book in the larger context of visionary leadership. We salute Gail as a statesman in the health care industry, one who has been at the forefront of integrated health care systems from the beginning and who knows firsthand the importance of aligning a system to achieve its most important focus. We also salute Bob King for his visionary leadership in recognizing the value of hoshin planning in Japan and in working to advance hoshin planning in America.

We are grateful to Gail O. Van Zyl, director of healthcare resources at First Care Health in Albany, Oregon. She provided us with a clear, concise example based on real-life experience that brings the how-to steps of hoshin planning to life.

Thank you, also, to the many people who contributed to this book through interviews and generous sharing of information about their organizations' hoshin planning experience – James Rieley of the Center for Continuous Quality Improvement at Milwaukee Area Technical College, William Thompson of SSM Health Care System, Eugenia Hamilton of Dartmouth-Hitchcock Medical Center, Dan Kratz of Minneapolis Children's Medical Center, David Demers of Fletcher Allen Health Care, Edward Schottland and Mary MacIntosh of The Miriam Hospital, Pat Cooksey of Bellin Hospital, and John Early of the Juran Institute, Inc.

We thank the many people throughout our careers and lives who have helped us discover the richness of strategic planning and hoshin planning. Thank you to our many original teachers and mentors for your vision and inspiration, including Joe Peters, Symond Gottlieb, James Webber, Bob Sigmond, Fred Schwettmann, Bob Tillman, Katsumi Yoshimoto, and Dr. Noriaki Kano. We also salute our colleagues in the quest for world-class strategic planning: Steve Kohlert, Ira Schlesinger, Marie Sinioris, and Clarence Teng, and other board, staff, and members of the Society for Healthcare Planning and Marketing of the American Hospital Association. Thank you, also, to Bob King, Joe Colletti, Michael Brassard, Ellen Domb, and the other GOAL/QPC hoshin planning instructors for significant contributions to hoshin planning in America and for sharing your contributions with us and others with such quality. We also express appreciation to Susan Soukup, Mike Cowley, Bill Cook, Spencer Graves, and Bruce Boles, our partners in learning.

We salute our clients and colleagues who advanced hoshin planning by creatively applying it to the real work of their organizations, including Jack Brown and Dave Lord at Procter & Gamble, Gerry Kaminski and Maureen Hollinbeck at Bethesda, Inc., Sandra Featherman and Bruce Gildseth at the University of Minnesota-Duluth, Michael Schmidt and the administrative council at Saint Joseph's Hospital, and the leadership team at SSM-Ministry Corporation. We are inspired by Sister Lois Bush, a role model of visionary CEO leadership.

Special kudos to Lois Gold of Hewlett-Packard, Marie Sinioris of Rush-Presbyterian St. Luke's Medical Center, and Richard Delano of Albany General Hospital, who made the time in their incredibly busy schedules to review the draft book and to suggest extremely helpful improvements. We are also indebted to the leaders who helped us shape the original direction of the book so it would provide real value: Ellen Gaucher, Gerry Kaminski, Phil Neubold, Marie Sinioris, and David Setzer. We also appreciate the contributions of Tara Hotopp for research on the case studies and of Aaron Collett for his insights and assistance during the early editing process.

And to all the other colleagues and leaders who in their own ways – both known and unknown to us – are working so hard to build organizations that are focused and aligned around what is most important to their customers and to their communities, we say thank you. You are an inspiration to us.

PART ONE

Introduction to Hoshin Planning

CHAPTER ONE

The Value of Hoshin Planning

> These are complex times. We are all doing the best we can, trying to do the right thing.
>
> –Sister M. Lois Bush, President, SSM-Ministry Corporation

This chapter discusses the value of hoshin planning. It begins by highlighting organizational needs that hoshin planning can help executives address. Then it identifies some of the organizations that use hoshin planning. Finally, it describes five benefits of hoshin planning.

What Needs Can Hoshin Planning Help Address?

Today change seems to be the only constant in our lives. The health care industry is a microcosm of this change. It is affected by the same market, competitive, and technological changes as many other industries, but, in addition, its fundamental purpose is changing dramatically. Health care organizations used to be in business to take care of people when they got sick. Today and tomorrow, health care organizations will be in business – and at risk – to improve the health status of a community. Some describe this as a shift from an illness industry to a health industry.

In the world of manufacturing, local consumers can now shop globally for products and services that have it all – quality, low cost, *and* reliability. Heightened competition has caused companies to employ radical new strategies, such as slashing new product introduction times or forming strategic alliances with their competitors. Meanwhile, the workforce continues to adapt to periodic resizing and reshaping forces and to the changing nature of work itself.

The field of education is also undergoing major change as it confronts the twin pressures of rising costs and increased competition. Informed consumers of education are comparison shopping and asking tough questions. Legislators and accrediting agencies are joining in the call for greater accountability, often linking funding to outcomes. New types of education are emerging, including whole-life learning opportunities.

Although these changes are sometimes invigorating, they can be enormously disruptive and even scary. Organizations are responding to or leading these changes with a multitude of strategies. One widespread strategy, in health care and in other industries, is to form integrated systems by merging or forming alliances with complementary organizations.

Leaders who are working hard amid much turmoil to develop integrated systems face some very tough questions:

- How do we *plan* a successful integrated system?
- What are the right things for people to *focus* on to ensure long-term success of the system?
- How do we *align* many different people, departments, and organizations to work together toward the success of the whole system?
- How can we increase employee *understanding* of the system's priorities and plans?
- How can we *balance* the need for organizational direction with opportunities for employee initiative and creativity?
- How can we promote *breakthrough thinking and results?*

There *is* a compass to help us answer these questions and to chart a successful course through the rough waters stirred up by change. That compass is called *hoshin planning.*

Hoshin planning is a management strategy that is really a return to the most important basics of strong leadership – basics such as focusing on what is most important, really listening to customers, and giving everyone a stake in the organization's success. Hoshin planning, also known as *hoshin management* or *policy deployment,* is a proven strategy that can help leaders to plan and align an integrated system.

Which Organizations Use Hoshin Planning?

Hoshin planning is relatively new to American industry. American companies that have found it to be a valuable management and planning strategy include Hewlett-Packard, Procter & Gamble, Florida Power & Light, Xerox, and at least four Baldrige Award winners: Motorola, Texas Instruments, Zytec Corporation, and the AT&T Transmission Systems Business Unit (TSBU). The TSBU recognizes the substantial contribution of hoshin planning to their selection as a Baldrige Award winner: "It was evident to the [Baldrige] examiners that the TSBU management system [hoshin planning, which they call policy deployment] was the process that led to the many dramatic operational performance improvements and the resulting increase in overall customer satisfaction. Only two and one-half years had passed between the first policy deployment [hoshin planning] workshop and the award announcement."[1] (Case studies of hoshin planning at AT&T and Hewlett-Packard are included in chapters 14 and 15, respectively.)

Hoshin planning has been a widely used business strategy in Japan for about 25 years. Dr. Noriaki Kano of the Japanese Union of Scientists and Engineers (JUSE), who is recognized as a major architect of hoshin planning and who has guided Florida Power & Light in its effort, notes that hoshin planning "is a marriage between the strengths of the East and the West: the strong leadership exercised by Western top management with the organizationwide consensus of traditional Japanese organizations."[2] Working extensively with Japanese and American leaders, GOAL/QPC has been instrumental in efforts to transfer and adapt learnings about hoshin planning to America.[3]

In American service industries, including health care, hoshin planning is in the early stages of implementation. Some of the early health care pioneers in hoshin planning include Bethesda, Inc., Dartmouth-Hitchcock Medical Center, Meadville Medical Center, The Miriam Hospital, Our Lady of Lourdes Medical Center, Sewickley

Valley Hospital, Southwest Texas Methodist Hospital, SSM Health Care System, SSM-Ministry Corporation, VHA of Pennsylvania, and Fletcher Allen Health Care. (Case studies of four of these health care organizations are included in part III of this book.)

What Are the Major Benefits of Hoshin Planning?

What benefits make hoshin planning worth considering, when our plate of management approaches is already overflowing? Hoshin planning can help you to do better the most important things you are already doing. It *builds on* the strengths of your current strategic planning and management efforts to integrate and leverage them and to develop them further. In addition, it offers five fundamental and powerful benefits:

1. *Focus:* Hoshin planning helps to focus the organization on the few vital priorities.
2. *Alignment:* Hoshin planning helps to align the organization – a system with multiple units and often organizations – so that all parts of the system work together to achieve a common vision.
3. *Collective knowledge:* Hoshin planning harnesses the collective wisdom of a system's employees and other stakeholders to achieve the organization's focus.
4. *Empowered employees:* Hoshin planning includes a system of accountability so that leadership and employees share the responsibility for achievement of breakthrough goals.
5. *Enhanced teamwork:* Hoshin planning encourages teamwork by providing a common focus to which every individual can make an important contribution.

The remainder of this chapter discusses each benefit in detail.

Benefit 1: Focus

Things which matter most must never be at the mercy of things that matter least.[4]

Many organizations have too few people and too many projects. Everything seems like a "priority." Signs of employee stress and burnout are evident to coworkers, to families, and even to customers. If the juggling act is sufficiently "advanced," workers can achieve a multitude of short-term goals, but at a terrible price. They sacrifice joy in their work, a balanced and healthy lifestyle, and longer-term goals – goals that are important but not urgent.

In some organizations, management efforts such as total quality management (TQM) have unintentionally added to the stress. Improvement teams often require so much time that team members and management feel there is not enough time to handle both team tasks and members' "real jobs." The Health Care Advisory Board describes this scattered approach in a report on TQM in health care. The board observes that in many institutions TQM is

> . . . *"a headless horseman"* lacking management direction. Even in hospitals with a long-term strategic plan, TQM often operates as a parallel entity with separate, vaguely stated objectives. [There is an] expectation that success will come by simply unleashing the TQM process; many organizations are training staff, forming teams, and waiting [and waiting] for quality improvement. . . . Without strategic direction, the TQM outcome [is] almost always disappointing: spotty, small-scale improvements with no discernible effect on long-term competitiveness.[5]

The Advisory Board recognizes that part of the answer to this common problem is to focus TQM on what is most important to the organization:

> Properly directed, TQM can be a potent tool for radically improving competitive position. Develop a long-term strategy and use it to drive TQM. . . . Tightly focus [your] TQM effort. Concentrating organizational energies on a handful of issues ensures that project results build on each other, producing noticeable improvements, [and] true competitive advantage.[6]

Other management strategies, such as benchmarking and reengineering, often suffer from similar problems: their potential power is only partially tapped because of unfocused implementation.

Most individuals occasionally–or constantly–experience some version of this organizational dilemma: too many diverse demands on our time and not enough focus. In his book *The Seven Habits of Highly Effective People*, Stephen Covey portrays this common dilemma graphically as a four-quadrant time management matrix that considers degree of urgency and importance of work. (See figure 1-1.)

> *Quadrant I* is both urgent and important [work]. It deals with significant results that require immediate attention . . . "crises" or "problems." Quadrant I consumes many people . . . it keeps getting bigger and bigger until it dominates you. It's like the pounding surf. A huge problem comes and knocks you down and you're wiped out. You struggle back only to face another one that knocks you down and slams you to the ground.
>
> *Quadrant II* is the heart of effective personal management. It deals with things that are *not urgent, but are important.* It deals with things like building relationships, writing a personal mission statement, long-range planning, exercising, preventive maintenance, preparation–all those things we know we need to do, but somehow seldom get around to doing, because they aren't urgent.[7]

Covey's advice to individuals is similar to the Advisory Board's for organizations: *Focus on what is most important.* "I believe that if you were to ask what lies in Quadrant II and cultivate the proactivity to go after it . . . your effectiveness would increase dramatically. In time management jargon this is called the Pareto principle–80 percent of the results flow out of 20 percent of the activities."[8]

Figure 1-1. Time Management Matrix

	Urgent	Not Urgent
Important	I Activities: Crises Pressing problems Deadline-driven projects	II Activities: Prevention, PC activities Relationship building Recognizing new opportunities Planning, recreation
Not Important	III Activities: Interruptions, some calls Some mail, some reports Some meetings Proximate, pressing matters Popular activities	IV Activities: Trivia, busy work Some mail Some phone calls Time wasters Pleasant activities

Hoshin planning offers a systematic way to focus on the few goals that are most important for the organization to achieve a breakthrough level of success. It helps executives to shift their efforts from Covey's quadrants I, III, and IV to more quadrant II activities. Hoshin planning recognizes that many goals are important and deserve to be included in the strategic plan and on your "To Do" list. But a few goals are so important at this time that they merit the concerted efforts and most intense energy of the entire organization.

Hoshin planning provides tools, techniques, and a system for top leadership to select an organizational focus based on what is most important to customers. It provides a structured approach to ensure that this focus drives work at every level of the organization. Fletcher Allen Health Care considers prioritization to be one of the most important benefits of hoshin planning. The medical center's vice-president claims that hoshin planning gives you the tools to pick one or two things that the organization can "come together around to create a breakthrough." At the medical center, three years of experience with hoshin planning has led the organization to "come together around" a new vertically and horizontally integrated health care system.

Hoshin planning can be thought of as the Pareto principle applied to leadership—80 percent of the key results come from 20 percent of the goals. An organization that focuses its resources on a few top priorities has a significant competitive advantage. The trick is to choose the right 20 percent to focus on. Choosing the focus in hoshin planning is similar to the game Pick Up Sticks—you must know which stick will move the most other sticks.

Hoshin planning helps ensure the right focus by basing it on customers. The leaders ask the people who shape the organization's success—its customers—what is most important to them. Customers themselves weight and rank their own needs and expectations. The leaders translate the highest-ranked expectations into organizational key success factors (KSFs) and then into breakthrough goals for the organization.

Following are examples of what different organizations chose to focus on through a hoshin planning process:

- AT&T Network Systems: Achieve 100 percent on-time delivery for all products in three years.[9]
- Motorola: Reduce total cycle time by 50 percent per year.[10]
- Bethesda, Inc.: Delight key customers by responding to their highest-priority demands for effective and low-cost health care.[11]
- Miriam Hospital: Be the highest-value health care provider.[12]
- SSM-Ministry Corporation: Promote the formation and development of integrated delivery networks (IDNs).[13]
- Our Lady of Lourdes Medical Center: Expand effective capacity.[14]
- Fletcher Allen Health Care: Develop a patient-focused integrated system of care.[15]
- SSM Health Care System: Provide information on demand for all customers.[16]
- Nissan Motor Company: Reduce the number of parts needed in its cars by 30 percent in three to five years.[17]
- Texas Instruments SC Group: Bring leadership products and/or product sets early to market.[18]
- 3M Corporation: Thirty percent of sales will be from products introduced within the past four years.[19]

An organization that focuses its collective energy on a few critical goals gains a significant competitive advantage. When the focus is based on key customer priorities, the organization is naturally more open to learning and positive change.

Benefit 2: Alignment

[Hoshin planning] enables business leaders to mobilize the organization toward a common destination, aligning all employees behind a common goal and a collective wisdom.[20]

By aligning the organization so people work to implement the plan in complementary ways, hoshin planning helps ensure that the right things are done right. *Align* means "to bring [parts or components] into proper coordination, to bring into agreement, close cooperation."[21] One of the key benefits of hoshin planning is that it brings employees throughout the organization into closer agreement and cooperation with the organization's focus–its top-priority goals.

James Rieley of the Center for Continuous Quality Improvement at Milwaukee Area Technical College describes the importance of alignment in hoshin planning as follows:

> Vertical alignment refers to the ability of everyone in an organization to be able to see the same picture, or in the case of the vision, everyone seeing the same future. . . . If the employees of a company were charged with building an automobile that attained exceptional mileage, it would be crucial for the people building the engine to know the parameters of the rest of the car. The exterior design of the car has a strong influence on the eventual mileage that the car will get. The design of the rest of the drive train will have a strong influence on the mileage as well. If all the workers in the company do not understand the "big" picture, the complete set of design parameters, they will design a car that will not get exceptional mileage. As a matter of fact, the component elements would probably not even fit together. . . .
>
> Without vertical alignment, different divisions or departments within an institution have a tendency to work at cross-purposes because they never see the entire picture. This is not necessarily intentional, but an outcome of each division or department seeing a different direction. The end result is a drain of resources and energy.[22]

Alignment is achieved in hoshin planning through an iterative, organizationwide process where targets are communicated and the means to achieve them are negotiated. This results, in AT&T's words, in a "Golden Thread." The *Golden Thread* is a set of interconnected targets and means that ties the whole organization together, as illustrated in figure 1-2. As described in the AT&T case study in chapter 14, the Golden Thread is "tied" from priority customer needs, to the organization's focus, to top leaders' targets and means. The Golden Thread is then tied to managers' targets and means, and ultimately to all employees' targets and means. "This links all our people to the key customer satisfiers."[23] This also links people throughout the organization to one another.

An example of a Golden Thread at AT&T is illustrated in figure 1-3 (p. 10). This Golden Thread originated with the need that AT&T Transmission Systems customers ranked as most important–the need for reliability. This customer need led to selection of the organization's focus: "Improve hardware quality and reliability." As illustrated, the Golden Thread continues as this focus is translated into "Reduce circuit pack returns" at the departmental level. At the section level, it becomes "Reduce transformer defects." For line supervisors and employees, the Golden Thread translates into teams working to "Reduce operations defects" in areas such as soldering, cover coat, and plating.

At Fletcher Allen Health Care, alignment through hoshin planning has been of value in two ways. In a way different from traditional planning, hoshin has helped the organization to build a shared vision, to engage stakeholders, and to gain commitment to a plan for the future. It has also helped in organizing work and creating linkages among departments and other business units.

Fletcher Allen Health Care is building alignment around its organizational focus: integrated delivery systems of care. This focus was translated into targets such as "Align medical manpower with the needs of a managed care environment." The people most involved with alignment of medical manpower were then linked to this target

Figure 1-2. Golden Thread: Linking All Levels of the Organization

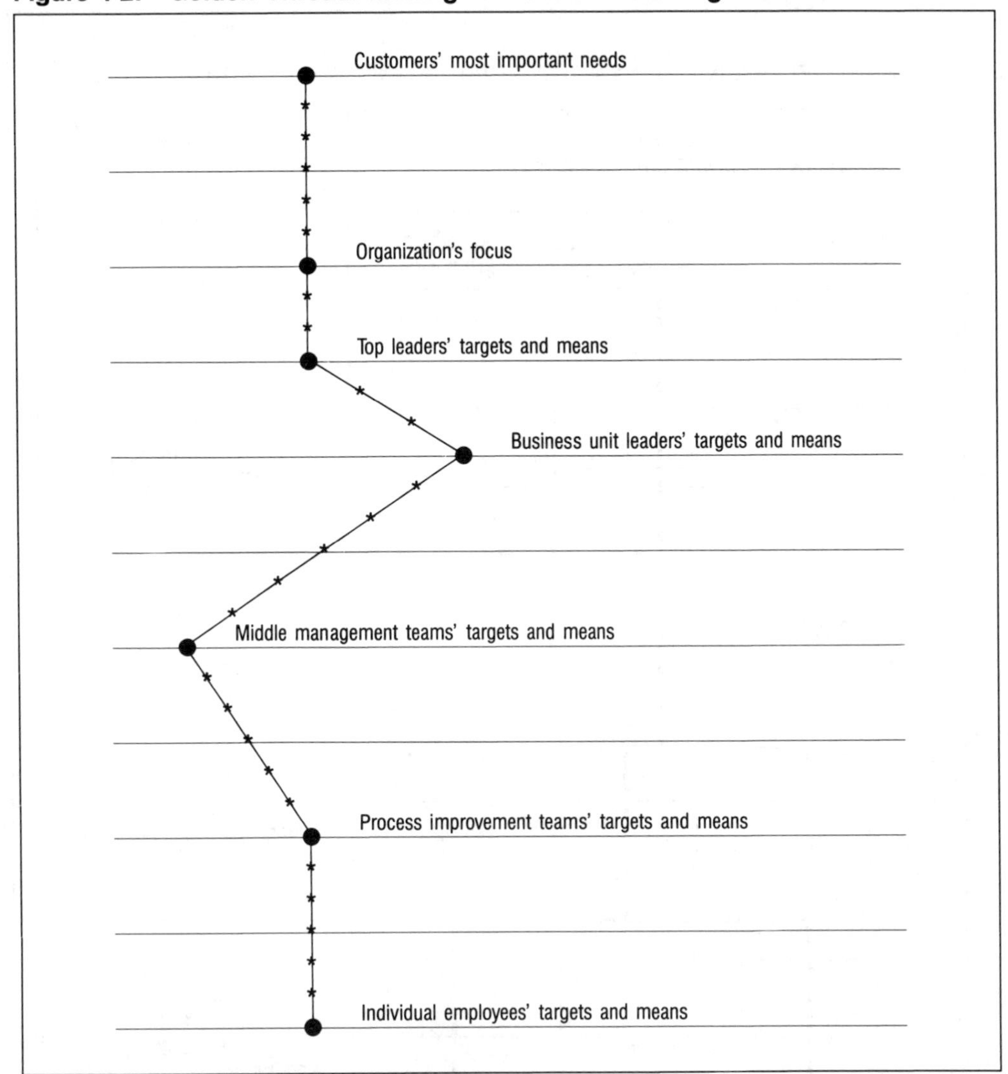

Reprinted, with permission, from Mara Melum & Associates, Inc. ©1994.

and to one another. For example, the president's means to contribute to this target include completing a medical manpower plan that outlines the size and mix of the physician panel. At the level of vice-president of planning, the means include developing a strategy to regulate the panel size, consisting of screening criteria and a screening process. At the business unit level, the means of the director of Vermont Managed Care include keeping the ratio of needed to actual medical manpower in balance with the plan. This was further translated and linked to the director of clinical systems, whose means include making decisions regarding applications to the medical manpower panel. (See figure 1-4, p. 11.)

Increased organizational alignment has also been a key benefit of hoshin planning at The Miriam Hospital, where hoshin planning "provided the link between employees and middle management and top management—so they all felt involved and understood their contributions to the organization's success."[24]

Benefit 3: Collective Knowledge

Hoshin planning taps the collective wisdom of employees throughout the system. Using an iterative process to develop targets and means that will achieve the organization's

Figure 1-3. Golden Thread

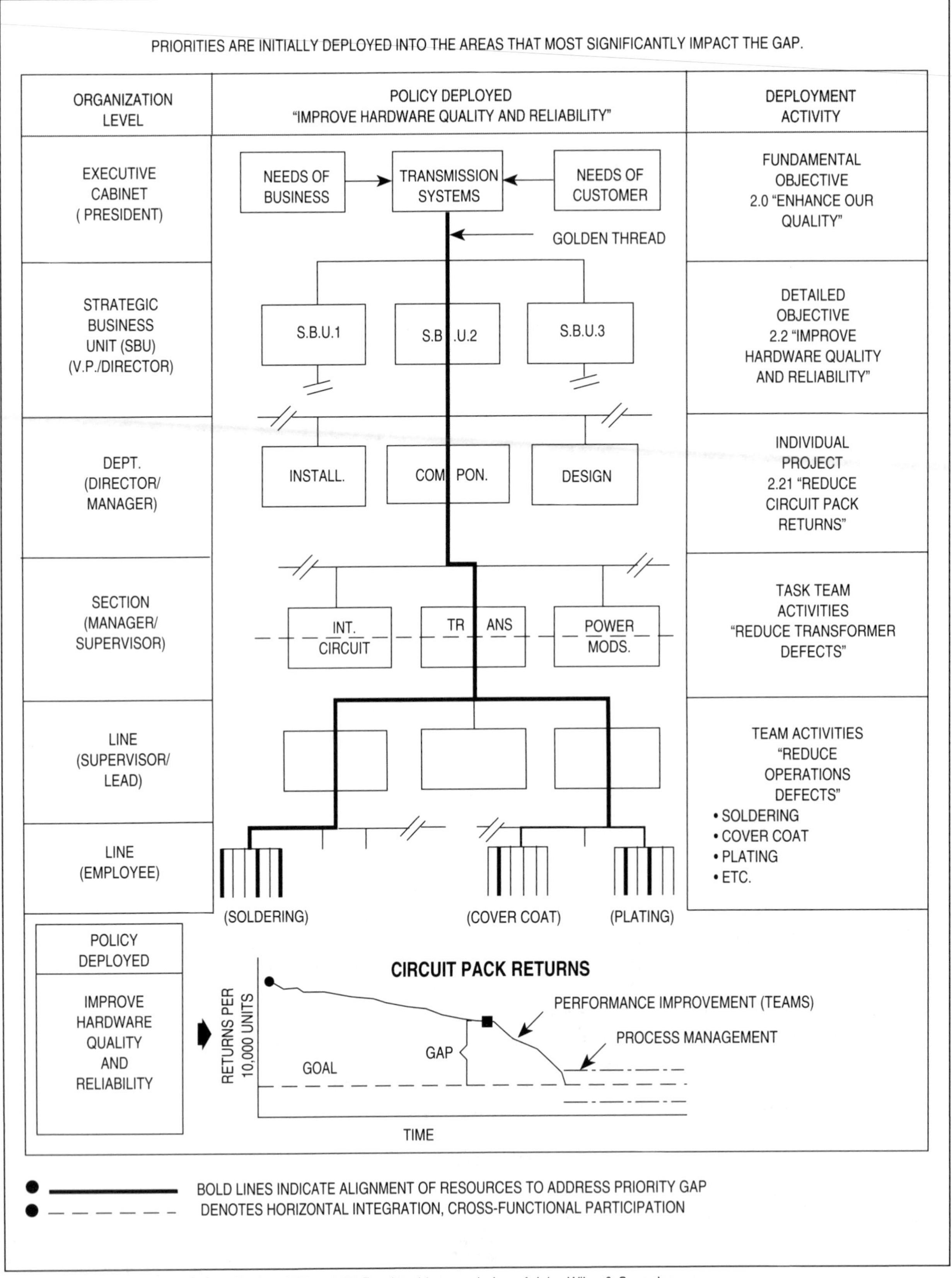

Source: *National Productivity Review*, Spring 1993, p. 165. Reprinted by permission of John Wiley & Sons, Inc.

Figure 1-4. Deploying Breakthroughs via Target/Means Matrixes

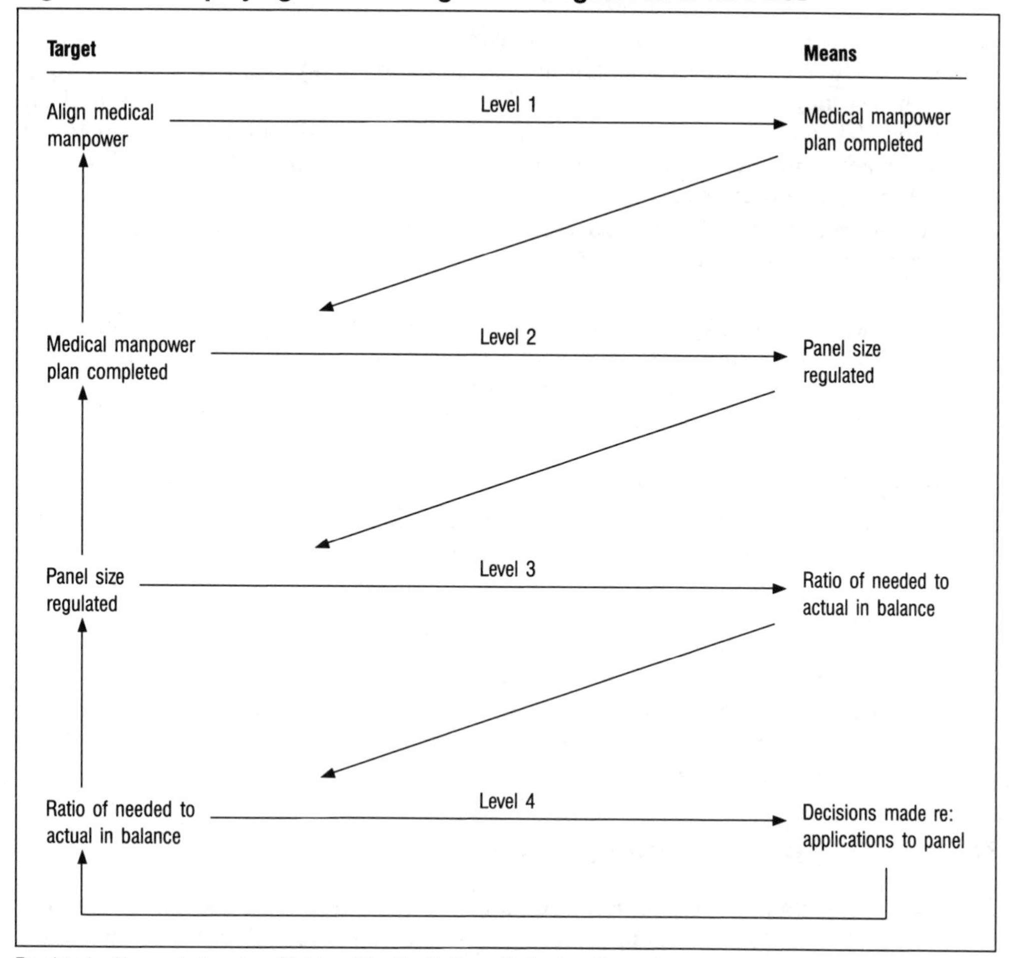

Reprinted, with permission, from Fletcher Allen Health Care, Burlington, Vermont.

focus, it helps people develop and implement plans collectively. The process proceeds in a top-down, horizontal, and bottom-up fashion. Particularly in the horizontal and bottom-up phases of this process, managers and top leaders assess how the proposed targets and means relate to one another. They work together to develop a synergistic plan. The result is that the collective knowledge of the organization–knowledge of customers, suppliers, competitors, technology, and interconnected job processes–is harnessed toward identifying the best ways to achieve the organization's focus.

Systems thinking is a discipline that emphasizes the importance of collective wisdom. As described by Peter Senge in *The Fifth Discipline:*

> You can only understand the system of a rainstorm by contemplating the whole, not any individual part of the pattern. Business and human endeavors are also systems. They, too, are bound by the invisible fabrics of interrelated actions, which often take years to fully play out their effects on each other.
>
> Systems thinking is a discipline for seeing wholes. It is a framework for seeing interrelationships rather than things, for seeing patterns of change rather than static "snapshots." . . . And systems thinking is a sensibility–for the subtle interconnectedness that gives living systems their unique character.[25]

This type of thinking results both in better plans and in stronger ownership of the plans by the people who helped to develop them and who see the "big picture."

Benefit 4: Empowered Employees

Some organizations define the "product" of strong leadership as "empowered employees." How do empowered employees benefit an organization? "Empowered employees know that they are shaping their own destiny. They have a greater sense of control and job ownership. They have a higher motivation to continually improve. Empowered employees act more often and more effectively with the organization's best interests in mind. They respond more quickly to customers."[26]

Empowerment is a widely used and sometimes abused concept. We define empowerment as providing employees with four things:

1. The appropriate *authority* to make changes within their sphere of responsibility
2. *Opportunities* to make decisions and correct problems
3. The *knowledge and skills* to act wisely and effectively
4. The *trust* of management that they will act responsibly[27]

Hoshin planning fosters empowerment because it gives the employee the opportunity to propose means to help achieve the organization's focus and targets. Also, when targets and means are approved, they are specific and include measures of success. This gives employees and teams a clear understanding of their responsibility. Hoshin planning encourages management trust in employees because, in addition to management's personal role in developing and approving the plan, hoshin planning includes clear lines of accountability. The accountability system includes assignment of specific targets and means to employees and teams, and periodic, structured evaluations of progress. The result is that the leadership and the employees share responsibility for the organization's achievement of breakthrough goals.

Benefit 5: Enhanced Teamwork

By encouraging empowered people throughout the organization to contribute in many ways to a common focus, hoshin planning builds a sense of the whole organization as one interconnected team working together. This is a vast improvement over situations where employees do not understand what the organization's purposes or priorities are, or do not see how they personally fit with the priorities.

In addition, hoshin planning fosters teamwork because the organization's focus is often deployed or handed off to cross-functional project teams that propose means to achieve it. Employees continue to gain experience serving on task-oriented teams that are critical to the organization. They are also exposed to a system of vertically and horizontally linked teams, which encourages their own systems thinking.

Summary

Hoshin planning is a back-to-basics approach to leadership whose time has come. It is particularly timely for executives who are developing and leading integrated systems. Hoshin planning has an impressive track record helping a core group of leading companies do five things that they want to do but often cannot do consistently and comprehensively:

1. *Focus* on what is most important
2. *Align* the organization to achieve the focus
3. *Tap into collective knowledge* of employees and other stakeholders
4. *Empower employees* to share the responsibility
5. *Enhance teamwork* so everyone contributes

Actions for Top Leadership

The following top leadership actions can help get hoshin planning off to a strong start and achieve strong demonstrated effects:

1. Assess whether the potential benefits of hoshin planning—particularly the benefits of focus and alignment—will significantly propel the organization toward meeting its needs and achieving its vision at this time.
2. Clearly communicate to the organization why hoshin planning is so important.
3. Begin to assess the organization's needs for training and continuing education about hoshin planning.
4. Be willing to articulate and to stand by an organizational focus, a "real direction" for the organization.

References and Notes

1. Monteforte, L., and Seemer, R. Winning more than the Malcolm Baldrige National Quality Award at AT&T Transmission Systems. *National Productivity Review,* Spring 1993, p. 158.
2. GOAL/QPC Research Committee. *Hoshin Planning: A Planning System for Implementing Total Quality Management (TQM).* Research Report No. 89-10-03. Methuen, MA: GOAL/QPC, 1989, p. 11.
3. GOAL/QPC's contributions include translating Japanese writings on hoshin planning into English, publishing a research report in 1989 that captured the best hoshin planning practices in American industry at that time, and providing seminars that share detailed information on hoshin planning theory and implementation.
4. Goethe, J. W. von. Quoted in Covey, S. *The Seven Habits of Highly Effective People.* New York City: Simon & Schuster, 1989, p. 146.
5. The Health Care Advisory Board. *Total Quality Management.* Vol. 1, *TQM: The Second Generation.* Washington, DC: The Advisory Board Company, 1992, pp. 16, 20.
6. The Health Care Advisory Board, pp. 15, 23, 29.
7. Covey, S. *The Seven Habits of Highly Effective People.* New York City: Simon & Schuster, 1989, p. 156.
8. Covey, pp. 154–55.
9. Monteforte, L., and Melum, M. Policy deployment at AT&T Transmission Systems: Case study of a Baldrige Award winner. Chapter 14 of this book.
10. AT&T Quality Steering Committee. *Policy Deployment: Setting the Direction for Change.* Indianapolis, IN: AT&T, 1992, p. 12.
11. Hotopp, D., with Kaminski, G. Bethesda, Inc., case study. Chapter 10 of this book.
12. Ed Schottland, executive vice-president, The Miriam Hospital. Personal correspondence to Mara Melum, June 15, 1994.
13. Bush, Sister M. L., and Beste, J. T. Sisters of the Sorrowful Mother Ministry Corporation case study. Chapter 12 of this book.
14. Hotopp, D., and McNally, O. Our Lady of Lourdes Medical Center case study. Chapter 11 of this book.
15. David Demers, vice-president of corporate planning, Fletcher Allen Health Care. Telephone interview by Mara Melum, Apr. 12, 1994.
16. William Thompson, senior vice-president, SSM Health Care System. Personal correspondence re 1994–96 strategic plan to Mara Melum, May 27, 1994.
17. Collins, B., and Huge, E. *Management by Policy.* Milwaukee, WI: ASQC Quality Press, 1993, p. 60.
18. Hayden, G. TQC starts with policy deployment. *TQC World,* June 1989, p. 13.
19. Owen McBride, marketing operations manager, 3M Corporation. Personal correspondence to Mara Melum, May 13, 1994.
20. AT&T.
21. *Webster's New World Dictionary,* 2nd college ed., s.v. "align."

22. Rieley, J. Closing the loop: An effective planning process in higher education. Unpublished paper, Center for Continuous Quality Improvement at Milwaukee Area Technical College, Feb. 1994, p. 7.

23. Monteforte, L. AT&T Quest for Excellence V Conference, Washington, DC, Feb. 14, 1993.

24. Edward Schottland, executive vice-president, The Miriam Hospital. Telephone interview by Mara Melum, June 15, 1994.

25. Senge, P. *The Fifth Discipline.* New York City: Doubleday, 1990, pp. 7, 68.

26. Melum, M. M., and Sinioris, M. K. *Total Quality Management: The Health Care Pioneers.* Chicago: American Hospital Publishing, 1992, p. 94.

27. Melum and Sinioris.

CHAPTER TWO

Definition of Hoshin Planning

You must be single minded. Drive for the one thing on which you have decided.

–Gen. George S. Patton, *War As I Knew It*

This chapter provides an overview of what hoshin planning is and how it works. First, it discusses the name and defines hoshin planning. Then it describes the complementary relationship between hoshin planning and other management strategies, such as management by objectives, total quality management (TQM), and strategic planning. The chapter also includes an overview of the four major steps of hoshin planning, which are described in more detail in chapters 6 through 9.

What Does the Term Mean?

The term *hoshin planning* comes from the Japanese phrase *hoshin kanri. Hoshin* means "shining metal compass" or "pointing direction." *Kanri* means "management" or "control." Hoshin planning is like a management compass that points everyone in the organization in the same direction, toward a common destination.

There are several English translations of *hoshin kanri.* Some companies, including Hewlett-Packard, use the translation "hoshin planning." The terms used at GOAL/QPC are hoshin planning and "hoshin management," to acknowledge that it helps a company to manage both the development and implementation of plans. Other organizations, such as AT&T and Texas Instruments, use the phrase "policy deployment." Zytec calls it "management by planning" (MBP). Closely related is what the Malcolm Baldrige National Quality Award program and Juran refer to as "strategic quality planning."

An alternative is just to *do* hoshin planning and not to call it anything special. Features of hoshin planning can be integrated into the existing strategic planning, accountability, and organizational learning systems to enhance them. This approach may be particularly effective where skeptical employees see any major new effort as another "flavor-of-the-month" management fad. However, leaders at Hewlett-Packard caution against this no-name approach. Their reasoning is that an organization needs creative tension to create and sustain significant change. By not giving a name to hoshin planning–or to any other change strategy–that creative tension may be diminished.[1]

How Is It Defined and What Are the Major Elements?

Hoshin planning can be defined as *a planning and management system that focuses and aligns the organization to achieve breakthroughs for customers.* There are other definitions, as well, including the following examples from these organizations:

- *AT&T:* An organizationwide and customer-focused management approach aimed at planning and executing breakthrough improvements in business performance
- *GOAL/QPC:* A top-down, bottom-up planning process for planning and executing strategic breakthrough
- *SSM-Ministry Corporation:* A system to identify and focus an organization on the most important direction it can take to move it forward in fulfillment of its mission
- *Juran Institute, Inc.:* The systematic process by which an entire organization sets and achieves specific long-term goals with respect to quality
- *Hewlett-Packard:* A process for annual planning and implementation that focuses on areas needing significant levels of improvement

Whatever hoshin planning is called, six key elements are constant components:

1. A *focus for the organization,* in the form of a few breakthrough goals that are vital to the organization's success. This focus is sometimes referred to as the organization's "hoshin."
2. A *commitment to customers,* including targets and means at every level of the organization that are based on meeting the needs and expectations that customers rank as most important.
3. *Deployment of the organization's focus* so that employees understand their specific contributions to it. This is referred to as the "Golden Thread" that links employees to what is important to customers and to one another.
4. *Collective wisdom to develop the plan,* through a top-down, bottom-up communication and negotiating process called "catchball."
5. *Tools and techniques* that make the hoshin planning process and the plan helpful, clear, and easy to use. These include the seven management and planning (7MP) tools (that is, the affinity chart, the relations diagram, the tree diagram, basic matrixes, decision matrixes, the process decision program chart, and the arrow or PERT diagram).
6. *Ongoing evaluation of progress* to facilitate learning and continuous improvement. The evaluation system emphasizes both results and the processes used to achieve results.

What Is the Relationship between Hoshin Planning and Other Management Strategies?

There are many similarities between hoshin planning and other management strategies, such as reengineering, benchmarking, critical paths, and continuous quality improvement. For example, most of these strategies emphasize the importance of:

- Process improvement
- Reduction of rework and other inefficiencies
- Meeting and exceeding customer expectations
- Employee participation
- Top management commitment

How do these strategies relate to one another? Hoshin planning is not a magic bullet that replaces all of these other management strategies. Rather, hoshin planning can help to leverage them and make them more successful by providing a compass for other management strategies. Reengineering, benchmarking, and others are specific *methods* that can help achieve the organizational focus developed through hoshin planning. For example, if the organization's focus is to become a "learning organization," leaders might decide to benchmark Motorola to learn about its world-class continuing education system.

In addition, once integrated goals are developed for related efforts such as benchmarking or reengineering, the hoshin planning catchball process can be used to align employees throughout the organization to work together to achieve those goals.

Management by Objectives and Hoshin Planning

Hoshin planning is sometimes viewed as a new form of management by objectives (MBO). Although hoshin planning and MBO are both systems to set and achieve objectives through employee involvement, there are important differences between the approaches, as noted in figure 2-1. For example, the primary purpose of hoshin planning relates to organizational performance, whereas MBO is oriented more to individual performance. Also, in hoshin planning, learning and improvement are based on reviews of both results and processes. In MBO, the emphasis is more strongly on results. An MBO-oriented organization that wants to evolve toward hoshin planning may go through transition stages similar to those described in figure 2-2.

Total Quality Management and Hoshin Planning

Hoshin planning is the vertical component of total quality management (TQM). It is the compass that sets the major direction for the organization's TQM efforts for everyone from the CEO to the front-line employee. The GOAL/QPC Wheel, in figure 2-3, illustrates that vertical alignment through hoshin planning is one of three major parts of a comprehensive system of TQM. (The other two parts are unit optimization through daily management and horizontal integration through cross-functional

Figure 2-1. Differences between Hoshin Planning (Policy Deployment) and MBO

	Hoshin Planning (Policy Deployment)	**MBO**
Main Purpose	Organizational problem solving for breakthroughs	Management of individual performance
Focus	Business capabilities in meeting customer expectations	Individual achievements
Execution Responsibility	Teams	Individuals
Methodology	Quality principles and tools	Not specified
Time Horizon	Annual activities aligned with long-term goal	Annual activities without long-term focus
Review	Periodic progress reviews on process and results	Final reviews on results
Objective Priority	Vital few for competitive advantages	Numerous
Decision Basis	Facts and data	Data not required

Policy Deployment Handbook: Setting the Direction for Change, p. 17. Reproduced with the permission of AT&T ©1992. All rights reserved.

Figure 2-2. The Transition from MBO to Hoshin Planning (MBP*)

MBO Stage	Interim Stage	Mature Hoshin Planning (MBP) Stage
Approach is from the company's perspective.	Approach is from the company's perspective.	Approach is from the customer's perspective.
All departments participate without regard to their potential for impact.	All departments participate without regard to their potential for impact.	Focus on participation. Those who can make a major contribution to this improvement effort participate. A prioritized approach for implementation is used.
Objectives are general.	Objectives are general. (Indicators and targets might exist but are not required.)	Contribution to improvement is based on analysis of methods to obtain objectives. Those who can actually have an impact on improvement are brought into alignment.
Quarterly status report.	Review structures are added but are perceived as punitive or an invasion of territory.	Review structures are added and are perceived as diagnostic and as an opportunity for support and progress.
Focus on quantity and cost.	Recognizes customers' needs as important.	Emergence of added structure—formalized customer input.
Each year is a new beginning and brings a new set of urgent objectives.	Problems gleaned from organization (objectives for improvement).	Opportunities for major improvement are determined by analysis of quality systems.

*MBP = Management by policy.

Reprinted, with permission, from *Management by Policy;* published by ASQC Quality Press, ©1993.

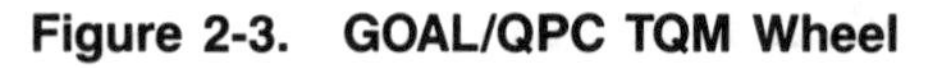

Figure 2-3. GOAL/QPC TQM Wheel

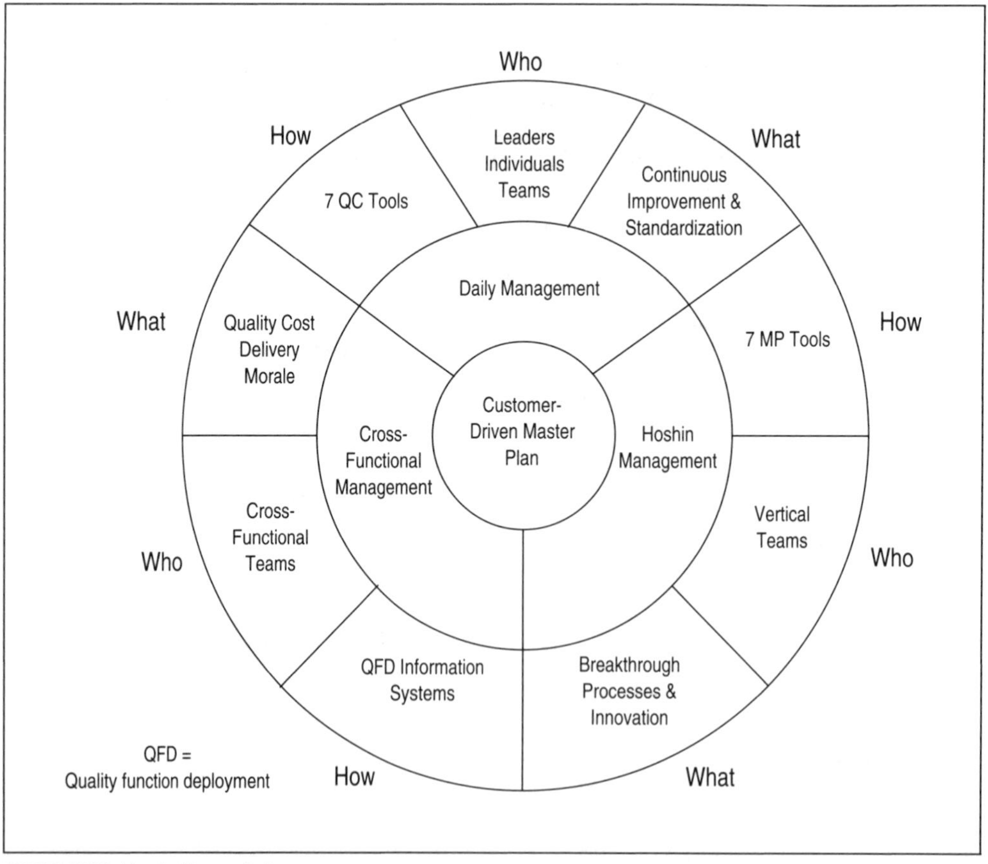

©GOAL/QPC. Used with permission.

management.) Hoshin planning, therefore, plays a critical role in shaping whether an organization's TQM strategy peaks with isolated improvement projects or evolves to become the overall approach to doing what is most important to the business.

Strategic Planning and Hoshin Planning

How does strategic planning relate to hoshin planning? At least two types of relationships can be observed in organizations today. In some organizations, such as SSM Health Care System, Dartmouth-Hitchcock Medical Center, Vermont Academic Medical Center, The Miriam Hospital, and Milwaukee Area Technical College, the hoshin planning process and the strategic planning process are one.

A second option exists for organizations with a strong strategic planning process. Often, multiple long-term goals emerge from strategic planning. The hoshin planning process can be used to identify which goals from the long-term plan will be addressed by the entire organization during that annual planning cycle. The assumption is that the long-term plan contains more than can be accomplished in any one year and that the hoshin process helps to focus on the vital few goals for that year. In some parts of AT&T, this relationship is described as follows: "Strategic planning points toward the direction that your organization should be moving and defines a strategy for your organization to create a sustainable competitive advantage. Policy deployment [hoshin planning] then becomes the method for implementing this strategy."[2] Both types of relationship between strategic and hoshin planning have in common the use of hoshin planning methodologies – such as catchball, management and planning tools, and ongoing reviews – to put a strategic plan into operation.

Whatever approach is used, the hoshin planning cycle should at least be integrated with the strategic planning cycle to maximize alignment of strategies and to minimize duplication of efforts. For example, hoshin planning tasks to select the organization's focus should be scheduled to follow or complement any strategic planning work on mission, vision, business and market assessments, and development of potential goals. Similarly, the hoshin planning annual reviews should be scheduled so they can provide input to the next year's strategic planning process. In addition, the entire hoshin planning annual cycle should precede budget decisions so that the budget can reflect the plan. (See chapter 3 for a discussion of lessons learned by The Miriam Hospital about integrating hoshin planning and budgeting.) At some point, either before launching into hoshin planning or after a year or two of experience, the senior leadership team also needs to decide if and when the two planning processes can be melded into one.

Whatever specific relationship is chosen, hoshin planning, in the words of SSM-Ministry Corporation leaders, "serves to extend the limits of more traditional planning processes, pushing the plan to the vertical and horizontal limits of the organization."[3] (See the SSM-Ministry Corporation and Hewlett-Packard case studies – chapters 12 and 15, respectively – for additional information on how these organizations relate strategic and hoshin planning.)

Overview of the Process

There are four fundamental steps in the hoshin planning process, as shown in figure 2-4: choose the focus, align the organization, implement the plan, review and improve. Where an organization starts in this process depends upon the organization's history, experience, and needs. For example, if an organization has already chosen its focus based on rigorous analysis of market, business, and environmental data, it may be appropriate to start with step 2 of hoshin planning, where the focus is deployed throughout the organization. However, if the organization previously chose a focus with minimal data and with little customer and employee input, it may decide to start somewhere in step 1. This would give the organization the opportunity to confirm and refine the focus through a more rigorous process.

Chapters 6 through 9 of this book discuss the four steps, along with useful tools and an example. Although the steps are described sequentially, hoshin planning is not a linear process. Rather, the four steps are interactive. The entire process can be visualized as a big check-analyze-plan-do (CAPD) cycle, with smaller CAPD cycles connecting individual steps. An overview of the steps follows.

Step 1: Choose the Focus *(or Hoshin Generation)*

The first step of hoshin planning results in the selection of an organizational focus that will lead to a breakthrough level of success. There is a strong emphasis on listening to customers to determine the appropriate focus.

Step 1 initially includes some tasks that are often found in strong strategic planning processes, such as analyzing the state of the business and the market and developing or refining mission and vision statements. Thus, an organization may choose to select from step 1 those tasks that will improve the current strategic planning process, rather than launching another, parallel process. For example, it might be helpful to beef up attention to the customer in the strategic plan, including analysis of data on how customers rank what is most important to them relative to the service. Or, hoshin planning tasks that identify and analyze critical processes may suggest refinements to an existing strategic planning process.

In the last tasks in step 1, the leadership team chooses from many goals the one goal or the vital few goals that the organization will focus on at this time. These focusing

Figure 2-4. Hoshin Planning Process

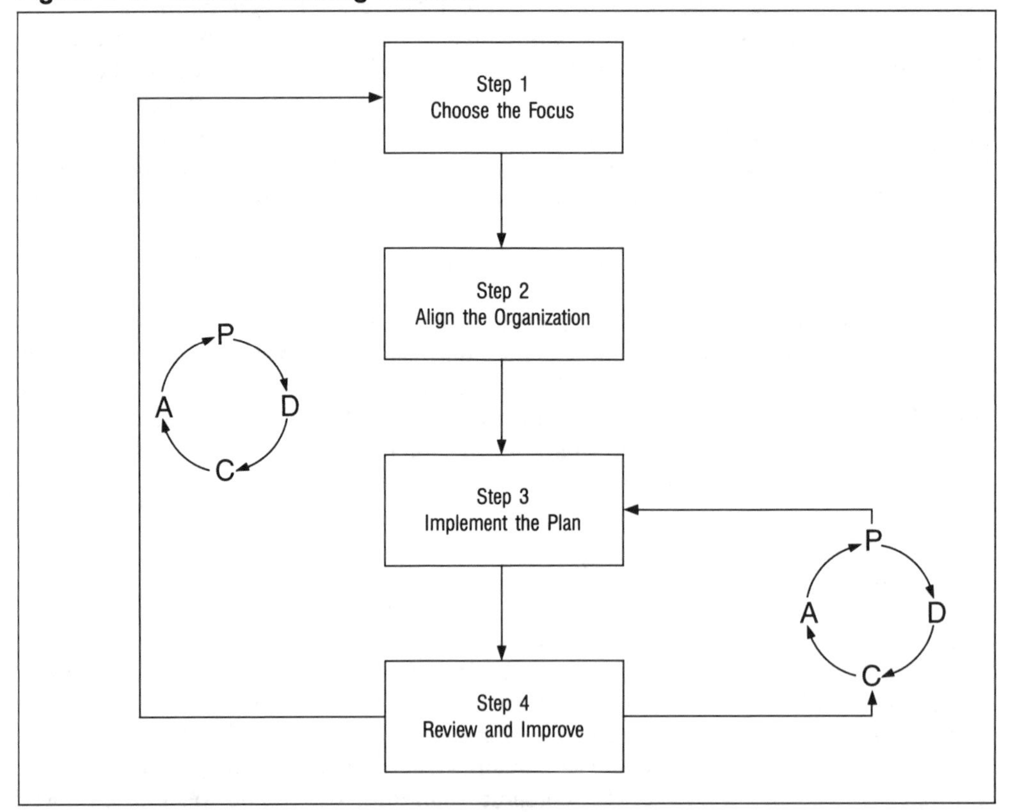

tasks may be a good place for organizations with strong traditional strategic planning processes to launch hoshin planning.

The major tasks in step 1, which are described in chapter 6, are as follows:

- Make the current state of the organization visible.
- Define what the organization wants to be in the future.
- Identify what the organization needs to focus on to achieve its vision.

Step 2: Align the Organization *(or Hoshin Deployment)*

In this step, which in many ways is the heart of hoshin planning, the organization builds the Golden Thread that weaves the organization together to achieve the breakthrough focus. Through a highly participatory but structured process, employees throughout the organization develop a sense of personal contribution to and ownership of the plan. There are four major tasks in step 2:

- *Develop annual targets:* The top leadership planning team first divides the organization's breakthrough focus into annual targets, with clear measures of success.
- *Develop means:* The planning team then shifts from *which* targets to achieve to *how* to achieve them. The team agrees to executive-level means, with measures of success.
- *"Catchball" the targets and means throughout the organization:* At this point, the richness of hoshin planning's deployment process becomes more visible. Through an iterative, organizationwide communication and negotiation process, the top leaders' targets and means are converted sequentially into business unit, team, and individual targets and means.

  This iterative communication and negotiation process is often referred to as catchball. In the catchball process, one level of management throws the ball – the task to be accomplished – to the next level of management or to a team and asks, "What are the most important things you can do (the means) to help to achieve this task, which is now your target?" This process continues down through the organization so that clear and interrelated targets and means are defined at every level by the people closest to the relevant customers and work processes. Then catchball is put into reverse. Each group throws the ball back up, level by level, and asks the succeeding group, "Will our proposed means sufficiently contribute to achieving the organization's focus?" "Are they feasible?" and " How do our proposed means fit with others throughout the organization?" (See figures 2-5 and 2-6.)

  Through this process, the organizational focus becomes more meaningful to employees because it is translated into actions they can do personally to help achieve the focus. Also, integration of the organization is enhanced when the "ball," consisting of targets and means to achieve them, is tossed down and across the organization, then back up to top leadership. (See chapter 13 – the case study of Southwest Texas Methodist Hospital – for a further discussion of catchball, including a sample catchball questionnaire and worksheet.)
- *Finalize the plan:* The plan is now made visible in an easy-to-understand format, so that it can again be communicated throughout the organization and so that progress can be easily tracked. This format includes a one- or two-page summary of the plan. The summary contains clear information on the organization's focus, targets, means, "owners" of targets and means, time lines, and a column to track progress on plan implementation.

Figure 2-5. Catchball

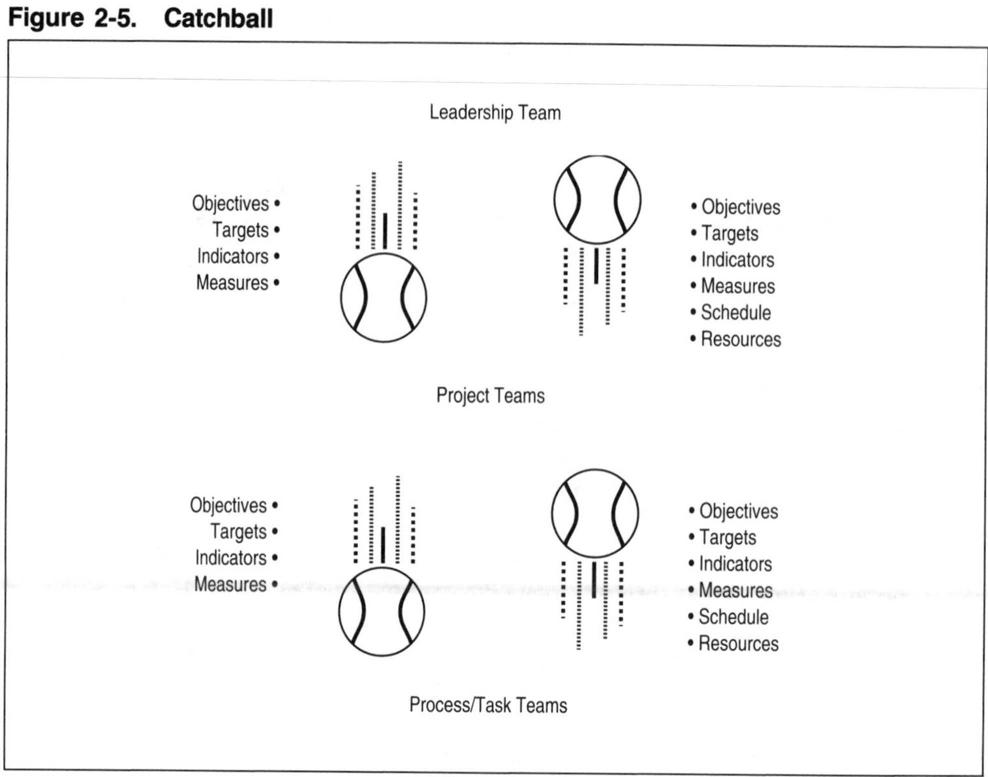

Source: *Policy Deployment Handbook: Setting the Direction for Change*, p. 61. Reproduced with the permission of AT&T ©1992. All rights reserved.

Figure 2-6. Hoshin Deployment

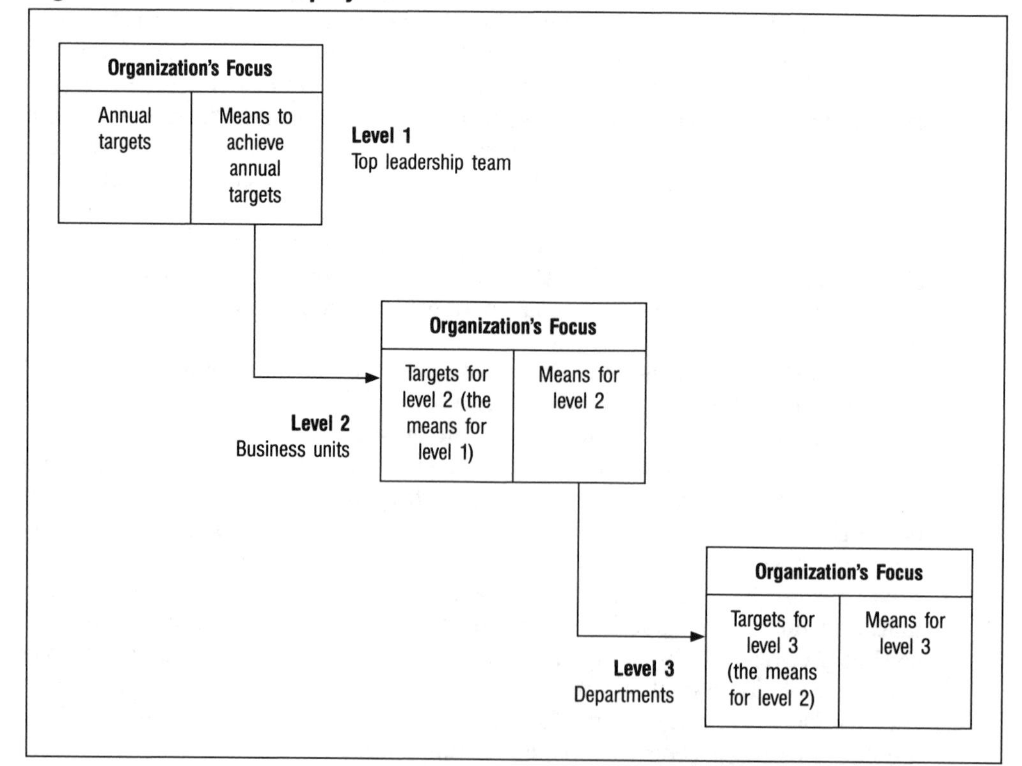

Step 3: Implement the Plan *(or Hoshin Deployment continued)*

In step 3, the plan is executed and relevant data are collected to feed into the review process. The two major tasks in this step are:

- Implement the plan.
- Monitor progress.

Each target and means is tracked as it is being implemented. This includes both quantitative tracking, where data are collected on the measures previously agreed to, and qualitative tracking, where patterns of comments and behaviors are noted.

Step 4: Review and Improve *(or Hoshin Review)*

The purpose of step 4 is to evaluate the process and outcomes of plan implementation to:

- Diagnose and correct problems as soon as possible, and at the level closest to the problem
- Disseminate learning throughout the organization
- Monitor and improve results, the plan, and the planning process
- Recognize and celebrate progress

Steps 3 and 4 are an interactive cycle, with lessons learned from the review incorporated into improved execution on an ongoing basis. In addition, lessons learned from the reviews are cycled back into steps 1 and 2, to improve future plans.

The review step may not seem as compelling as other aspects of hoshin planning. Yet the review step is essential to long-term, sustainable results. This step, in particular, is where the organization benefits from ongoing learning and from ongoing improvement based on that learning.

The reviews can be done efficiently. At The Miriam Hospital, for example, the hoshin planning review process has not added any more meetings. Reviews of progress on both the organization's focus and departmental targets are integrated into existing management meetings on a regular basis.

Although the frequency may vary by organization, there are usually at least three types of review, which take place in a bottom-up cycle:

- *Team reviews:* These reviews are conducted by the individual teams on a frequent basis, such as monthly. The primary purpose is to diagnose problems as soon as possible and to prevent or to correct them.
- *Review by next level or levels of management:* These reviews, which might take place quarterly or bimonthly, focus on cross-functional problem solving, sharing lessons learned, and monitoring progress on plan implementation.
- *Top management review:* This organizationwide review takes place quarterly or at least every six months. Top management reviews three things: the process, the results, and key lessons learned. Then the process is improved for the next cycle.

At first glance, these reviews may sound similar to what the organization is already doing. To tap the value-added potential that hoshin planning brings to reviews, it is important to:

- Again use a catchball-type dialogue process to evaluate progress.

- Use a simple standard evaluation format that takes minimal time and makes it easy to track progress on implementation of the Golden Thread. (See chapter 3, figure 3-8, and chapter 9 for examples.)
- Resist the temptation to review only results; instead, put equal emphasis on evaluating the process to learn about what worked, what did not work, and why.

(See the case studies of Bethesda, Our Lady of Lourdes, and Hewlett-Packard – chapters 10, 11, and 15, respectively – for examples of the review process, including sample review worksheets.)

Summary

Hoshin planning is a planning and management system that focuses and aligns the organization to achieve breakthroughs for customers. It does not replace other management strategies, such as benchmarking, reengineering, and continuous quality improvement. Rather, hoshin planning helps an organization to focus on a breakthrough direction and on annual targets. The other management strategies can be a means to help accomplish the targets and to progress in this direction.

In some organizations, the hoshin planning process and the strategic planning process are one. In others, hoshin planning is used to focus on and rigorously deploy a vital few priorities from within the strategic plan. Whatever the relationship, hoshin planning "serves to extend the limits of more traditional planning processes, pushing the plan to the vertical and horizontal limits of the organization."[4]

There are four fundamental steps in the hoshin planning process:

1. Choose the focus.
2. Align the organization.
3. Implement the plan.
4. Review and improve.

As described in more detail in chapters 5 through 9, an array of tools and techniques helps make this process efficient, creative, and effective.

At AT&T's Transmission Systems Business Unit, hoshin planning looked complex at first, but "with thorough training up front and ongoing communication on the job, people now say they've never had a clearer idea of why they're doing what they're doing and how what they do furthers the most important goals of the organization."[5]

Actions for Top Leadership

In the awareness-building stage of hoshin planning, leadership should:

1. Determine whether this effort will have a special name and, if so, select a concise and memorable name and definition.
2. Communicate the major elements of hoshin planning to the organization, including why they are important and how the organization will address them.
3. Clarify how hoshin planning will fit with TQM, strategic planning, and other major management efforts currently under way. Make this fit visible in graphical form, and communicate it widely throughout the organization.
4. Gain an understanding of the four basic steps of the hoshin planning process sufficient to: (a) introduce the four steps to employees, (b) ensure that the process does not get overly complicated and burdensome and that existing meetings are used as much as possible, (c) begin to identify the types of

supportive resources – such as people, systems, and education – that will be needed to do hoshin planning well.

5. Keep the reasons for implementing hoshin planning visible to the leadership team to keep the effort on track and in perspective.

References

1. Lois Gold, vice-president Citibank, N.A, Citicorp. Personal communication to Mara Melum and Casey Collett, May 24, 1994.
2. AT&T Quality Steering Committee. Policy Deployment. Morristown, NJ: AT&T, 1992, p. 14.
3. Bush, Sister M. L., and Beste, J. T. SSM-Ministry Corporation case study. Chapter 12 of this book.
4. Bush and Beste.
5. Monteforte, L. AT&T Quest for Excellence V Conference, Washington, DC, Feb. 14, 1993.

CHAPTER THREE

Hoshin Planning Key Success Factors

> Never tell people *how* to do things. Tell them *what* to do and they will surprise you with their ingenuity.
>
> –Gen. George S. Patton, *War As I Knew It*

The results of hoshin planning, like any change strategy, are proportional to the commitment and capabilities an organization brings to the effort. The purpose of this chapter is to discuss six key factors that contribute to successful hoshin planning–hoshin planning that leads to increased organizational focus and alignment. The chapter also discusses the evolution of hoshin planning in an organization. Additional factors that have been key to the success of individual case study organizations are described in chapters 10 through 15 of this book.

These six key success factors[1] (KSFs) are a guide–a lighthouse beacon amid foggy seas:

1. Ability to prioritize
2. Customer-based plan
3. Leadership champions
4. Deployment of the plan throughout the organization
5. Foundation of planning and process improvement skills
6. User-friendly process and tools

Not every organization will be equally strong in all factors. Some organizations may see the need to substantially improve in all six factors but will decide to embark on hoshin planning anyway. The important thing is to work for continuous improvement in these six areas–and in other areas key to the organization's customized version of hoshin planning.

KSF 1: Ability to Prioritize

It is difficult for most CEOs and leadership teams to narrow down the long list of "things we must do" to a very short list of the *vital few* organizational goals. This was the case at Fletcher Allen Health Care, where one of the toughest hoshin planning challenges was identified as "integration at the top central level–reconciling the trade-offs that had to be made to select a focus."[2] Top leadership must develop a rigorous process to select the vital few organizational goals. Then leadership needs to have the courage to say no, for now, to the other priority goal candidates.

Hoshin planning provides a process to prioritize and choose the focus. In this prioritization process, the top leadership team serves as the planning team. It gets input from internal and external customers and suppliers. As described in more detail in chapter 6, hoshin planning includes three basic tasks to prioritize and choose the organizational focus:

1. The planning team first makes the *current* state of the organization visible. To do this, the leadership reaffirms or refines the organization's mission and values; identifies major customer, supplier, and competitor trends; and analyzes the current state of the business.
2. Then top leadership, often including the board, defines the vision of what the organization will be in the *future.*
3. Top leadership identifies what the organization needs to *focus* on to achieve its vision. This third task includes listening to customers to determine the most important customer expectations relative to the vision. Then these customer expectations are translated into organizational key success factors. Next, the leadership team may do a gap analysis to assess where the organization stands on each success factor. Finally, top leadership chooses the organization's breakthrough focus.

Figure 3-1 illustrates this process of choosing a focus with a health care example.

There are many helpful planning and management tools that can be used to analyze data and narrow the list of potential goals. (See chapter 6 and appendix B for more information on helpful tools.) But there is no easy formula for making the final choice of an organizational focus. This is where the art of leadership merges with a fact-based decision-making process. Leadership judgment prevails.

Leadership can consider three additional guidelines as it chooses the focus:

1. Limit the number of breakthrough organizational focuses to a vital few. How many are a "vital few"? Ideally, an organization will start with only one breakthrough focus. As it gains experience, it may expand this to two or three. SSM-Ministry Corporation found it helpful to use a "rule of twos" in its first year of hoshin planning. The corporation has one organizational focus and, in the first year of hoshin planning, limited targets and means to two at every level of deployment. For organizations starting out on hoshin planning, GOAL/QPC's Research Committee advises the following: "Recognizing that the organization is on a learning curve, the planning team should choose a limited number of objectives (i.e., two maximum)."[3]

   Dr. Noriaki Kano warns against chasing "too many rabbits" and notes, "It is very common for a company introducing [hoshin planning] to set up too many policies, and I often caution companies about this. This caution, however, is generally neglected or forgotten during the first year, and as a consequence, the results are inadequate. Then management pays attention to focusing its efforts from the second year on."[4]
2. At the point of difficult decisions, ask a magnitude question about each alternative: "Is this focus really a breakthrough, or is it continuous improvement of a more moderate nature?" For example, will "reducing all waiting times" significantly help the organization leap toward a market leader position? Or are

these smaller (albeit important) changes that the organization needs to make to maintain its current strong position in the face of more demanding customers? If so, can the organization implement this change in a more limited way, instead of targeting the full power of the organization on it?

3. Keep the time element in mind. As the leadership team is searching for the most important focus for the organization, it may want to organize the potential focuses into a multiyear matrix. This type of matrix can help clarify when it is most important to work on a specific focus, including whether there is a critical path that should be followed. A multiyear matrix also visibly "saves" the list of other opportunities for future reference, thereby preventing the dampening of sponsors' enthusiasm.

A strong prioritization process results in a top leadership team that is focused on Stephen Covey's quadrant II: goals that may not be urgent, but are important—that is, goals that are important for the long term. For information on how certain organizations have selected their focus, see the case studies of Our Lady of Lourdes Medical Center, AT&T, and Hewlett-Packard in chapters 11, 14, and 15, respectively.

Figure 3-1. Choosing the Focus: A Health Care Example

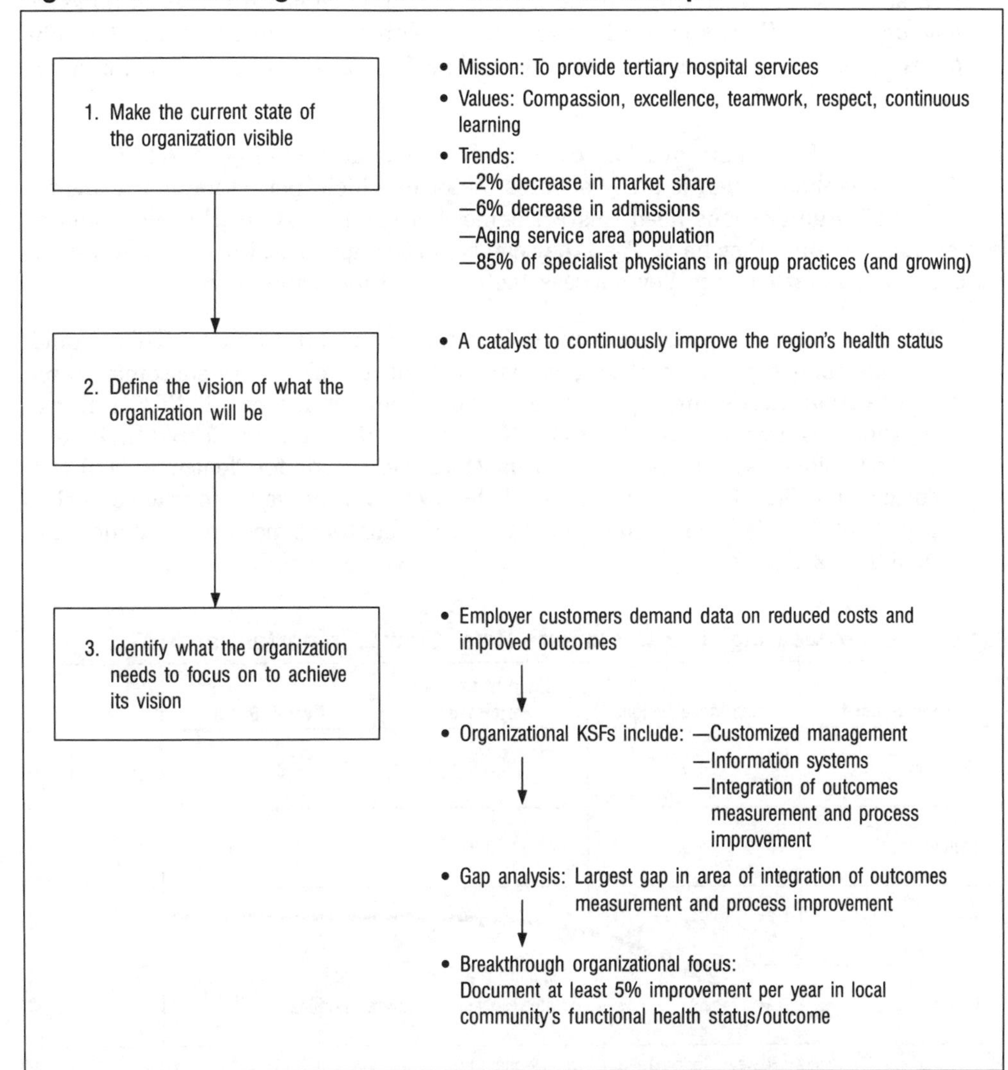

KSF 2: Customer-Based Plan

When hoshin planning is done well, success is almost ensured. One reason is that the entire hoshin planning process is based on a rigorous understanding of customer needs and expectations. But many organizations are in a situation similar to that of Fletcher Allen Health Care, which identified one of its two toughest hoshin planning challenges as "developing a profound base of customer knowledge." Even Baldrige Award winner AT&T Transmission Systems, at the start of its hoshin planning efforts, faced the problem of insufficient customer data.

> Customer needs were known in the general sense, but not specifically in many cases. In addition, the customers' weighting of specific needs was not known and . . . performance in meeting the needs was not well understood or quantified. Many performance measures were internally focused and did not have the customers' viewpoint.
>
> To overcome this information shortcoming, the management team tentatively spoke for the customer by developing an initial list of specific needs and ranking their importance. Next they developed indicators to determine existing . . . performance levels for each one.
>
> At first glance, this approach appears to be in direct conflict with the TQM principle of management with facts. However, developing this information through formal market research would have taken at least nine months. *It was either start now or wait until next year.* Management developed a list of deployment candidates by collecting sufficient marketing and performance data to validate preliminary conclusions.[5]

(See chapter 14 for a more detailed case study of hoshin planning at AT&T.)

A customer-based plan is a key success factor in which "perfection is the enemy of the good." Organizations need to start somewhere and build on whatever foundation of customer data they have. Then they can begin to improve it. For example, organizations can strengthen this key success factor in the following ways:

- Measure how customers rate what is most important to them. This should include some type of weighting system, so that it is clear how customers rank their various needs and expectations. As illustrated in figure 3-2, AT&T's Transmission Systems Business Unit (TSBU) found that customers scored their need for "reliability" (4.8) as more important than their needs for "features" (4.5) and "price" (4.4). The TSBU then assessed the need to improve performance in this area (5.0). This led to a high score of 24 for the customer need of reliability ($4.8 \times 5.0 = 24.0$).

Figure 3-2. Measuring How Customers Rate What Is Important at AT&T

Customer Need	Importance Weight	× Need to Improve Performance	= Overall Score	
Reliability	4.8	5.0	24.0	→ Priority
Features	4.5	3.2	14.4	
Price	4.4			
Others				

Legend: 1 = low 5 = high
Note: Highest scores are priorities.

Source: *National Productivity Review,* Spring 1993, p. 154. Reprinted by permission of John Wiley & Sons, Inc.

Figures 3-3 through 3-7 (pp. 31–35) illustrate the approach used by the Center for Continuous Quality Improvement at Milwaukee Area Technical College (MATC) to identify and prioritize customer needs. Customers of the college include students, business and industry, taxpayers, K–12 districts, employees, the Wisconsin technical college system, universities, labor, the North Central Association accrediting organization, the media, and advisory committees. The college ranked customer needs both through the strategic planning steering committee and through town meetings with customers. The top four customer needs identified are "quality education and services," "training," "treated with respect," and "accountability." The strategic planning steering committee then developed the customer needs matrix shown in figure 3-7 to clarify which needs are most important to which MATC customers.

- It may also be helpful to measure three levels of customer expectations—expected quality, requested quality, and exciting quality:[6]
  - *Expected quality:* These are the baseline traits that the customer assumes, often unconsciously, that the product or service will have.

    For example, a hospital patient assumes that medical staff has the appropriate technical knowledge and that the surgeon has the information to operate on the correct knee. An HMO member assumes she will be billed correctly for any copayments. Health care providers do not get points for meeting these expectations, but they do get disappointed customers when they do not meet them.
  - *Requested quality:* These are the product or service traits that the customer specifically asks for.

    For example, the hospital patient may request a private room or a clear explanation of treatment options from the physician. The HMO member may request that she be able to see any physician of her choice in case of an emergency or a life-threatening illness.

Figure 3-3. Customer Needs

Note: These numbers are for classification only and do *not* indicate any prioritization of needs.

1. Quality education and services
2. Training
3. Treated with respect
4. Accountability
5. Needs met in a timely manner
6. Transfer of technology
7. Career laddering
8. Articulation (up and down)
9. Accessibility
10. Skills for employment
11. Equity
12. Cost-effective
13. Economic development
14. Counseling
15. Leadership for innovation
16. Stable environment
17. Community involvement and participation
18. State-of-the-art technology
19. Qualified teachers, staff, and administrators
20. Easy registration process
21. Variety of offerings
22. Efficiently kept statistics
23. Return on investment
24. Clear plan
25. Alternative delivery
26. Faculty, staff development
27. Up-to-date curriculum
28. Functional equipment
29. Operational facilities
30. Safe, clean environment
31. Professionalism
32. Evaluation of teaching
33. Positive mentoring
34. Reasonable work load
35. Relevant education
36. Positive self-image
37. Andrological teaching models
38. Outlet for opinions
39. Sense of purpose and security
40. Effective leadership
41. Open entry, open exit
42. Improved college image
43. Target marketing (high skills, high pay)
44. High expectations
45. Focus on achievement
46. Effective communications
47. Flexible systems
48. Access for seniors

Figure 3-4. Milwaukee Area Technical College Customer Needs, As Ranked by the Strategic Planning Steering Committee

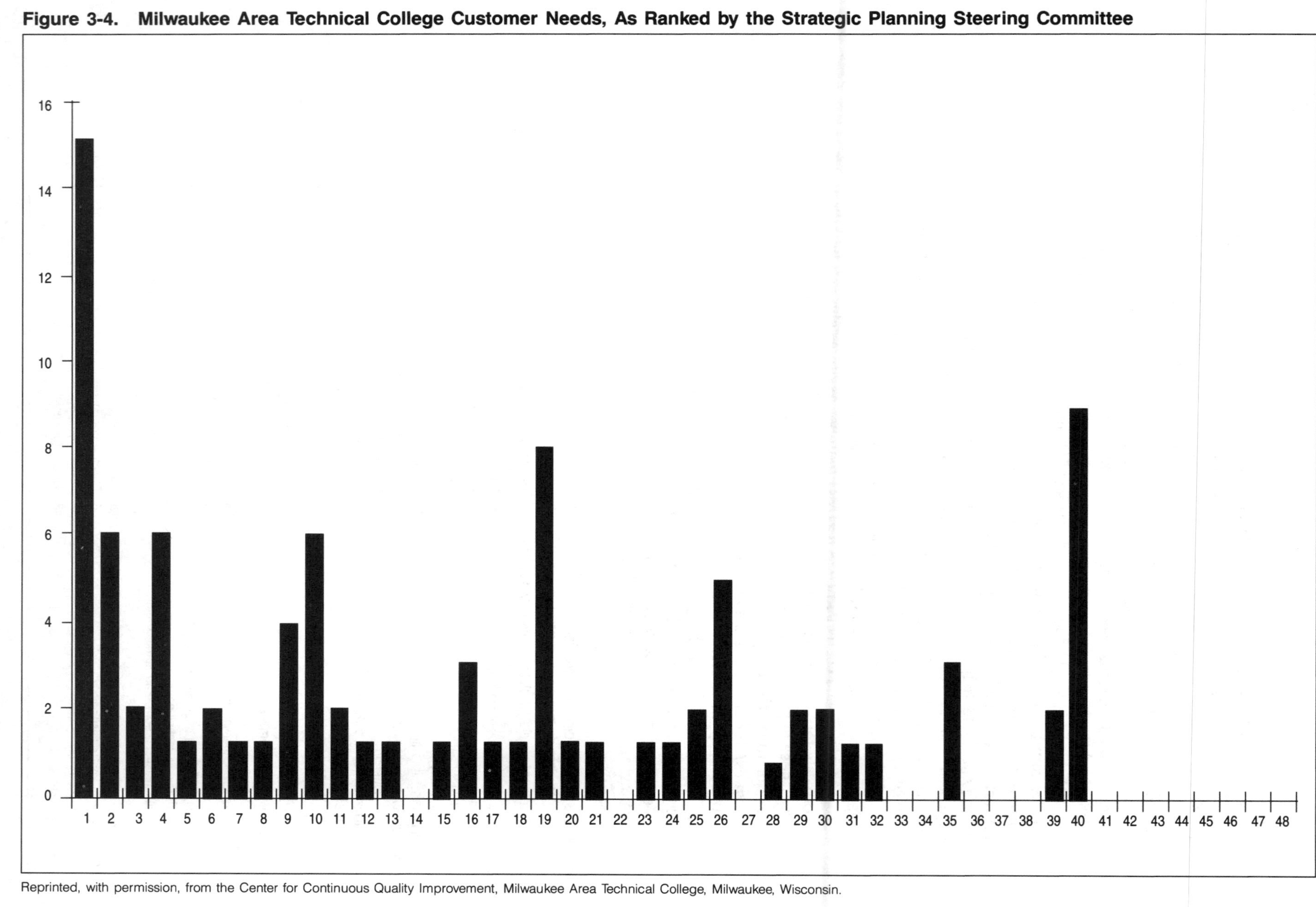

Reprinted, with permission, from the Center for Continuous Quality Improvement, Milwaukee Area Technical College, Milwaukee, Wisconsin.

Figure 3-5. MATC Customer Needs As Ranked at Town Meetings

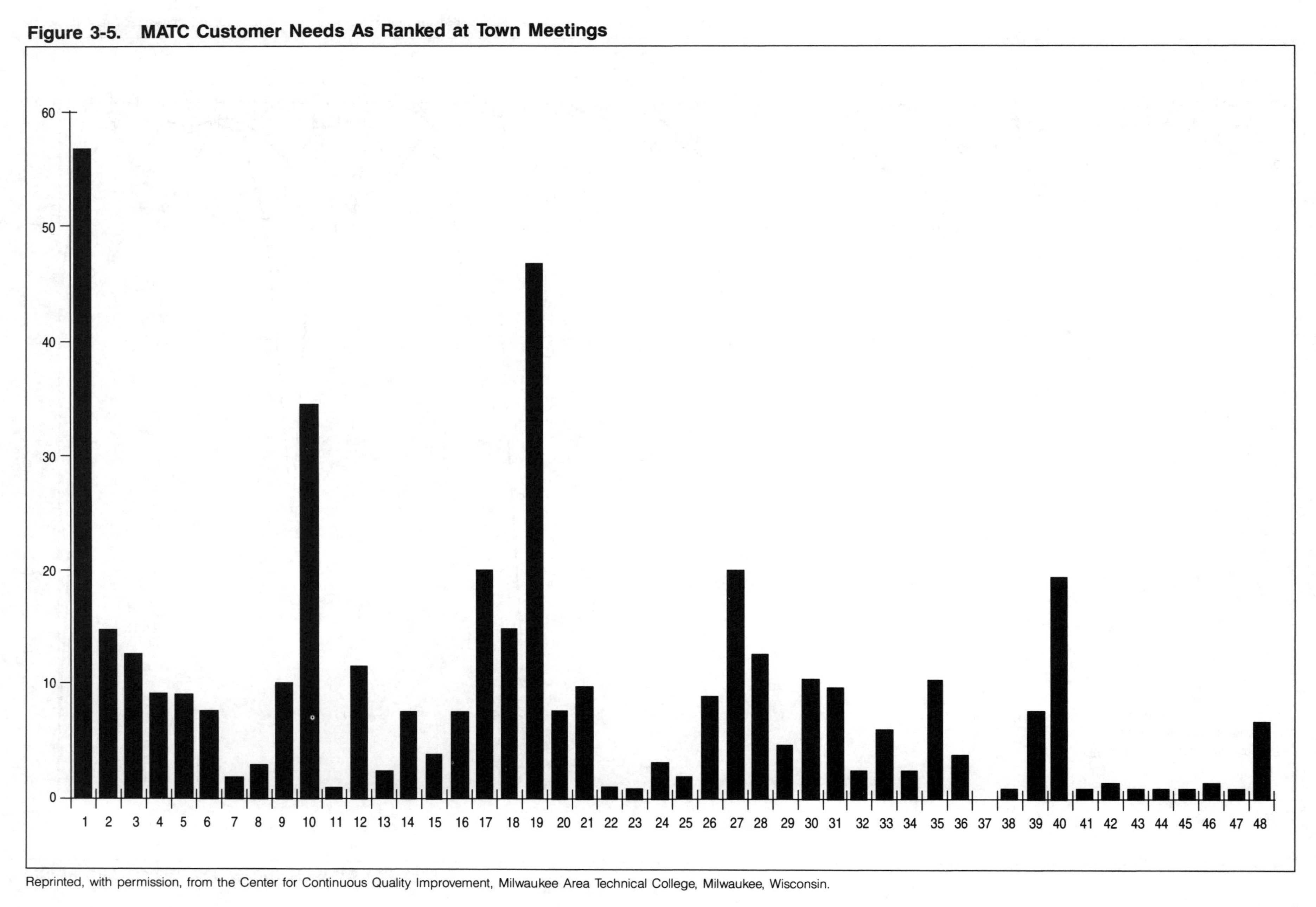

Reprinted, with permission, from the Center for Continuous Quality Improvement, Milwaukee Area Technical College, Milwaukee, Wisconsin.

Figure 3-6. Customer Needs/Relative Ranking

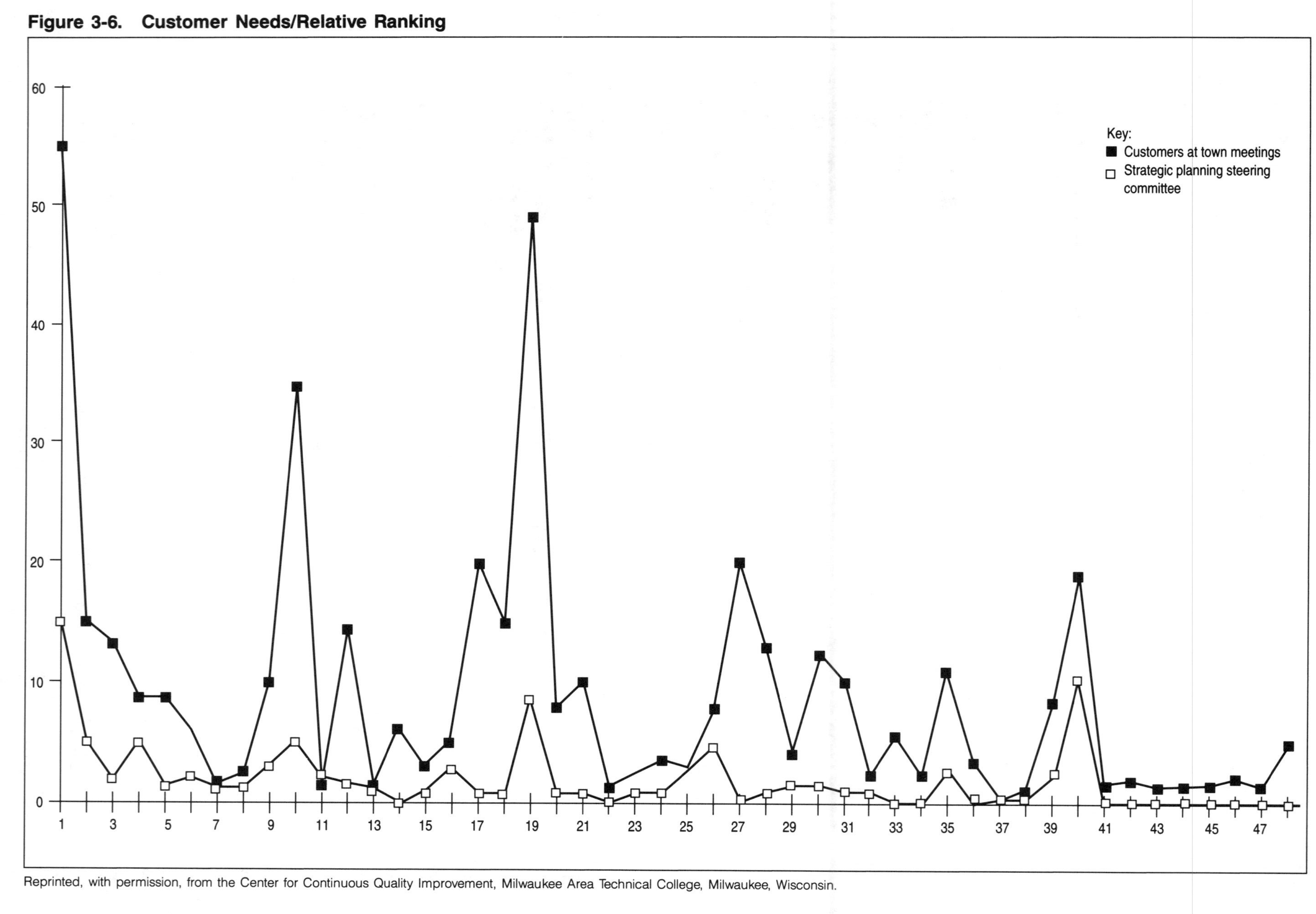

Reprinted, with permission, from the Center for Continuous Quality Improvement, Milwaukee Area Technical College, Milwaukee, Wisconsin.

Figure 3-7. Customer Needs Matrix, Strategic Planning Steering Committee

Legend
⊙ Strongest
○ Stronger
△ Strong

	Students	Business and Industry	Taxpayers	K–12 Districts	Employees	WI VTAE	Universities	Labor	NCA	Media	Advisory Committee
Quality Education and Services	⊙	△		○							
Effective Leadership			△								
Qualified Teachers, Staff, and Faculty	○						⊙		△		
Training		⊙						⊙			
Accountability			○							○	○
Skills for Employment	△					△		○			
Community Involvement and Participation				△						⊙	⊙
Up-to-Date Curriculum				⊙			○				△
State-of-the-Art Technology		○						△			
Treated with Respect					△						
Functional Equipment											
Cost-Effectiveness			⊙			○					
Faculty, Staff Development				△	⊙	⊙			⊙		
Accessibility										△	
Stable Environment					○						
Relevant Education							△		○		

Reprinted, with permission, from the Center for Continuous Quality Improvement, Milwaukee Area Technical College, Milwaukee, Wisconsin.

–*Exciting quality:* These are product or service traits that will surprise and thrill the customer. This is often the breakthrough area of quality, where organizations need to truly see life through the eyes of the customer and anticipate his or her needs.

In a hospital, exciting quality might be finding that there is no admissions process to go through – that, instead, all necessary data are already online at the bedside, in the patient's automated medical and related records. An HMO member might be thrilled to find that the HMO has worked with her employer to set up easily accessible exercise and health status testing facilities at her company.

If the organization wants to achieve dramatic performance breakthroughs, it is likely that it will have to meet both expected and requested quality expectations and to strive to achieve exciting quality.

- A technique called quality function deployment (QFD) may also be useful to strengthen an organization's customer focus. *Quality function deployment* is designed to listen to the "voice of the customer" and to translate it into business decisions. First, customers identify, in their own words, their expectations for the product or service offered. The customers' words can then be translated into the language of the company. Then the company identifies a work process that affects a customer expectation and sets a related goal. For example, if health care customers describe their expectation as "convenience," this can be translated into the company language of "short wait times." This focus can be turned into a goal the organization can control, such as "to reduce all scheduled wait times within the organization to less than 15 minutes."

Staying close to what is most important to customers is hard but essential work. The CEO of Motorola asserts that "fame is a fleeting thing." He understands that each day customers expect more than they did the day before and "you'd better find ways to be better."[7]

KSF 3: Leadership Champions

All major changes require leadership support and participation to succeed long term. In the case of hoshin planning, top leaders are likely to be natural champions. That is because hoshin planning helps top leaders focus on the issues *they* determine to be the *most important issues* for the organization's success. Because hoshin planning is a kind of management compass, it supports the direction-setting role of top leaders.

As champions, the CEO and other senior leaders play a number of roles. For example:

- Senior leaders need to make the decision that hoshin planning will be the central way the organization plans its major directions, not an extra "flavor-of-the-month" program. This means that hoshin planning is closely integrated with—or in some cases *is*—the strategic planning process. This decision needs to be clearly communicated throughout the organization.
- The senior leadership team needs to personally go through a rigorous planning process that includes determining the organization's vision, really listening to the voice of the customer, and biting the bullet to select the organization's focus—the vital few organizational goals.
- To reinforce the importance of the organization's breakthrough focus and to ensure deployment throughout the organization, a senior leader should serve as "focus champion" for each focus. The role of the focus champion is to ensure achievement of the focus, including:
  - Assessing and quantifying current performance relative to the focus
  - Serving as coach and catalyst to the teams at various levels of the organization that are working on the focus
  - Cutting through bureaucracy, as needed, and reducing other barriers to cross-functional progress on the focus
  - Tracking team progress and serving as liaison to keep the CEO and the top leadership team informed

  At AT&T every team working on priority projects has a senior executive champion. "These are no figureheads; the executive champions are ultimately accountable for the team's results."[8] Hewlett-Packard says that it is important to identify a single owner for each focus. "If more than one person is assigned ownership, there may be confusion around who is accountable for what."[9]
- Senior leaders need to deploy the plan through a "catchball"-type process that depends on others to propose the best means to achieve the targets. This requires

substantial trust in both the process and in employees. It is likely to require a major change in management style for senior leaders who are used to directing others on both what targets to achieve and how to achieve them.

- Another important role of senior leaders is to champion learning and improvement by conducting ongoing reviews of progress on plan implementation. This includes making clear to employees the importance of evaluating both the results and the means used. It also means incorporating lessons learned in the next cycle of hoshin planning.

The president of SSM-Ministry Corporation describes the roles and responsibilities of a president in hoshin planning as follows:

- To ensure [implementation of] training programs
- To allow mistakes and confusion while switching the process
- To let go of what doesn't promote the hoshin [the focus][10]

Hewlett-Packard emphasizes that "management must create the appropriate environment for planning and conducting reviews. If a safe and comfortable environment for sharing poor performance data has not been established, people may distort or hide their data for fear of reprisal. Focus on process improvement and not fault finding throughout your planning and reviewing. Use the opportunities for cross-functional planning to improve teamwork."[11]

More detailed discussion of the role of leaders in hoshin planning can be found in the case studies of Bethesda, Inc. (chapter 10), Our Lady of Lourdes Medical Center (chapter 11), SSM-Ministry Corporation (chapter 12), AT&T (chapter 14), and Hewlett-Packard (chapter 15). In addition, chapters 6 through 9 describe the role of top leaders in each of the four basic steps of the hoshin planning process and chapter 4 includes a leaders' hoshin planning implementation worksheet (pp. 63–64).

KSF 4: Deployment of the Plan throughout the Organization

Deployment of the plan means converting the organizationwide focus into specific operational plans throughout the organization. The SSM-Ministry Corporation notes that:

> Deployment [is] a series of carefully engineered, inseparably linked plans, each of which is integral to the future structure, stability, and success of the organization. [It] can be thought of as a repetitive process, at each level within the organization, of collectively defining (or acknowledging) the desired outcomes, then deciding how they are to be achieved and who will be held responsible for the planned actions.[12]

The deployment process often used in hoshin planning is referred to as catchball, which is defined in chapter 2 and discussed in detail in chapter 7. Catchball is an extremely powerful process to ensure that there is broad understanding and ownership of the plan. The Juran Institute has found that "feedback from companies using this process suggests that it outperforms the process of unilateral goal setting by upper managers."[13] When it is done well, ultimately everyone in the organization understands how he or she contributes to achieving the organization's most important goals. Catchball is the essence of good, effective communication. It is an important building block of strong support for the plan.

It is critical to carefully decide as to whom the ball will be thrown in catchball. At this point, the organization is determining who is in the best position to propose means to achieve the target and who will be accountable to achieve the target. As discussed in more detail in chapter 4, deployment channels can be either functional teams (that is, existing departments or other business units) or cross-functional teams. The primary criterion should be to select the group of people who are closest to the processes associated with the specific target and means.

The Miriam Hospital is an example of an organization whose "big hoshin planning mistake in year one" related to catchball. "We gave the annual objectives to each VP and said, 'Meet with your direct reports and identify what to do to achieve them.' They proceeded to propose means for everyone else but themselves to implement!"[14] Now top management at The Miriam Hospital asks vice-presidents to figure out what they personally can do to achieve the annual objectives (targets) and to figure out who else should work with them.

Catchball is also likely to be most effective if simple worksheets and matrixes are used to make the relationship between various levels of the plan visible and clear. People can thus more easily trace the Golden Thread that ties their targets and means to the organization's focus.

In the first years of hoshin planning, it is not unusual to find a combination of catchball at the higher levels and more traditional top-down planning further down in the organization. For example, in the first year of hoshin planning in a multihospital system, there might be strong catchball between the system senior leadership team and the hospitals' senior leaders. However, the hospital senior leaders might then go back to directing middle management teams as to both what they should do to contribute to the system's focus and how they should do it.

Although not ideal, this is a natural phase as organizations wrestle with how much change they can introduce at one time and still efficiently manage the organization on a daily basis. "Crazy time," when the organization lives with both old and new ways of doing business, is a natural – albeit tumultuous – phase in most change processes. It should be acknowledged for what it is, not misread as a lack of management commitment. There should, however, be a plan to increase both the amount and the effectiveness of catchball as the organization gains comfort with hoshin planning. The deployment process and catchball, including a sample catchball worksheet, are described in more detail in the case studies on SSM-Ministry Corporation (chapter 12), Southwest Texas Methodist Hospital (chapter 13), AT&T (chapter 14), and Hewlett-Packard (chapter 15).

KSF 5: Foundation of Planning and Process Improvement Skills

An organization will more easily succeed at hoshin planning if it already is familiar with the tools and techniques of good strategic planning and process improvement. This includes an understanding of what a mission and vision are and a comfort level with setting organizational and personal goals that can be measured. Minneapolis Children's Medical Center puts it more strongly: "An organization's hoshin planning effectiveness is directly related to its success with strategic planning. A strong foundation of strategic planning fosters an ability to say not everything is equal – and that a limited number of efforts are more crucial to the organization now than others."[15]

In addition, it is helpful if an organization has some experience with process improvement methodologies such as total quality management (TQM) and continuous quality improvement (CQI). Much of the work of hoshin planning applies the plan-do-check-act (PDCA) cycle to processes. Such TQM/CQI tools and techniques as flowcharts and matrixes help make hoshin planning work well. An organization that is comfortable with the concept of processes and with these tools can concentrate on using them to identify the best targets and means and on achieving them. The importance of this experience is elaborated upon in the Bethesda and Hewlett-Packard case studies in chapters 10 and 15, respectively.

It is important for organizations at all levels of experience to develop just-in-time continuing education programs to facilitate continuous learning. An organization with less experience in process improvement is likely to need a customized training program early in the hoshin planning effort to build a foundation of skills.

To build knowledge and skills to successfully implement the four steps of hoshin planning, a continuing education effort could, for example, address the following needs:

- *Step 1: Choose the focus.* It can be helpful to provide education for leaders in the philosophy of hoshin planning, how it differs and fits with more traditional strategic planning, the seven management and planning tools (see appendix B), and the specific responsibilities of leaders in hoshin planning.
- *Step 2: Align the organization.* Everyone who will be involved in catchball is likely to benefit from a short, just-in-time course on hoshin planning. This course should clearly communicate the organization's focus, emphasize the individual's role in deployment, introduce the time line, and include specific instructions on how to select the best means and measures and how to fill out any worksheets.
- *Step 3: Implement the plan.* Everyone involved in implementing and monitoring the plan should receive specific, just-in-time instructions about his or her role. This should include information on how to collect, record, study, and report data.
- *Step 4: Review and improve.* Reviewers need education on the organization's approach to reviews in hoshin planning. This could include information on interviewing skills, techniques such as "Asking 'Why?' Five Times," and coaching skills.

The AT&T case study in chapter 14 describes in more detail one leading organization's approach to education and training related to hoshin planning.

Although the tools, techniques, and skills called upon in hoshin planning are critical, organizations need to avoid the common pitfall of getting lost in the tools. It is important to continue to remind yourself that the tools are simply means to an end, not ends in and of themselves. The Center for Continuous Quality Improvement at Milwaukee Area Technical College recommends continually asking, "Does this make sense here?" And if something does not make sense, "change the decision to fit common sense, not to fit the tools."[16] Chapter 4 elaborates on options regarding when an organization should embark on hoshin planning.

KSF 6: User-Friendly Process and Tools

Hoshin planning is a structured approach that systematically and rigorously translates organizational priorities into front-line work. Its structure includes strong accountability systems and a range of planning and management tools.

One challenge facing organizations embarking on hoshin planning is to incorporate the strengths of this systematic approach while avoiding the common traps. Some organizations find that hoshin planning – or any planning and management process – can become an end in itself, rather than a means to an end. Organizations need to prevent hoshin planning from becoming overly bureaucratic, rigid, and driven by paperwork and tools. For example, the Juran Institute provides organizations with a planning-for-deployment worksheet to help identify and prevent some of these potential problems. This worksheet notes, "One of the important tactical issues in strategic quality planning is how to involve many levels in the organization without (1) causing excessive delay and (2) creating too much paperwork. What are your concerns with respect to these two issues? What would be some ways to deal with them?"[17]

In the first year of hoshin planning at The Miriam Hospital, for example, the top management team found itself overwhelmed by paperwork as it attempted to review plan implementation reports from every department. Middle managers and other employees became frustrated by the "hurry-up-and-wait" syndrome, where they rushed to submit their reviews and then often waited three weeks while top management struggled to evaluate progress on 79 pages of plans. But hospital management learned what to look for in hoshin planning reviews and developed a simple review worksheet that "facilitates true delegation. Now the entire review process takes top management only about three hours, and it usually takes only about five minutes to fill out each review form."[18] The review form used at Miriam, shown in figure 3-8, is part of an exception-based review process in which managers simply fill out one of three sections for their part of the plan:

1. Task is completed and measure was or was not met.
2. Task is in progress and the completion date is expected to be met.
3. Change is needed to the task, measure, and/or completion date and the change has been approved by the appropriate VP.

As The Miriam Hospital recognized, hoshin planning needs to strike a balance between structure and creativity–and to be user-friendly. Following are some of the characteristics that give hoshin planning the potential to be user-friendly:

- Hoshin planning provides a new level of clarity about the targets that teams and individuals are held accountable to achieve.
- It employs numerous planning and management tools, such as matrixes and tree diagrams and flags, which are ingredients of a creative, user-friendly process. Joe Colletti of GOAL/QPC and the Woodledge Group notes that the appropriate use of tools can provide three important benefits:
  – *Visibility:* The tools provide the capability to make plan details, development, and discussions "visible." "Seeing" the plan enhances communication and understanding.
  – *Neutrality:* The tools separate ideas from the originating individuals. They minimize biases that can compromise discussions.
  – *Compatibility:* The tools have been used before in a variety of different forms. The "learning curve" on the tools is minimal.[19]

  For example, in the review step, the same plan summary previously used to deploy the plan can be used again. A simple technique called a "flag" can be incorporated to make visible the progress on the target. The team colors a portion of the flag to illustrate the percentage of the target (or means) that has been achieved, or writes this percentage in the flag. For example, as seen in figure 3-9, VHA of Pennsylvania achieved 90 percent of its target B: "Continue the development and implementation of the health assessment model for meeting community health needs."
- Another user-friendly characteristic in hoshin planning is that the organization is encouraged to make the top level of the plan visible on one page, as shown in figure 3-10.

  Sample plans from Fletcher Allen Health Care and The Miriam Hospital are included in appendix C, and additional plans are shown in the case studies in part III, chapters 10 through 15, of this book.
- Still another user-friendly aspect of hoshin planning is the ongoing feedback loop, from the review step to improvements in plan implementation. Leaders at Dartmouth-Hitchcock Medical Center appreciate that there is no need to repeat the entire planning process each year. Instead, "the plan can just be readjusted, based on changes in the environment and relevance of the organization's vision. In addition, the emphasis can be on creating more synergy among the strategies."[20]

Figure 3-8. Sample Review Self-Assessment Form

HOSPITAL-WIDE OBJECTIVES-- HOSPITAL-WIDE TARGETS Administrative Means [Primary or Secondary Resp.]	Relation. to Hospital-Wide Objectives	Responsibility				1.Task Completed		2.In-Progress	3.Change Needed			
		Primary	Secondary	Measure	Exp. Completion Date	Date	Measure Met (Y/N)	Expect to Meet Compl. Date	Revised Task	Revised Measure	Revised Compl. Date	VP Appvd
LIMIT INCREASE IN COST PER ADJUSTED DISCHARGE — HAVE COST ACCOUNTING SYSTEM WITH COST/CASE BY PAYOR												
Obtain Cost/Case by Payor From Curr. System (CQMS, SMS) [Primary – SC, Secondary–ES]	3/1/4											
Task 1		Name	Name	Measure	Date	Oct 31	Yes					
Task 2		Name	Name	Measure	Date	Oct 31	Yes					
Task 3		Name	Name	Measure	Date	Oct 31	Yes					
LIMIT INCREASE IN COST PER ADJUSTED DISCHARGE — ALLOW NO INCREASE IN SUPPLY COST/CASE (CASE MIX ADJUSTED) FROM 93												
Apply Value Analysis to All New Purchases [Primary–RB, Secondary–JM, CM]												
Task 1		Name	Name	Measure	Date			X				
Task 2		Name	Name	Measure	Date			X				
Task 3		Name	Name	Measure	Date			X				
LIMIT INCREASE IN COST PER ADJUSTED DISCHARGE — HAVE LOWEST PRICE FOR SELECTED PRODUCT LINES (CVD, ORTHOPEDICS, ONCOLOGY)												
Realign Charge Structure [Primary–SC]												
Task 1		Name	Name	Measure	Date				Revised Task			Yes
Task 2		Name	Name	Measure	Date					Revised Measure		Yes
Task 3		Name	Name	Measure	Date						Revised Compl. Date	Yes

MANAGERS TO FILL IN SECTION 1, 2 OR 3 FOR EACH TASK ON MONTHLY BASIS

etc ...

Source: The Miriam Hospital.

Figure 3-9. 1993 Market Share Increase: Final Summary

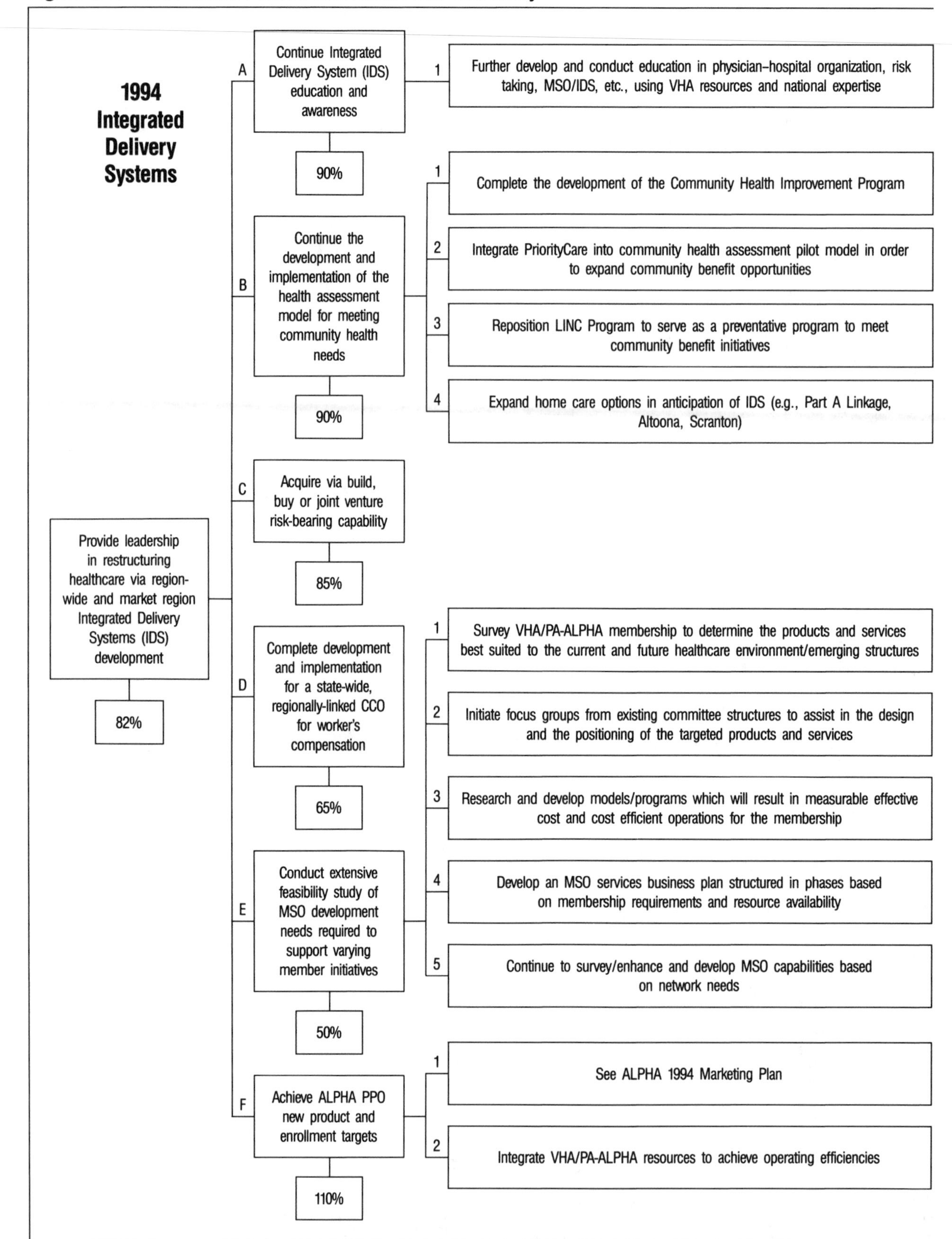

1994
Integrated
Delivery
Systems
Provide leadership in restructuring healthcare via region-wide and market region Integrated Delivery Systems (IDS) development
82%
A
Continue Integrated Delivery System (IDS) education and awareness
90%
1
Further develop and conduct education in physician-hospital organization, risk taking, MSO/IDS, etc., using VHA resources and national expertise
B
Continue the development and implementation of the health assessment model for meeting community health needs
90%
1
Complete the development of the Community Health Improvement Program
2
Integrate PriorityCare into community health assessment pilot model in order to expand community benefit opportunities
3
Reposition LINC Program to serve as a preventative program to meet community benefit initiatives
4
Expand home care options in anticipation of IDS (e.g., Part A Linkage, Altoona, Scranton)
C
Acquire via build, buy or joint venture risk-bearing capability
85%
D
Complete development and implementation for a state-wide, regionally-linked CCO for worker's compensation
65%
E
Conduct extensive feasibility study of MSO development needs required to support varying member initiatives
50%
1
Survey VHA/PA-ALPHA membership to determine the products and services best suited to the current and future healthcare environment/emerging structures
2
Initiate focus groups from existing committee structures to assist in the design and the positioning of the targeted products and services
3
Research and develop models/programs which will result in measurable effective cost and cost efficient operations for the membership
4
Develop an MSO services business plan structured in phases based on membership requirements and resource availability
5
Continue to survey/enhance and develop MSO capabilities based on network needs
F
Achieve ALPHA PPO new product and enrollment targets
110%
1
See ALPHA 1994 Marketing Plan
2
Integrate VHA/PA-ALPHA resources to achieve operating efficiencies

Source: VHA of Pennsylvania.

A1 IDS education and awareness conferences/seminars included: four education sessions held for hospital physicians, trustees and senior management in each PA region; one managed care conference for hospital physicians and CEOs in California with over 200 attending.

B1 Completed the development of the VHA/PA program. Communicated availability of Program to membership. Also developing an educational "train-the-trainer" manual to support member hospitals in their community health improvement initiatives.

B2 Implementation of plan to expand PriorityCare to all member HCOs and transition Program into a VHA/PA Older Adult Services Network (OASN) as part of the community health assessment model is underway; a January kickoff meeting for the OASN, including a Medicare Risk Contracting seminar is scheduled. A second seminar on Community Health Improvement, in conjunction with VHA, Inc. will be held in June 1995.

B3 The LINC Program was terminated due to the lack of participation by VHA/PA member hospitals.

B4 Provided facilitation and technical assistance to LHHS in the development of a concept paper on integrated home care opportunities.

C *Southwest Market Region:* Provided educational consulting, technical assistance, and staff support to SIDN development. Significant accomplishments include Business Plan development, market assessments, ALPHA assessment and staff support for HMO license filing.

Central Market Region: Provided technical assistance and consulting to the region for completion of HMO license application. Continue to provide technical assistance via managed care modeling and market analysis.

Mountain Market Region: Provided additional managed care demand modeling for network development. Provided technical assistance with regard to integration of modeling into financial plan.

Northeast Market Region: Provided additional managed care modeling to assist in the development of strategic plan.

Northwest Market Region: Provided additional managed care demand modeling for network development.

D Butler, St. Clair, Sewickley, Harrisburg, Allegheny Valley, Wyoming Valley and St. Margaret contracted to participate in the CCO. Application will be finalized and submitted in December 1994. The ALPHA Care Workers' Compensation managed care program has been implemented in participating hospitals. Marketing of program to employees and payors has been initiated mid-year. First contract with County of Butler. In the northeast a full service of occupational health and workers' compensation services is being jointly marketed with Wyoming Valley.

E1–5 A business plan for implementing a MSO is currently under development. Eighty percent of customer interviews (represented by physicians, CEOs, managed care executives) have been completed. Preliminary evaluation of MSO service needs by region, with time frames for implementing, is being completed. Final recommendations will be made following completion of the interview process, and within 60 days of receipt of the BDC Business Plan.

F1 ALPHA exceeded projected growth targets of 15%. New products and enrollents grew by 18%.

F2 VHA/PA and ALPHA integration accomplished to achieve managed care, advertisers/public relations, quality and physician services initiatives.

Figure 3-10. Hoshin Plan Executive Summary

ORGANIZATIONAL FOCUS ______________________________

Targets	Means	Measure of Success	Responsibility (Deployment Channel)		Resources/ Budget	Comments/Priorities	Timeline	Evaluation		
			Owner/ Leader	Team			Qtr 1 2 3 4	Re- viewer	Review Dates	% of Means Achieved
										[: : :]
										[: : :]
										[: : :]
										[: : :]
										[: : :]
										[: : :]
										[: : :]
										[: : :]

Hoshin planning has a wealth of techniques that make it easier to do this job well. The case studies in chapters 10 through 15, including those of the SSM-Ministry Corporation and the Southwest Texas Methodist Hospital, include examples of user-friendly techniques and plan formats.

Surviving the Growing Pains of Hoshin Planning

Organizations that invest in hoshin planning deserve to get a return on their investment. These key success factors represent ways to maximize that return. Each factor includes a whole continuum of behaviors that should grow stronger with experience and confidence. Figure 3-11 illustrates this continuum, as organizations develop through five stages of maturity with hoshin planning.

Even the strongest and most committed organizations will face challenges and setbacks on their hoshin planning journey. The Center for Continuous Quality Improvement at Milwaukee Area Technical College identified these problems as the major causes of failure in hoshin planning:

- Senior management is not committed.
- Purpose and objectives are not clearly defined.
- Responsibilities of each manager are not clear.
- Scope of process is limited to certain divisions.
- Plan lacks measures, timetables, responsibilities.
- Education does not include tools.
- Problems are seen as excuse not to use TQM rather than a focus of TQM.
- A common language is lacking.

Figure 3-12 lists some of the problems faced by hoshin planning pioneer Florida Power & Light, as well as their actions in response. These problems will sound familiar to leaders in every industry – from "weak understanding of customer needs" to "executives unable to effectively address problems that crossed department lines."

The Miriam Hospital identified two primary problems with its hoshin planning process in the first year: (1) not enough time – the process was too rushed and budgeting had to be done at the same time – and (2) not enough information provided to employees about the process.[21] In addition, in the first year of hoshin planning, the hospital's top management "thought we had made a tremendous mistake by choosing a hoshin priority (to be the highest-value health care provider) that went too far."[22]

The Miriam Hospital, Milwaukee Area Technical College, and Florida Power & Light stayed the course with hoshin planning and addressed their problems. At The Miriam Hospital, the time problem was significantly reduced in the second year of hoshin planning by improving integration of the planning and budgeting processes. Now hoshin planning takes place in the first quarter of the year, leading into the budgeting process, which occurs in the second quarter. The communication problem is being addressed through increased time for the process, improved instructional materials, and technical assistance sessions. The vice-presidents are also providing more specific one-on-one guidance to their staff. As for the choice of organizational focus, "It has meaning to everyone. There isn't anything more important to the organization."[23]

As shown in figure 3-13, results in the first four months of hoshin planning at The Miriam Hospital are noteworthy: 111 of 119 assigned means were completed. Florida Power & Light's impressive results achieved through the hoshin planning process are summarized in figure 3-14.

Figure 3-11. Stages of Hoshin Planning Evolution in an Organization

CLASSIFICATION	EVALUATION LEVELS (STAGES) 1	2
Overall control system quality policy, QC policy, *Hoshin Kanri* system, QA system	• No overall control system (not clear) • No *Hoshin Kanri* • Unclear quality, QC (promotion policy—QA policy only plan of QC circle promotion) • Poor interdepartmental relationships	—Effort for overall control—*Hoshin Kanri*—quality assurance system —Partly clear quality policy. QC policy. • Need for cross-functional management • No problem extraction • No match to improvement measures
Management strategy and long/medium-term plan company motto basic concept management strategy long/medium-term plan	• Company motto exists but not alive • Insufficient strategy • Long/medium-term plans (5-yr. and 3-yr.) are not there • No long-term vision	—Company motto exists (basic concept is clarified) —Long/medium-term policy based on strategy is there. Information is being collected • Plans of department are not streamlined No companywide policy is clear
Planning of policy-plan on self-inspection	• No self-inspection of last year (collection and analysis of information) • Theme is sporadic • Only results are evaluated • No process-oriented concept	—Self-inspection of last year is done —Some policy-plan is clear • Collection of data, type, and quantity are insufficient • Weak work on critical problems, weighing a study of factors
Analysis capability Problem solution capability	• Haphazard and no plan	• Abstract policy-plan, weak base of target-means • Budget control is separated from *Hoshin Kanri*
Setup of control items	• No items are set • No understanding of control items (definition)	—Each job sets control items • Control value of item is abstract • Same items for supervisor and subordinate, of tunnel type
Coordination and deployment policy-plan control item	• No coordination between superior and subordinate • Loosely set policy-plan and control items • No consistency and thoroughness	—Some coordination —Some relation between supervisor and subordinate • Poor relationship with self-inspection of last year (check and analysis of critical problems)
Check-action of policy-plan	• No check of policy-plan (progress) • Handling of emergency is sporadic • Revision and issue of standards are few	—Difference between target and actual is studied (no analysis) —Standards are being issued • Review of policy-plan is not done • QC diagnosis is not done (diagnosis, hereunder) • Revision of standard is inactive
Model actions by supervisor and participation Annual *Hoshin Kanri*	• Negative attitude to *Hoshin Kanri* (no understanding) • Same as above for clerical, sales, and engineering depts.	—Positive attitude among superiors of production department —Partial participation at clerical, sales and engineering depts. • Policy-plan cannot be set unless data from bottom is submitted, in general

Figure 3-11. (Continued)

EVALUATION LEVELS (STAGES)		
3	**4**	**5**
—Overall control—*Hoshin Kanri*—QA systems are there with actions —Clear quality, QC policies, plan —Effort on cross-functional management • Problems out of above systems are there but not enough corrective measures	—System chart for each system is there with good correlationship —System of function is there —Long/medium quality—QC policies and promotion plan are there —Problems are extracted and properly dealt with	—Challenging work for excellence in all department/functions is there —Top-director-department/section heads with good leadership —System among functions and administration rules are there with PDCA
—Deployment of basic concept is done —Strategy is clear (long/medium-term plan) —Basic target-means are clarified • Analysis of environment, long/medium-term, is weak	—Strategy is based on company motto and concept —Strategy and long/medium-term plan are compatible • Long/medium-term policy and annual policy-plan are not well related	—Leadership is strong for plan of strategy and plans —Rules for planning are there with PDCA —Good match between plan and policy —Above is based on quality-supreme concept
—Critical problems and factors are studied based on self-inspection —Target and means are set for problem solution —Integration of *Hoshin Kanri* and budget control is planned	—QC story is there for self-inspection and analysis —Policy-plan (target means) are planned in relation to critical problems —Supervisor's and subordinate's policy-plan are well related	—Rules and system for planning of policy-plan based on self-inspection is there (system) —Control with emphasis on *Hoshin Kanri* is there and well related to budget control
• Weak in QC analysis and solution of problems • Policy-plans are mostly formality only • Weak connection between superior's and subordinate's policy-plan	• Still budget-control oriented, weak relation with profit plan	—Proper, timely correction of policy-plan against charges —Long/medium-term plan is related policy-plan
—Connection between items for jobs is studied —Target value of items is clear • Handling limit of item is not clear	—Target value-handling limit of items are clear —Connection with policy-plan (target means) is good • Setting up of items of daily control is good	—Rules for items of *Hoshin Kanri* and daily control is there —Revision is properly handled
—Setup based on supervisor policy-plan and control items —Related to self-inspection of last year • No check of relation to related departments	—Policy-plan, control items are set up with good check with related departments —Supervisor's policy-plan, items are used for setup • Coordination and deployment not system-like	—Rules for coordination of policy-plan and control items are there (system) —Consistency in deployment of policy-plan and control items
—Analysis of target/actual if QC —Regular QC diagnosis —Revision of standards is active • Feedback of check results to next year policy-plan is insufficient	—Feedback to next year is good, re: policy-plan QCD —Not enough standards revision —Diagnosis (*Hoshin Kanri* audit) is done • Upstream check-action is insufficient • Control items are used and emergency handling is done	—Check-action procedures are ruled re: policy-plan (system) —Check-action at upstream is done
—Leadership of top of prod. dept. is there for *Hoshin Kanri* —Engineering dept. is getting active • Relation with and deployment to related company, dealers, etc. are weak • *Hoshin Kanri* at clerical-sales depts. is separated from daily control	—Production and engineering depts. are both active for *Hoshin Kanri* —Engineering top is exhibiting good leadership for *Hoshin Kanri* —Clerical and sales are getting to be positive • Process-oriented view is insufficient	—Roles of supervisors for *Hoshin Kanri* are ruled —Clerical and sales are active in *Hoshin Kanri* —*Hoshin Kanri* is related to related companies (or group companies as well) —*Hoshin Kanri* is working in practice

Figure 3-12. Chronology of Florida Power & Light Hoshin Planning (MBP) Implementation

Year	Actions
1986	
• Weak understanding of customer needs	1. Customer needs survey
• Employees unclear on what needed improvement	2. Initiated midterm and short-term plans
1987	
• Improvement and control activities not clearly tied to customer needs	3. Initiated corporate system of indicators
1988	
• Executives unable to effectively address problems that crossed department lines	4. Formalized cross-functional management
• Corporate and department quality/delivery activities did not link	5. Introduced quality/delivery and cost management systems
• Management unable to confirm that department functions aligned with company objectives	6. Initiated levels 1, 2, and 3 reviews
1989	
• Employee safety activities did not link to the FPL management system	7. Introduced the employee safety system
• Activities to improve corporate citizenship not clearly tied to FPL management system	8. Introduced the corporate responsibility system

Reprinted, with permission, from *Management by Policy;* published by ASQC Quality Press, ©1993.

Figure 3-13. The Miriam Hospital 1994 Hoshin Statistics (Oct. 1993–Feb. 1994)

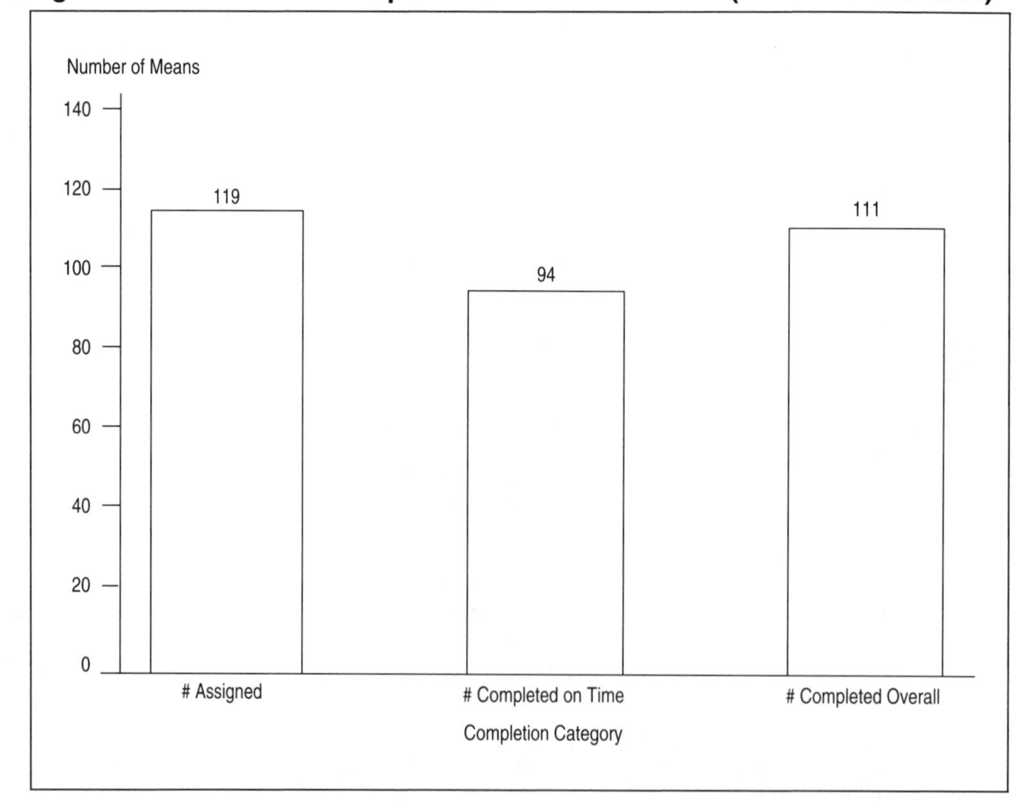

Figure 3-14. Florida Power & Light's Results

Short-Term Plan	Indicator
Improve reliability of electric service	Customer minutes interrupted per customer served 1983 — 78 minutes; 3/90 — 44 minutes Number of unscheduled transmission outages 1985 — 950; 12/89 — 660
Improve customer satisfaction	Florida Public Service Commission complaints per 1000 customers 1984 — 0.90; 12/89 — 0.22
Improve employee safety	Lost-time injuries per 100 FPL employees 1986 — 1.20; 12/89 — 0.39
Control price and provide competitive services through cost reductions and improved system utilization	Total megawatt peak demand reduction capability Started in 1988; 12/89 — 793 megawatts
Continue to emphasize safe, reliable, and efficient operation of nuclear power plants	Automatic trips per 1000 hours of operation 1985 — 0.77; 12/89 — 0.20
Establish fossil unit reliability, availability, and maintainability targets, and develop a program that achieves those targets	Equivalent forced outage rate 1987 — 14.0%; 1989 — 3.62%

Reprinted, with permission, from *Policy Deployment: The TQM Approach to Long-Range Planning*; published by ASQC Quality Press, ©1993.

Summary

At least six factors can help an organization to tap the rich benefits of hoshin planning, particularly the benefits of increased focus and alignment. These key success factors are:

1. Ability to prioritize
2. Customer-based plan
3. Leadership champions
4. Deployment of the plan throughout the organization
5. Foundation of planning and process improvement skills
6. User-friendly process and tools

In addition, other factors may be key to success in an organization's specific market. To do hoshin planning well, build up the key success factors in a way that is unique to your organization.

Actions for Top Leadership

As top leaders begin to shift from gaining a basic understanding of hoshin planning to decisions about how to make it work in their own organizations, the following actions are suggested:

1. Develop a customized list of hoshin planning key success factors. This list can be developed based on a review of the six factors described in this chapter and of the case studies in chapters 10 through 15, consideration of the organization's internal and external environments, and, if desired, discussions with other organizations experienced with a hoshin planning process.
2. Assign a senior leader to "champion" each key success factor with the CEO. The champion's tasks may include tasks 3 and 4 listed below.
3. Evaluate the gap between where the organization is now on each key success factor and where it wants to be. (See the radar chart in appendix B, "Hoshin Toolbox," for information on one technique to do this.) In addition to estimating the relative size of the gaps, identify likely root causes.
4. Develop work plans to strengthen those KSFs judged by the leadership team to be most critical to the success of hoshin planning and to the organization. This should include regular reviews of progress on each factor.

References and Notes

1. In chapter 6, the term *key success factor* will again be used but in a different context. As the hoshin planning steps are described in chapter 6, some of the tasks include determining the *organizational* KSFs needed to meet customer expectations and to achieve a vision. Chapter 3 describes *hoshin planning* KSFs that will contribute to successful hoshin planning regardless of specific customer expectations or organizational vision.
2. David Demers, vice-president, Fletcher Allen Health Care. Telephone interview by Mara Melum, Apr. 12, 1994.
3. GOAL/QPC Research Committee. *Hoshin Planning: A Planning System for Implementing Total Quality Management (TQM).* Research Report No. 89-10-03. Methuen, MA: GOAL/QPC, 1989, p. 33.
4. Kano, N. A perspective on quality activities in American firms. *California Management Review,* Spring 1993, p. 24.
5. Monteforte, L., and Seemer, R. Winning more than the Malcolm Baldrige National Quality Award at AT&T Transmission Systems. *National Productivity Review* 12(2):153–54, Spring 1993.
6. These three levels of customer expectations are often referred to as the Kano model, developed by Dr. Noriaki Kano of Tokyo Science University and the Japanese Union of Scientists and Engineers.
7. Henkoff, R. Keeping Motorola on a roll. *Fortune* 129(8):70, Apr. 18, 1994.
8. Monteforte, L. AT&T Quest for Excellence V Conference, Washington, DC, Feb. 14, 1993.
9. Hewlett-Packard Corporate Quality. *Hoshin Planning Reference Guide.* [Internal company document.] Hewlett-Packard, Oct. 1991, pp. 2–8.
10. Sister M. Lois Bush, President and CEO, SSM-Ministry Corporation. Personal communication to Mara Melum, July 12, 1994.
11. Hewlett-Packard, pp. 2–9.
12. Bush, Sister M. L., and Beste, J. T. SSM-Ministry Corporation case study. Chapter 12 in this book.
13. Juran Institute, Inc. *Strategic Quality Planning.* Wilton, CT: Juran Institute, July 1993, pp. 49–50.
14. Edward Schottland, executive vice-president, The Miriam Hospital. Telephone interview by Mara Melum, June 15, 1994.
15. Dan Kratz, senior vice-president, Minneapolis Children's Medical Center. Telephone interview by Mara Melum, Apr. 25, 1994.
16. James Rieley, coordinator for the Center for Continuous Quality Improvement at Milwaukee Area Technical College. Telephone interview by Mara Melum, Apr. 19, 1994.
17. Juran Institute, p. 59.
18. Schottland.
19. Colletti, J. *Hoshin Kanri.* GOAL/QPC course manual. Methuen, MA: GOAL/QPC, 1994, p. 16.
20. Eugenia Hamilton, senior vice-president, Dartmouth-Hitchcock Medical Center. Telephone interview by Mara Melum, June 4, 1994.
21. The Miriam Hospital. Internal memo to Operations Group, Dec. 2, 1993.
22. Schottland.
23. Schottland.

CHAPTER FOUR

Organizing and Customizing Hoshin Planning

Nothing is particularly hard if you divide it into small jobs.

—Henry Ford

The purpose of this chapter is to assist leaders to successfully start implementing hoshin planning. The top leadership team needs to prepare for success by taking the time to organize the effort and customize hoshin planning to the unique needs of the organization. The chapter discusses three questions that should be addressed up front by the CEO and other members of the senior leadership team:

- Why are we implementing hoshin planning?
- When should we start to implement it?
- How will we implement it?

Why Are We Implementing Hoshin Planning?

In hoshin planning, as in any major change effort, an organization must articulate why it has chosen this course. On one level, the motivation is obvious and likely to apply to every organization: to focus on what is most important. But what motivates the organization to be willing, even excited, to take on the hard work of focusing through hoshin planning—hard work that includes choosing one breakthrough focus from many good options and deploying the plan through the "catchball" process?

The motivator may fit into the category of "pain" (such as poor teamwork or shrinking volume) or of "gain" (such as to become the market leader). Often the motivators are a combination of both pain and gain. Currently, a common motivator in the health care arena is a desire to successfully integrate disparate organizations such as hospitals, clinics, home health companies, and HMOs into a seamless delivery system with a shared vision. Milwaukee Area Technical College was motivated by the desire to "increase customer satisfaction, decrease entropy, and improve financial stability."[1] Hewlett-Packard wanted "a way to align decentralized organizations that had to cooperate to conquer new markets or to remain industry leaders."[2] SSM Health Care System wanted to incorporate the best of continuous quality improvement (CQI) principles into its strategic planning process.[3]

Clear and honest expression of the motivators will help in a number of ways. For example, as:

- *A reality check:* to test whether hoshin planning really has the potential to do what the organization hopes it will do
- *A consensus check:* to determine the extent to which the top leadership teams see the state of the organization through the same lens and are willing to invest in similar types of change efforts
- *A communication tool:* to express in a compelling and unified way to others throughout the organization why this effort is worth their time and hard work
- *"Glue" during bad times:* to remind everyone in the organization, when the going gets tough, why it is so important to stick it out and make hoshin planning work

When Should We Start to Implement Hoshin Planning?

To determine when to start hoshin planning, an organization needs to consider at least two issues. First, hoshin planning has to be timed to be relevant to market and internal organizational needs. For example, a strong new competitor or changing customer expectations may require the type of highly focused organizationwide response that hoshin planning can provide. As organizations consolidate or form other strategic alliances, hoshin planning can help provide "glue" and a shared direction.

Second, an organization must determine when it is likely to have the start-up conditions needed to successfully implement hoshin planning. It can be helpful for executives to consider both optimal and minimal conditions for starting hoshin planning. Some of these conditions are described in the following subsections.

Minimal Start-Up Conditions

Some organizations incorporated hoshin planning techniques in early stages of their quality management efforts and found them to be valuable. Examples include SSM-Ministry Corporation (subject of the case study in chapter 12) and Milwaukee Area Technical College.

The following components of the longer-term KSFs discussed in chapter 3 can be considered minimal start-up conditions for a successful hoshin planning effort:

- *Commitment to a focus:* A strong top leadership commitment to focus on only one or a very few organizational priorities for the first cycle of hoshin planning.
- *Commitment to deploy the plan:* Leadership commitment to deploy the organizational focus throughout the organization, using a catchball process as much as possible. This includes leadership commitment to empower those people most knowledgeable about specific targets to propose the best means to achieve them. It also includes recognizing that top leadership's role in deployment is primarily to (1) develop the organizational focus, top-level targets, and top-level means; and (2) ensure the integration and collective effectiveness of the means proposed by others throughout the organization.
- *Education:* A customized, just-in-time continuing education program on hoshin planning and related process improvement tools and techniques.
- *Commitment to ongoing reviews:* A commitment to review plan implementation on an ongoing basis includes design of a work plan for a user-friendly review process that readily integrates learnings and facilitates improvement.
- *Communication:* A communication system that effectively communicates to the organization what hoshin planning is, why the organization is doing it, the

organization's overall hoshin planning work plan, employees' personal roles in hoshin planning, and where to go for assistance.

- *Infrastructure:* A start-up infrastructure to support the effort, including information systems and trained facilitators and team leaders, and a commitment to continue to improve the infrastructure.

In addition to these minimal conditions, an organization is likely to be in a stronger hoshin planning start-up position if it is working to identify and measure the performance of its critical processes and if it is continuously refining its database of customer needs and expectations.

Optimal Start-Up Conditions

Many experts consider it optimal for an organization to have a strong foundation in the following before embarking on hoshin planning:

- Quality management, including process improvement
- Strategic planning

The GOAL/QPC Research Committee hoshin planning team, which included representatives from Dow Chemical, Procter & Gamble, Hewlett-Packard, and IBM, identified the optimal prerequisites for successful hoshin planning as shown in figure 4-1. They include factors in the areas of knowledge and experience, the manager's role, motivation, and organization. For example, knowledge and experience factors include widespread understanding and use of total quality management (TQM), the plan-do-check-act (PDCA) cycle, daily management, and process improvement tools and techniques.

Figure 4-1. Hoshin Planning Optimal Prerequisites

Knowledge and Experience	Manager's Role	Motivation	Organization
• Widespread understanding of the basics of TQM, including where hoshin planning fits. • Understanding of PDCA model. • Widespread knowledge and use of the seven basic QC tools. • Some specialized knowledge of the appropriate seven tools for management and planning. • Widespread understanding of daily management/control.	• Set direction: —Provide a clean focus. —Establish priorities. —Communicate it to everyone. • Support people's efforts: —Provide resources. —Create horizontal coordination. —Remove system barriers. —Teach and coach. • Provide a focus on the process: —Practice PDCA. —Demand data. • Reinforce and recognize employees' efforts.	• Clear and compelling answer to the question "Why do Hoshin Planning?" (Find a burning issue.) • Desire on management's part to narrow and/or coordinate the focus.	• Leadership demand from the top. • Develop steering teams at different levels of deployment to coordinate problem solving. • Facilitators (preferably bosses) in place. • Champion/sponsor in a highly visible, influential management slot. • A coordinating mechanism (team, committee, or individual) to integrate plans across functions and departments. • A system for making daily management/ control work.

Source: GOAL/QPC 1989 Research Report, *Hoshin Planning: A Planning System for Implementing Total Quality Management (TQM)*, pg. 7. Used with permission.

Organization factors include steering teams at different levels of deployment to coordinate problem solving; a champion in a highly visible, influential management slot; and a coordinating mechanism to integrate plans across functions and departments.

A phased approach, in which hoshin planning follows work on process improvement, has important advantages. In particular, this approach maximizes the odds that an organization will be able to focus on the essence of hoshin planning, rather than getting bogged down in new terminology, unfamiliar tools, uneasiness about the emphasis on processes, debates about whether customers really know what they need, and so on. In other words, the organization will be better able to concentrate on its strategic direction, rather than on mechanics. There is also more likely to be a base of customer-oriented data at this point, which can be tapped to make hoshin planning decisions.

Bellin Memorial Hospital is an example of an organization that recognized its need for a firmer grasp of quality improvement principles and tools before an organizational focus could be deployed through catchball. Bellin decided to shift direction to build this base of knowledge and experience. Before proceeding with hoshin planning, the organization provided additional education and support for each department to improve its daily work processes.[4]

The nature of the transition from the existing system to hoshin planning depends on the existing system. The "maturity pyramid," a self-assessment worksheet developed by the executive director of GOAL/QPC can help determine an organization's current position. This worksheet, shown in figure 4-2, may be a useful tool for leaders to assess the magnitude of change that hoshin planning will call for, and thus the appropriate timing.

How Will We Implement Hoshin Planning?

These how-to questions cover issues that fall into four categories – start-up, pace, operations, and human resources. This section discusses some of the issues that the leadership team needs to address as it organizes the hoshin planning effort.

Issue 1: Should We Start with a Pilot Project or Roll Out Hoshin Planning Full-Scale to the Entire Organization?

In the *full-scale* option, everyone begins the process of learning about and implementing hoshin planning at approximately the same time. The advantage of this approach is that it makes a strong statement to employees that the organization is very serious about hoshin planning. It may also be possible to achieve a more comprehensive and challenging goal with the entire organization engaged and aligned. The disadvantages include the concentrated costs of educating everyone at once and the common risks of implementing any major change on a grand scale without learning on a smaller, pilot-test scale first.

Organizations that have started full-scale on hoshin planning include Florida Power & Light, Milwaukee Area Technical College, SSM-Ministry Corporation, and Our Lady of Lourdes. At Dartmouth-Hitchcock Medical Center, three organizations – the hospital, the clinic, and the medical school – chose a hoshin planning type of process for their first comprehensive effort at joint planning.

The *pilot project* approach to hoshin planning has been used at Hewlett-Packard and Vermont Academic Medical Center. Vermont Academic Medical Center started its hoshin planning effort with pilot projects in the areas of rehabilitation and mental health services. The advantage of this approach is that problems and risks are contained on a small scale. Also, learnings can then be applied to the larger organization, to maximize chances of success when the effort is rolled out further. Pilot tests can

Figure 4-2. Hoshin Planning Readiness Self-Assessment Worksheet

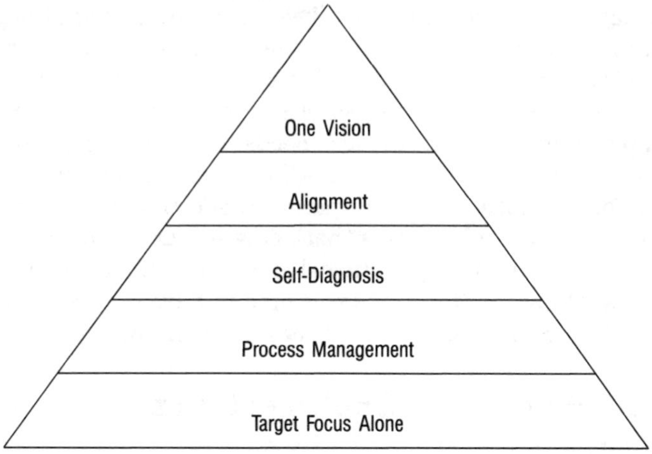

Some of the following kinds of questions may help determine the organization's position.

	Strongly Agree			Strongly Disagree	
1. Targets are announced with no plan of how to reach them.	5	4	3	2	1
2. Each year a new plan is developed from a clean sheet of paper.	5	4	3	2	1
3. If a target is not met, a major effort is made to determine why it was not met.	5	4	3	2	1
4. Appropriate data are gathered and analyzed so that people know what is going on.	5	4	3	2	1
5. People have a clear idea of what to expect of other people and what other people expect of them.	5	4	3	2	1
6. Basic problem-solving tools are regularly used to decide how the organization can be improved.	5	4	3	2	1
7. Each manager has two or three written goals and reviews progress on them each month.	5	4	3	2	1
8. Each manager evaluates his or her own missed goals to understand problems and make adjustments.	5	4	3	2	1
9. Each manager uses learnings about past problems to help set better goals for the future.	5	4	3	2	1
10. Managers are generally aware of the key goals of others in the organization.	5	4	3	2	1
11. Managers do not consciously select goals that will adversely affect other managers in the organization.	5	4	3	2	1
12. Managers from various departments get together every one or two months to coordinate efforts on quality, cost, and delivery of products and services.	5	4	3	2	1
13. The top two or three priorities of the organization are posted and described thoroughly in the organization's magazine, and so forth. Everybody knows the strategy to accomplish.	5	4	3	2	1
14. Everybody knows the organization's top priorities.	5	4	3	2	1
15. Every person has his or her own top two or three priorities, which are tied to those of the organization.	5	4	3	2	1

Source: Robert King, GOAL/QPC. Used with permission.

also help to develop support, inasmuch as a track record can begin to be built, with accompanying champions. Disadvantages of the pilot project approach include the appearance that this may just be another short-lived program, a lack of organizationwide alignment around one focus, resistance to eventual increased standardization of the process, and duplicate or even conflicting efforts in different parts of the organization.

Regardless of whether the pilot project or full-scale start-up approach is used, the scope of hoshin planning in later stages also needs to be addressed. For example, after three years of hoshin planning at Fletcher Allen Health Care, two *organizationwide* hoshin planning focuses currently are in place. In addition, every strategic business *unit* is asked to choose two unit focuses that address four key areas identified by the organization: customer satisfaction, clinical outcomes, financial performance, and process complexity. Other organizations continue to have only one organizationwide focus even after they gain experience with hoshin planning.

Issue 2: What Will Be the Implementation Time Line/Schedule?

Hoshin planning is a substantial change strategy, not a quick fix. Dr. Yoji Akao suggests that hoshin planning can "bubble up" in an organization over a 1½- to 2½-year period. Based on his research, the executive director of GOAL/QPC, Robert King, has developed the four- to five-year hoshin planning model shown in figure 4-3. The annual hoshin planning timetables from Hewlett-Packard, Florida Power & Light, and The Miriam Hospital are shown in figures 4-4 through 4-6 (pp. 58–61).

The Research Committee of GOAL/QPC estimates that, after the organization's vision is refined or affirmed, the individual steps of hoshin planning take approximately the following amount of time:

- *Assess gaps and narrow down list of three- to five-year objectives (targets):* periodic meetings over two months
- *Develop annual objectives (targets):* periodic meetings over a one- to two-month period (which would include an intensive month of internal reviews)
- *Deployment:* one to two months
- *Implementation:* depends on complexity and time schedule of plan
- *Reviews:* one hour per plan per month
- *Quarterly reviews:* four to eight hours per organizational unit
- *Annual review:* one to one and a half months[5]

(For sample hoshin planning time lines, see the case studies of Bethesda, Our Lady of Lourdes Medical Center, and AT&T, in chapters 10, 11, and 14, respectively.)

Issue 3: What Channels of Deployment Will Be Used to Align Everyone with the Organization's Focus?

An important issue facing leaders is how to deploy an organizational priority throughout the organization so that everyone understands and contributes to it. Hoshin planning stresses the importance of such deployment to achieve organizational alignment. Channels through which the organizational focus can be deployed include functional work units (that is, existing departments), cross-functional teams, and individuals.

To determine the most appropriate deployment channel for a specific organizational focus and annual target, leaders should assess which processes significantly affect achievement of the focus and target. If the target is strongly linked to individual work or to a single process, deployment to functional work units or occasionally to individuals may be appropriate. Milwaukee Area Technical College deploys its organizational focus primarily to individuals.

Figure 4-3. Sample Phase-In Time Line for Hoshin Planning

Steps	1	2	3		4	5	6	Added Dimension
			Deployment					
	Vision	1-Year Plan	Individual	Align	Execution (Process Management)	Monthly Diagnosis	Annual Diagnosis	Developmental Learnings
Phase 1						●		Management by facts
Phase 2			●		●	●		Self-diagnosis
Phase 3		●	●	●	●	●		Align —3 goals each
Phase 4	●	●	●	●	●	●	●	Understand new direction
Tools:	**Aim**	**Plan**	**Do**	**Do**	**Do**	**Check/Act**	**Check/Act**	
QC:								
Fishbone	●		●			●	●	
Pareto	●			●		●		
Line	●				●	●	●	
Flow	●		●			●	●	
Check Sheet	●					●		
Histogram	●					●		
Control	●				●	●		
7M:								
KJ	●	●						
ID	●	●					●	
Tree	●	●	●					
Matrix	●	●					●	
MDA								
PDPC					●			
Arrow					●			
Alignment Tools:								
Flag		●		●		●	●	
Target/Means				●				
Cascading				●				
T/M Tree								
QFD		●		●				

Source: Robert King, GOAL/QPC. Used with permission.

Figure 4-4. Hewlett-Packard MPG Hoshin Planning Process Time Line

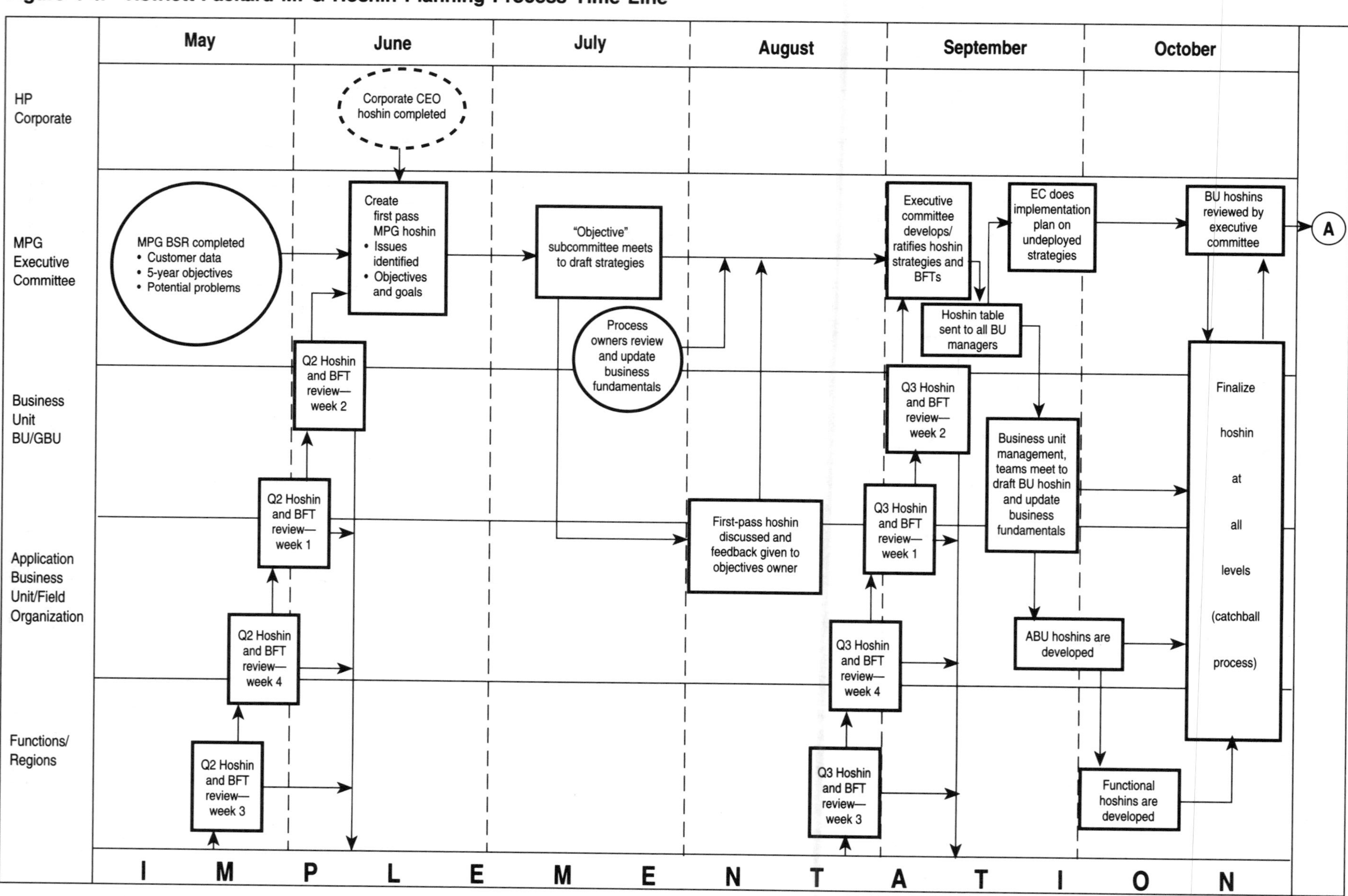

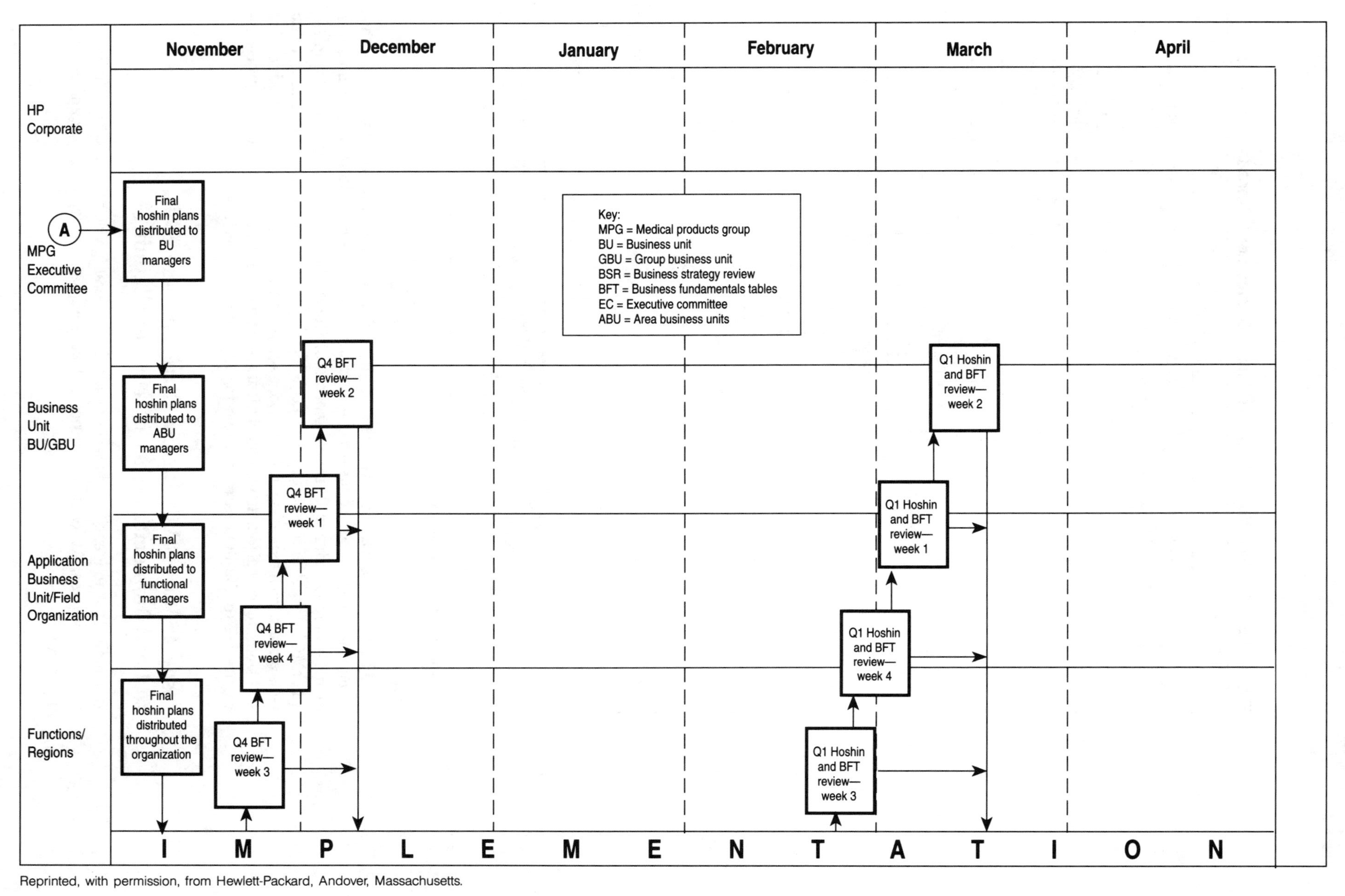

Reprinted, with permission, from Hewlett-Packard, Andover, Massachusetts.

Figure 4-5. Florida Power & Light's Policy Deployment Process Time Line

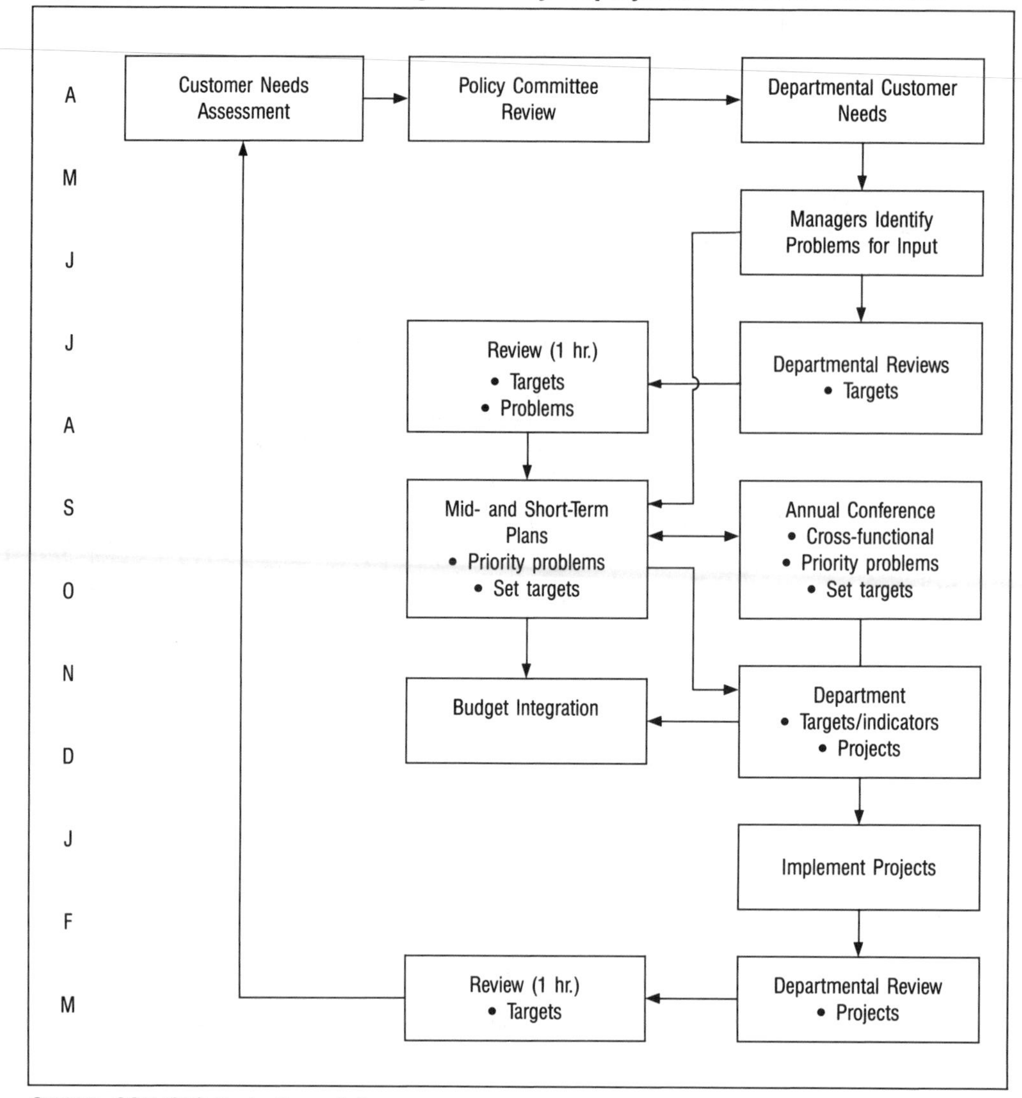

Many targets will, however, be strongly linked to several processes. In that case, it may be most effective to have a collaborative effort by a cross-functional team whose members are familiar with many aspects of the different processes. For example, if an HMO's target is to reduce heart attacks of members by 25 percent, it might convene a team with expertise in nutrition, exercise, screening for risk factors, education, and smoking cessation, as well as clinical experts in the relevant treatment processes. Figure 4-7 (p. 62) illustrates options for deploying objectives.

Issue 4: What Will Be the Structure and Roles to Lead Implementation of Hoshin Planning?

It is important to identify who will provide the leadership critical to a successful hoshin planning process. At least four types of leadership at the top of an organization are important:

1. CEO
   - Determine and communicate the purpose and pace of the hoshin planning effort
   - Lead the top leadership team
   - Ensure continued focus, for example, through ongoing progress checks (both formal and informal), consistent guidance, and linkage of hoshin planning to reward and other management systems
   - Provide wisdom, balance, and clear vision through the hard times
2. Top leadership team
   - Select and communicate the organizational vision and focus
   - Develop the high-level plan
   - Ensure efficient deployment of the plan
   - Provide resources for carrying out the plan
   - Model and reward good planning and review practices
3. Top-level cross-functional management teams
   - Create coordinating mechanisms to integrate plans across departments
   - Remove system barriers

Figure 4-6. FY 1995 Hoshin Planning Process and Time Line

Activity	Exp. Dates	# Weeks
Administrative review of annual objectives, targets, and means.	3/2 (Wed)-3/7 (Mon)	1
Planning department develops FY 1995 hoshin planning workbook.	3/8 (Tue)-3/9 (Wed)	—
Planning department sends workbook package to VPs, managers, and clinical chiefs with instructions.	3/9 (Wed)-3/10 (Thu)	—
VPs hold QMT meetings to review objectives, targets, and means; answer department director questions; provide direction.	3/11 (Fri)-3/15 (Tue)	—
VPs, department directors, and chiefs fill out packages indicating FY 1995 departmental targets (activities) [catchball]. **Note:** Hoshin department targets requiring incremental resources should be submitted as new program and/or capital equipment requests.	3/11 (Fri)-3/31 (Thu) **Note:** New prog. and cap. equip. requests send to mgrs. 3/25	3
Planning department updates strategic planning committee on 1994 YTD results, FY 1995 objectives, targets, and means.	Date TBD	—
Planning department schedules and holds technical assistance sessions with each department director, chief.	3/15 (Tue)-3/28 (Mon)	—
VPs hold QMT meetings to review/approve department director *or* department managers obtain individual VP feedback/approval.	3/29 (Tue)-3/31 (Thu)	—
VPs, department directors, and chiefs submit packages to planning department.	4/1 (Fri)	—
Planning department summarizes catchball results.	4/4 (Mon)-4/8 (Fri)	1
Planning meets with clinical management team to review workbook results.	4/6 (Wed)	—
Administrative review of FY 1995 plan.	4/11 (Mon)-4/15 (Fri)	1
Planning department incorporates administrative comments, revisions.	4/18 (Mon)-4/22 (Fri)	1
Planning department sends out package to VPs, managers, chiefs, other affected parties.	4/26 (Tue)	—

Source: The Miriam Hospital. Used with permission.

Figure 4-7. Options to Deploy the Focus throughout the Organization

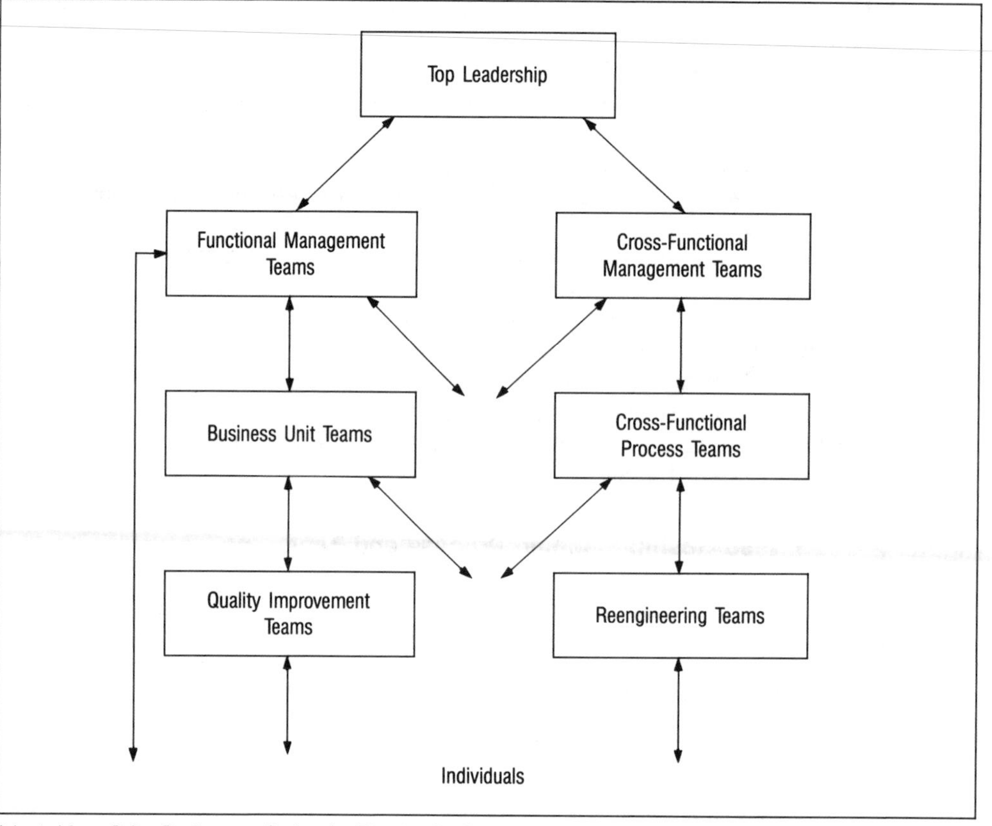

Adapted from *Policy Deployment: Setting the Direction for Change.* Reproduced with the permission of AT&T ©1992. All rights reserved.

4. Focus or target leaders
   - Assess and quantify current performance relative to the focus
   - Serve as coaches and catalysts to the teams at various levels of the organization that are working on the focus
   - Cut through bureaucracy, as needed, and reduce other barriers to cross-functional progress on the focus
   - Track team progress and serve as liaisons to keep the CEO and the top leadership team informed

Regardless of how their roles are defined, it is essential that these leaders do *not* delegate hoshin planning. The top leadership team *is* the organization's planning team in hoshin planning. How can it be any other way when hoshin planning is about focusing on what is most important to the future of the organization?

These leadership roles are discussed in chapter 3 and in chapters 5 through 9 of this book. In addition, specific examples of the role of CEOs and other top leadership in hoshin planning can be found in the Bethesda, Our Lady of Lourdes Medical Center, and SSM-Ministry Corporation case studies, in chapters 10, 11, and 12, respectively.

Implementation Worksheet

A more comprehensive list of questions that leaders should address as they organize the hoshin planning effort is included in the leaders' hoshin planning implementation worksheet shown in figure 4-8.

Figure 4-8. Leaders' Hoshin Planning Implementation Worksheet

Implementation Issue	Responsibility	Deadline	Priorities	Summary of Decision
I. *Why* are we implementing hoshin planning?				
A. What are the major reasons?				
B. How will we communicate them?				
II. *When* should we start to implement it?				
III. *How* will we implement it?				
A. *Pace Issues*				
1. Should we start with a pilot project or go organizationwide?				
2. How many organizational focuses (hoshins) do we want: first year and long term?				
3. How far down in the organization will we deploy the plan: first year and long term?				
4. What will be the implementation time line/schedule?				
B. *Direction Issues*				
1. What criteria will be used to select the organization's focus?				
2. How will we evaluate the success of hoshin planning?				
3. How will hoshin planning relate to our current strategic planning process?				
4. How will hoshin planning fit with our other management efforts (e.g., TQM, reengineering)?				
5. What will be the major barriers to hoshin planning and how can we minimize them?				
6. How can we ensure that the plan is based on our customers' priorities?				
C. *Operational Issues*				
1. What channels of deployment will be used?				
• Functional work units				
• Individuals				
• Cross-functional teams				

(Continued on next page)

Figure 4-8. (Continued)

Implementation Issue	Responsibility	Deadline	Priorities	Summary of Decision
2. What will be the structure and roles to lead implementation?				
• CEO				
• Leadership team				
• Cross-functional management				
• Planning staff				
3. How will catchball take place?				
4. What will be the common format of action plans?				
5. What will be the format, timing, and process for reviews?				
6. What units will be used for analysis and planning?				
• Critical processes				
• Strategic business units				
• Product or service lines				
7. What resources will we allocate to hoshin planning?				
• Budget				
• Management information systems				
• People				
D. *Human Resource Issues*				
1. What types of continuing education will maximize success?				
2. How will the process and plan be communicated?				
3. How will we recognize and reward efforts to achieve the hoshin plan?				
4. Who is likely to resist these changes and why? How can we gain their support?				

Summary

There are at least three categories of concern that the top leadership team should address before it launches a hoshin planning effort. First, leaders must clearly and honestly identify and communicate the reasons the organization is implementing hoshin planning. Second, they have to decide when hoshin planning will be implemented. This decision should weigh market needs and the current strength of the organization's process improvement and planning capabilities. Strengths in those areas will facilitate successful hoshin planning. Third, leaders need to customize how the organization will implement hoshin planning.

Actions for Top Leadership

Leadership actions to enhance the start-up and long-term success of hoshin planning include the following:

1. Schedule a top leadership meeting to organize and customize the hoshin planning effort. Do not just start with an off-the-shelf model. The leaders' hoshin planning implementation worksheet in figure 4-8 (p. 63) suggests an agenda of issues to be addressed.
2. Identify and broadly communicate why the organization is embarking on hoshin planning.
3. Determine how hoshin planning will be rolled out in the organization, including whether it will start organizationwide, with multiple organizations, or with a pilot test.
4. Develop and communicate at least two clear work plans with time lines:
   - A *multiyear work plan* should illustrate the overall timing of how hoshin planning will be rolled out throughout the organization. This time line should indicate how far down and across the organization hoshin planning will be deployed each year as the organization works toward full deployment. The time line should also clarify when and how hoshin planning capabilities, such as process improvement techniques, will be strengthened through continuous education.
   - An *annual hoshin planning work plan* should include information on how hoshin planning will be coordinated with any different strategic planning, performance review, and budget cycles.
5. Determine the channels through which the plan will be deployed, including whether it will be deployed primarily through business unit and department managers or through cross-functional teams.
6. Identify the critical leadership roles in hoshin planning and agree on who will carry them out. This includes assigning senior leaders to be focus champions for each organizational focus. The role of focus champion is described in chapter 3 and in the AT&T case study in chapter 14.

References

1. James Rieley, coordinator for the Center for Continuous Quality Improvement at Milwaukee Area Technical College. Telephone interview by Mara Melum, Apr. 19, 1994.
2. Lois Gold, vice-president Citibank, N.A, Citicorp. Personal communication to Mara Melum and Casey Collett, May 24, 1994.
3. William Thompson, senior vice-president, SSM Health Care System. Telephone interview by Mara Melum, May 27, 1994.
4. Pat Cooksey, vice-president, Bellin Hospital. Telephone interview by Mara Melum, June 22, 1994.
5. GOAL/QPC Research Committee. *Hoshin Planning: A Planning System for Implementing Total Quality Management (TQM).* Research Report No. 89-10-03. Methuen, MA: GOAL/QPC, 1989, pp. 31–46.

PART TWO

How Hoshin Planning Works

CHAPTER FIVE

Introduction to Process and Implementation

Hoshin planning can be made difficult, but it's really a very user-friendly system.

–David Demers, vice-president of corporate planning, Fletcher Allen Health Care

In part I, chapters 1 through 3 described the background and theory of hoshin planning. Chapter 4 discussed ways to organize and customize hoshin planning to prepare for a successful launch. Now, in part II, chapters 5 through 9 tell how to make hoshin planning work. These chapters will be useful for those who are charged with the task of implementing hoshin planning for the first time or for improving an existing system.

Chapters 6 through 9 discuss the hoshin planning process step by step, including tools and methods that the reader may find useful. Each step of the process covers pertinent leadership issues, strategies, lessons learned, and key roles and responsibilities.

Some steps of the process closely resemble traditional strategic planning. Other steps can be conducted in a variety of ways. In addition to providing a basic explanation of steps, tools, and methods, these chapters also give the reader some more detailed information and, where appropriate, alternative approaches. Appendix A expands on the concepts of establishing mission, values, and vision statements; and appendix B, "Hoshin Toolbox," contains instructions and tips on tools.

Initiating Hoshin Planning

As you read the following chapters, imagine you have decided to take a well-deserved vacation somewhere new and exciting to you. You know your starting point, your destination, and that you will be driving. You have a good map, clearly marked with a primary route and various points of interest that will allow you to explore new territory. You even have travelogues written by others who have gone before you and lived to tell about it! The trip promises to be an enticing combination of the known and the unexpected.

Initiating hoshin planning is a bit like taking this trip. You know your current management system and that you want to add hoshin planning to it. The route map is a four-step hoshin process that you can follow. (See figure 5-1.) In that process, you choose the focus, align the organization with that focus, implement the plan, and review and improve. Chapters 6 through 9 describe each step of the process in detail, along with some choices you can make to vary the route and to maneuver unexpected bends in the road. Later, in part III (chapters 10 through 15), a travelogue in the form of hoshin case studies will help you learn from the experiences of others who have taken the journey before you.

Like taking a successful journey, making hoshin planning work in your organization will require both discipline and creativity. The discipline begins when the top leadership team maps out a hoshin planning process and commits itself to following it. Creativity is required to negotiate the unexpected turns in the road – the issues that arise as the hoshin process and the organizational culture adapt to each other over time.

Some of the issues associated with particular steps of the hoshin process will be addressed later, but two global issues bear mentioning now. These are organizational readiness to do hoshin planning well, and the time required.

Organizational Readiness to Do Hoshin Planning Well

Two measures can determine whether an organization is ready to proceed with hoshin planning. During the first year of planning (year zero), preparatory work (leaders' commitment, education, review and information systems, and so forth) must be in place to ensure optimal start-up conditions, as must dissemination of communications materials (review forms, resources for information, a time line). Also, a system of time management must strike a balance between time and creativity. These measures are discussed below.

Figure 5-1. Hoshin Planning Process

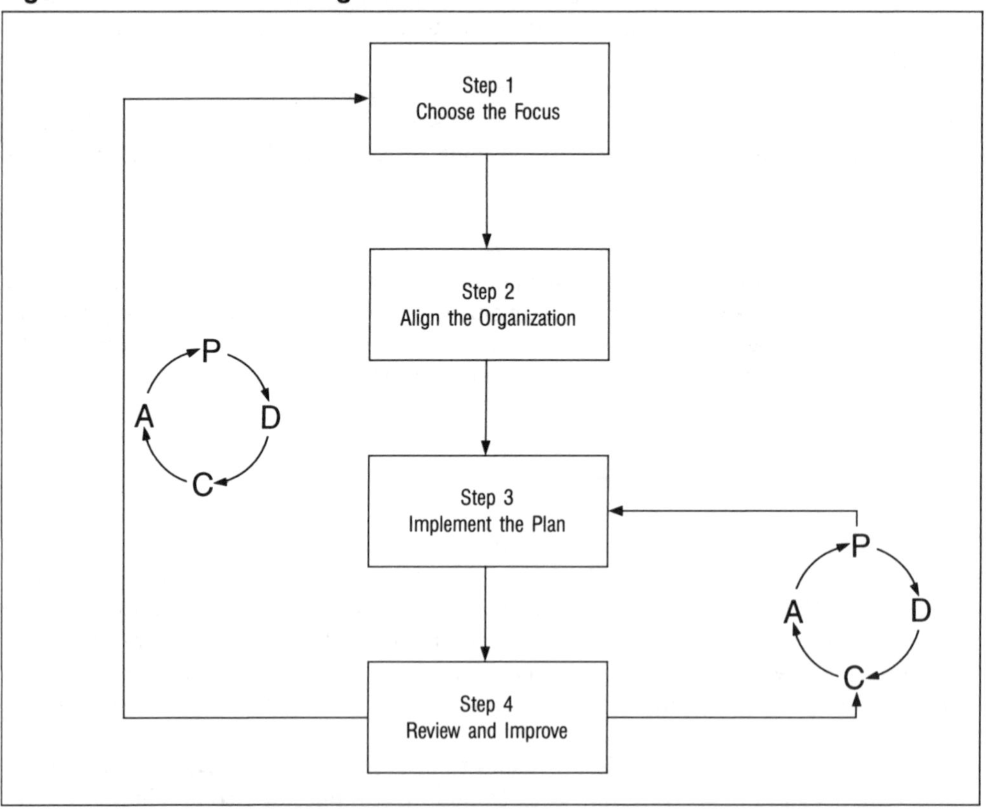

Year Zero

The first year of the hoshin planning process is one of tremendous learning. Whether leaders decide to implement parts or all of a hoshin system, considerable work must be done to prepare the organization to succeed at hoshin planning. As mentioned in chapter 4, minimal start-up conditions include committed leadership, education plans, review schedules, information systems, and trained facilitators. Optimal start-up conditions include additional experience with process improvement tools and techniques.

The use of systematic techniques and tools to maintain and improve vital work processes is known as daily management. An organization with an effective daily management system has developed the capability to identify and track the work processes that are vital to achieving organizational objectives and satisfying customers.

Daily management is a pervasive activity. Every person in the organization can think of work and talk about work as processes – processes that can be diagrammed, measured, studied, maintained, and improved. When daily management is practiced over time (years), three things happen:

1. People collect and study data from the processes that emerge as most important. These critical processes determine organizational success.
2. Patterns and anomalies appear in the process data.
3. These patterns and anomalies help people locate weak spots or undesirable trends – both of which are opportunities for process improvement.

The longer people practice daily management, the more familiar they become with process thinking and process improvement tools and techniques. The capability to track and improve processes is useful in all four steps of the hoshin process.

- *Step 1: Choose the focus.* Daily management data help the organization locate and choose the correct focus.
- *Step 2: Align the organization.* When the plan is being developed, the means to achieve specific hoshin targets often involve improving familiar daily management processes.
- *Step 3 and step 4: Implement the plan and, review and improve.* These steps are easier if the organization is already proficient at implementing, reviewing, and making the incremental improvements associated with daily management plans.

Organizations must resolve issues concerning quality and accessibility of data on markets, customers, and processes. They also need time to establish measurement and data collection systems, gain control of critical processes, and obtain necessary resources. If these preparatory activities take a significant portion of the first year, it may be wise to designate "year zero"[1] as the time to build the infrastructure to make hoshin planning succeed.

Materials to Develop and Publish

When hoshin plans are first developed, it is a good idea to publish the following materials:

- Standard planning and review forms
- Definitions of every term on the forms
- Clear, concise instructions for filling out the forms
- Examples of forms filled out correctly
- Places to go for help
- A calendar to guide the planning process

See the Bethesda and Hewlett-Packard case studies in chapters 10 and 15, respectively, for examples of planning and review forms.

Time

Time is an issue on two levels of significance. During a given year, leaders must devote adequate time to each step of the process to ensure that the focus is satisfactorily selected, planned for, and carried out. On a longer-term basis, the whole hoshin process is like any new skill: it takes time to perfect, time that may be measured in years.

By applying a balance of discipline and creativity, the top leadership team guides evolution of the hoshin planning process. Over time, the entire organization develops a sense of ownership of a successful planning process and its results. The long-term payoff of a hoshin planning system is that the organization spends more time doing the right things – that is, focusing on what is truly important to the organization and its customers.

Summary

The hoshin planning process can be summarized in four steps:

1. Choose the focus.
2. Align the organization.
3. Implement the plan.
4. Review and improve.

Chapters 6 through 9 present tools, methods, and tips for each step of the hoshin planning process, along with key leadership issues and roles.

Actions for Top Leadership

As top leaders implement a hoshin planning process, the following actions are suggested (in addition to those set forth at the conclusion of chapter 4):

1. Gain a thorough understanding of the hoshin planning process that your organization will use so that you can answer questions about the process's:
   - Purpose
   - Timing
   - Structure
   - Fit with other management systems
2. Learn the methods and tools you will need to conduct planning and deployment better than anybody else. Be familiar enough with the methods and tools others will use so that you can ask good coaching questions.
3. Read what other organizations have published about their hoshin planning journeys. Pay special attention to the bumps in the road and how they got past them.
4. Ask lots of questions about the progress of the plan as well as what it is accomplishing. Look for patterns in the responses and take those patterns into account as you improve and develop the hoshin planning process.
5. Recognize teams and individuals for their use of a good process – and help team members be patient as they wait for the process to produce good results!

Note

1. The term *zeroth year* was coined and defined by Ellen Domb, PhD, of the PQR Group in Upland, CA. Dr. Domb confirmed this fact in a personal communication to Casey Collett, Apr. 1994.

CHAPTER SIX

Step 1: Choose the Focus

The first step in the hoshin planning process, choosing a focus, has a dual purpose: to create a unified, compelling vision for change – the "pull factor" that will power and guide the rest of the hoshin planning process; and to select the organization's focus using a solid, fact-based decision-making process.

Expected outcomes from this step are as follows:

- A clear statement of the organization's priority
- Endorsement of that priority at the executive level
- Ability to communicate the priority with consistency

Leadership Issues

In carrying out the first step of the planning process, the top leadership team must deal with four issues:

1. Agreeing on a focus
2. Ensuring a good process for choosing the focus
3. Determining the extent of change needed for breakthrough
4. Communicating the organization's focus

These issues are detailed in the following subsections.

Issue 1: Agreeing on a Focus

Immediately, the hoshin planning process distinguishes itself from traditional strategic planning by requiring leaders to agree on a focus and stick to that agreement for the life of the hoshin plan. Agreement may take hours or days, depending on the diversity of leadership opinions on two questions: "What is the focus for our organization?" and "How much of a change is needed to achieve breakthrough [significant change]?"

To reach agreement, leaders must hold frank discussions on the issues facing the organization, considering factual and opinion data. Leaders need to consider all potential focus items and the pros and cons of choosing each. Consensus discussion or a tool such as a prioritization matrix (appendix B) may help the leadership team to decide on a focus and to eliminate or postpone others.

To maintain agreement, leaders may need to hold periodic, frank discussions on the progress of the plan and issues that arise. These discussions may coincide with formal reviews or they may be spontaneous. In either case, airing and resolving concerns *within* the leadership team will help leaders maintain unity and consistency throughout the life of the plan.

Issue 2: Ensuring a Good Process for Choosing the Focus

Agreeing on the area of focus means saying yes to something and no to a lot of other things. It means looking at all of the important strategic objectives and isolating the one that can make the biggest contribution to achieving the organization's vision. Even though the organization's focus is a stretch goal that may be quite visionary, the choice of the focus is based on solid facts and a healthy decision-making process.

The leadership team may want to standardize and document a decision-making process that works well so that it can be replicated in each hoshin planning cycle. The following is an example of one such process:

1. Compile a book of relevant strategic and operational data for leaders to read.
2. Leaders meet to generate potential focus items.
3. Leaders see if focus items could be sequenced over a multiyear period.
4. If there are still multiple potential focus items for next year, leaders use tools such as a prioritization matrix, interrelationship digraph, or force field analysis to select the best focus. (See appendix B for discussion of tools.)
5. Leaders come to consensus.
6. Leaders plan communication of organization's focus.

Issue 3: Determining the Extent of Change Needed for Breakthrough

Setting breakthrough targets may seem more an art than a science. Some guidance comes from inside the organization itself. If the organization sets a breakthrough goal that is easy to achieve using current systems, the goal may not be stretchy enough. (See figure 6-1.)

Guidance from outside comes in the form of benchmarking other organizations, looking for examples of excellent performance to use in setting goals. Leaders need to assess the capability of the organization to produce breakthrough change as they set the goal and time line. Leaders can rely upon performance data from past change efforts to test their tentative goal. Or they can solicit opinions from a wider circle of employees, even at this early stage of planning. The focus should produce a breakthrough without breaking the back of the current organization.

Issue 4: Communicating the Organization's Focus

By the time the focus is chosen, the leaders have grappled with it so long that they understand it well. Now they must put themselves into the shoes of others who need to hear and understand the focus so that they can participate in developing the plan. The leaders must communicate the focus clearly and convincingly. They also must communicate the process by which the focus was chosen. For example, the yearly hoshin process can include a standard communication format that recaps current issues, outlines the process for selecting the focus, and announces the new focus, including its potential impact on the strategic plan.

Figure 6-1. Breakthrough or Continuous Improvement?

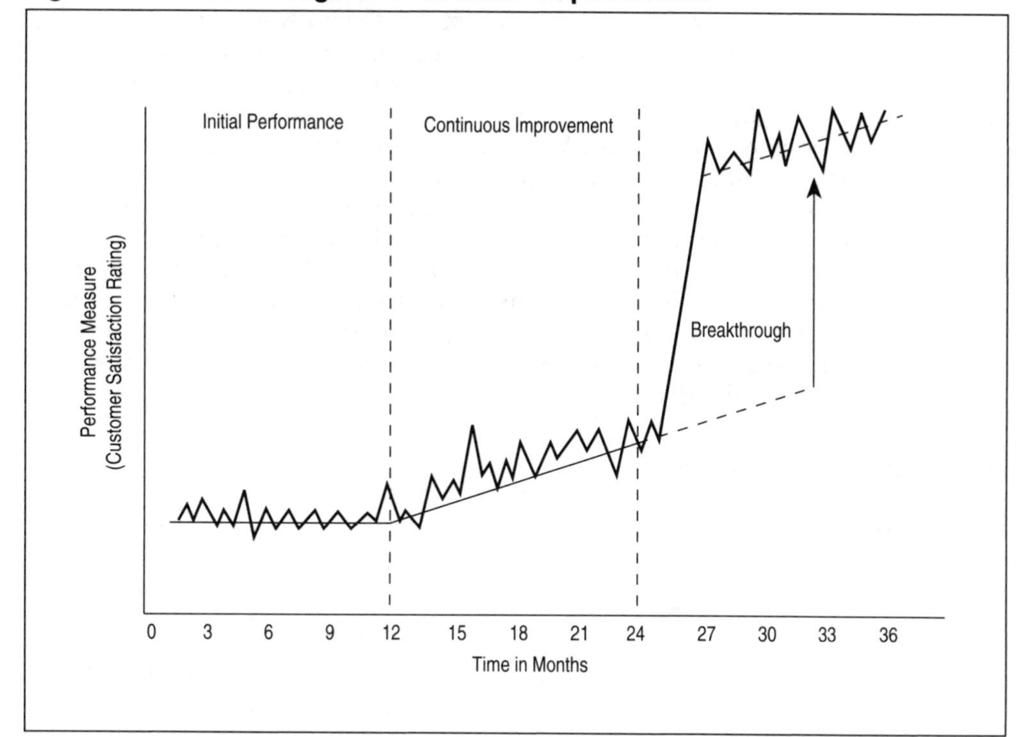

Implementation Tasks

The first step in the hoshin process is about focus. The top leadership team becomes the planning team and carries out a series of tasks, shown in figure 6-2 as substeps:

1. Make the current state of the organization visible.
2. Define what the organization wants to be in the future.
3. Identify what the organization needs to focus on to achieve its vision (such as listening to customers, identifying KSFs, and conducting gap analysis of KSFs)

Much of the methodology in tasks 1 and 2 is covered in traditional strategic planning. Therefore, the following section provides only a brief outline. (For a detailed explanation of these tasks, see appendix A.) This section *does* include a complete discussion of task 3, however, the point at which the hoshin planning process begins to distinguish itself from traditional strategic planning.

Task 1: Make the Current State of the Organization Visible

This procedure requires the top leadership team to collect and analyze relevant data that will enable the team to select the most appropriate hoshin focus. Obtaining the relevant information requires the following actions:

- *Revisit why the organization exists: mission and values.* The top leadership team defines, refines, or reviews the mission and values of the organization. These stable documents remind the leadership team of the purpose and character of the organization.

- *Identify trends regarding the major customers, suppliers, and competitors.* The team collects important trend and anecdotal data on key customers, suppliers, and competitors. It searches the data for patterns of weaknesses and strengths. The hoshin focus may be designed to address significant weaknesses and to enhance strengths.
- *Analyze the current state of the business.* The team examines the external forces affecting the business, including global, national, regional, and industrywide trends. It examines the internal environment by looking for trends in critical processes within and across business units and/or product lines.

  To identify trends in critical processes, an activity that is a part of the daily management system, businesses must first identify which processes are vital to the success of the business. As those processes are measured and tracked over time, trends become apparent. The team may also analyze competitive advantages and disadvantages.

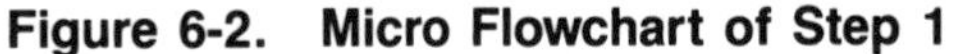

Figure 6-2. Micro Flowchart of Step 1

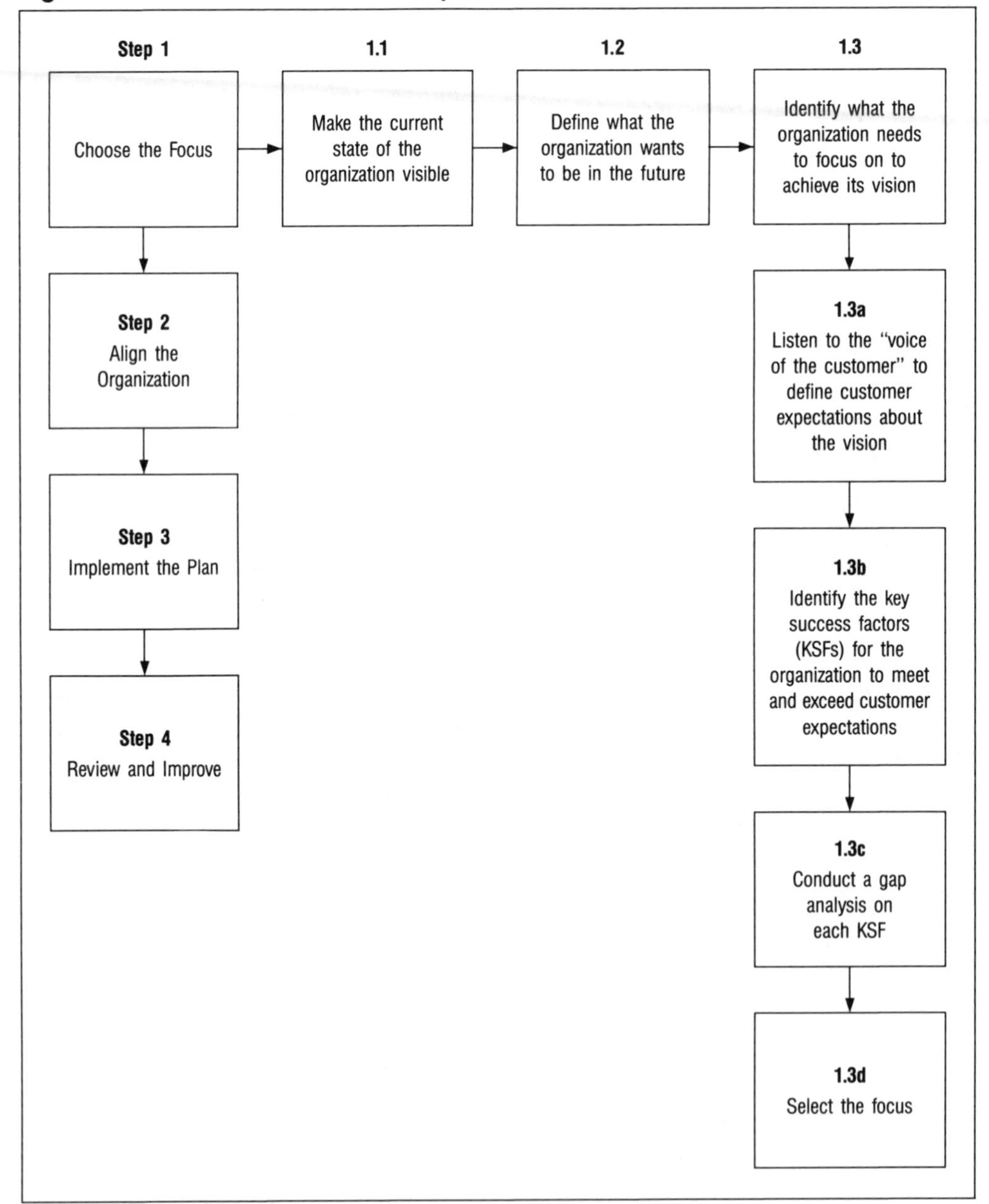

Task 2: Define What the Organization Wants to Be in the Future

This procedure is usually referred to as defining or refining a vision. The vision, or dream of what the organization will be, is colored heavily by what the customers need, both currently and in the future. As the top leadership team progresses through tasks 1 and 2, it may wish to collect its findings on a worksheet such as the one represented in figure 6-3.

Task 3: Identify What the Organization Needs to Focus on to Achieve Its Vision

At this point, hoshin planning really begins to distinguish itself from traditional strategic planning. This is the part of the hoshin planning process that forces the top leaders to declare a focus – a customer-based focus. The leaders emerge from this procedure with a clear view of the vital few things the organization must do to achieve its customer-oriented vision. To complete task 3, top leaders must follow a four-step process, as shown in the micro flowchart in figure 6-2 (p. 76):

- Listen to the "voice of the customer" to define customer expectations about the vision.
- Identify the key success factors (KSFs) for the organization to meet and exceed customer expectations.
- Conduct a KSF gap analysis to assess where the organization stands on each KSF.
- Select the focus.

Listen to the "Voice of the Customer"

To begin to identify what the organization needs to focus on to achieve its vision, the top leadership team works to form a clear picture of the future needs and expectations

Figure 6-3. Worksheet: Data Collection and Analysis for Selection of the Focus

Column 1	Column 2	Column 3	Column 4
Observations about the current state of the organization Include themes, observations, or issues about: • Current strategy • Customer needs • Supplier data • Competitor data • External environment • Internal environment	Observations about the future Record "short list" of future customer needs Record future demands/issues related to: • Competitors • Suppliers • External environment • Internal environment	Key Success Factors (KSFs) 5–6 or fewer The few important things the organization must do well to meet customer needs and to achieve the vision	Ideas for potential breakthrough (focus) Record ideas for possible hoshin focus items
Examples: Strategy: Tertiary care Customer base aging (*B) Two new competitors (*A)	Anticipate increased local competition for recruiting geriatric care specialists	Retraining, reallocating workforce Understanding and meeting needs of the specialists	New levels of specialist recruitment/retention

***Note:** You can use an "A, B, C" system to indicate the impact of each observation you write in columns 1 and 2:
A = High impact item B = Medium impact C = Minimal impact

of the organization's customers. These future needs will highlight opportunities for delighting customers or for exceeding the competition's ability to anticipate customer needs and expectations.

When the leadership team reviewed trends in customer data (in the example in appendix A, step 1.1), it looked at historical evidence of what customers wanted, did, and believed. Even current information from surveys, focus groups, and interviews about customers' future preferences will, at best, yield ideas for evolutionary change.

Hoshin is about revolutionary (breakthrough) change. The most potent source of breakthrough ideas is the voice of the customer projected into the future. The top leadership team has two options for anticipating the future needs and expectations of the customer.

- *Option A:* To work "inside-out"–that is, to ask the organization to paint a clear picture of future customer needs and then to validate that picture with the customers
- *Option B:* To go straight to the customers and ask them to paint their own picture

Option A: Organization Paints Picture of the Future and Validates It with Customer Data

In the first part of this option, the organization has to ask, "What will our customers need?" Discussions take place at various levels. The internal perception check may begin with a top leadership team discussion of future customer needs at a global level. Later discussions conducted at departmental levels may address specific customers or products and services. The ideas that arise in these discussions may be recorded, summarized, and used later to formulate lists of future needs.

There are two types of questions to ask in these discussions–direct and indirect:

- *Direct questions:* These types of questions will elicit ideas for *evolutionary* change. The discussions may begin with straightforward questions such as the following:
  - –Who will our customers be in the future?
  - –What will they need?
- *Indirect questions:* Ideas for *revolutionary* change are more likely to come from questions such as the following:
  - –What problems are customers trying to solve–now and in five years? What are their visions?
  - –If you could do anything for our customers in five years–no constraints–what would it be?
  - –What could we do that would thrill our customers?
  - –What would our customers do differently if they ran our business?

After the questions have been asked and answered, the information from the discussions has to be organized. Data from the internal discussions of future customer needs and expectations can be segmented into several types of lists:

- A macro list of customer needs and expectations, expressed at a high level and very strategic in nature
- Lists broken out by key strategic customers
- Lists broken out by key products, services, or work units in the current organization

The second part of option A involves validating those lists. This is done, before any plans are made, by asking customers to validate the organization's perception.

- *Conduct a "$100 test."* One method of testing how well the organization projected future customer needs is to conduct a $100 test. In this test, representative samples of customers receive a list of projected needs and an imaginary $100. They have to weight the importance of the needs listed using their money as the weighting factor. The results of this test can be displayed on a matrix, as shown in figure 6-4. This simple test will reveal how a given customer weights the needs and how much diversity of opinion exists among customers. This activity also gives customers the opportunity to critique and modify the list of needs generated by the organization.
- *Create a short list of customer needs.* By comparing the lists developed from discussions within the organization (the macro list, for example) with the results of the $100 tests conducted with selected customers, the top leadership team can create a short list of future needs. The team may record the short list of future customer needs in column 2 of the data collection worksheet (shown earlier in figure 6-3, p. 77).

Example of Option A

Firstcare Health is now an integrated system (hospital, physicians' group, and philanthropic foundation) offering a coordinated approach to medical services in a community of 30,000 and a geographic area of 100,000 persons. Over the past decade, the hospital has adapted to a significant shift in its patient population. Now providing equal amounts of inpatient and outpatient care, the hospital has an average length of stay of three and a half days.

More recently, hospital and physician leaders in the community began to look for ways to respond to growing demands from local businesses to provide lower-cost care. They were also searching for the best way to organize to meet ongoing managed care pressures from the national level. One response was to form Firstcare Health and to create a "clinic without walls," which would represent the majority of primary care physicians in the community. The top leadership team at Firstcare Health used a hoshin planning approach to develop a plan for the clinic without walls.

Using option A, described in the preceding text, the leaders did a thorough analysis of the needs of five key customers (the patient, physician, employer, insurer, and the hospital). For each key customer, they created a short list of needs. For example, this is the short list of needs for the physician group:

- Healthier patients
- Prevention of acute episodes

Figure 6-4. $100 Test: How Important Are the Needs to These Customers?

Short List of Needs:	Customers A	B	C	D	E	Totals
1	20	0	0	0	0	20
2	20	30	0	20	0	70
3	10	30	0	10	45	95
4	50	0	100	70	30	250
5	0	30	0	0	5	35
6	0	10	0	0	20	30
Totals	$100	$100	$100	$100	$100	$500 Grand Total

Note: Customers "spend" their money based on the importance they place on each of the needs they are asked to assess.

- More direct patient care time
- Ability to offer new and different services
- Ability to keep practice in same office in small town
- Potential to contract as managed care organization and maintain patient population

After creating a list of needs for each key customer, the leadership planning team conducted interviews and surveys to validate the lists.

Option B: Organization Asks Customers to Paint the Picture of Their Future Needs and Expectations

The second option for listening to the voice of the customer is to go straight to the customers themselves and to ask them to paint their own picture of the future. The way to do this is to survey the customers and create a customer data table, and then to use data from that table to create a customer need/measures matrix.

- *Customer data table:* A good way to start is by surveying the customers and recording their responses on a customer data table. (See example in figure 6-5.)

  Ask customers to describe their future needs and expectations, and record their responses verbatim in column 1 of the table. Customer responses may be clustered or categorized. Then, in column 2, "translate" or categorize the customer responses into organizational language (for example, technical or clinical terminology). Columns 3 through 6 on the customer data table allow the interviewer to probe for things the customers did not think to express on their own.

  Breakthrough ideas often result from unexpressed needs and expectations. In column 7, the organization lists measures or indicators to track important customer needs – at macro and micro levels. It may be necessary to complete customer data tables for several key customers and to consider them separately and collectively to look for trends in responses.

Example of Option B

Firstcare Health interviewed all of its key customers to determine their future needs and expectations for a clinic without walls. In column 1 of the customer data table, the interviewer recorded the fact that several physicians said they needed "the ability to offer new and different services."

Figure 6-5. Customer Data Table

Column 1	Column 2	Column 3	Column 4	Column 5	Column 6	Column 7
Customers' Words: What they say they need/want in a product/service (P/S)	**Customers' Words: Translated into organizational language**	**Who will use the P/S?**	**How will they use the P/S?**	**When will they use?**	**Where will they use?**	**Potential Measures or Indicators**
We need the ability to offer new and different services	Spectrum of services	All physicians in clinic without walls	To gain networking opportunities	—	—	Number of formal networking opportunities
Instructions: Interview customer. Record verbatim responses in column 1. Translate customer words into organization language in column 2. Continue to probe customer need with questions in columns 3 through 6. Record possible measure in column 7.						

Source: Firstcare Health.

This need was grouped with similar thoughts expressed by other key customers and was eventually translated (column 2) into the term *spectrum of services.*

As the interviewers probed the physicians' responses (column 4), they learned that physicians hoped to use the clinic as a networking opportunity, to share ideas and to develop new services in collaboration with leading employers in the community. Therefore, a possible measure (column 7) might be the frequency of formal networking opportunities built into the new clinic system.

- *Customer need/measures matrix:* The top leadership team may use the results of columns 2 and 7 on the customer data table to create a customer need/measures matrix, similar to the one shown in figure 6-6. A few primary customer needs/expectations are translated into the language of the organization. These needs are displayed down the vertical axis of the matrix. Across the top of the matrix are all of the possible measures that were listed in column 7 of the customer data table. These measures help track the satisfaction level of customer needs.

  The boxes inside the matrix may be filled in with the symbols shown on figure 6-6. (See appendix B, "Hoshin Toolbox," for tips on using a matrix diagram.) These symbols display the degree to which the needs and the measures are related to one another. The patterns of symbols in the rows and columns of the matrix are important. For example, a nearly empty row says that the organization has no strong measures for a particular customer need. On the other hand, a column full of double circles says that the indicator is strongly related to several important customer needs and is a particularly powerful measure.

Creating the customer data table and the customer need/measures matrix is the beginning of a method called quality function deployment (QFD). Often used in product and service design and development work, QFD is a method of carrying the voice of the customer all the way through the design/development/production process. In a full QFD system, the customer need/measures matrix (also known as the A-1 matrix) is the foundation upon which many design decisions are based.

Figure 6-6. Customer Need/Measures Matrix

	Measures		
Customer Need	**Cost per Procedure**	**Wait times**	**Etc.**
Provide a spectrum of services	○	○	
Satisfy patients	⊙	⊙	
Meet regulatory requirements	△	○	
Use clinically effective practices	⊙	⊙	
Provide services at reasonable cost	⊙	⊙	
Ensure timely access	○	⊙	

Strength of relationship: ⊙ Strong ○ Medium △ Weak

Source: Firstcare Health.

Identify the Key Success Factors for the Organization

During this step, the leadership team considers the following sources of data:

- The short list of what the customer wants (described in the preceding text)
- Competitive data (such as the emergence of a new competitor or the development of new products or services by an existing provider)
- Internal process data (such as current wait times in key service areas)
- Other factors external to the organization (including trends in the requests made by employers or national trends that are bound to affect the organization)

The team compiles data from all of these sources into a list of critical issues facing the organization. It translates the issues into organizational responses expressed as "key success factors." The team goes through the following steps in this translation:

1. Identify issues to address in the future.
2. Prioritize issues (if necessary).
3. Develop key success factors to address the priority issues.
4. *(Optional)* Check the KSFs against the short list of customer needs.

Identify Issues to Address in the Future

Two methods can help a leadership team identify issues to be addressed in the future. They are the affinity diagram method and the worksheet method.

- *Affinity diagram method:* In substep 1.2 ("Define what the organization wants to be in the future") of the hoshin planning process illustrated in figure 6-2 (p. 76), the leadership team may have used an affinity diagram to generate the organization's vision. (See appendix A for the vision generation process. See appendix B, "Hoshin Toolbox," for affinity diagram instructions.) This vision is based on customer needs—not on the isolated needs of one customer, but on the blended needs of all key customers. The vision is also based on ideal responses to competitive pressures, internal process improvements, and forces from the external environment.

  If the planning team used an affinity diagram as a means of generating a vision for the organization, it has a head start in identifying key success factors. The affinity process produces categories that help formulate the vision. Each separate affinity category represents an issue that could be developed into a KSF.

Example

Firstcare Health combined the needs of all five key customers in the affinity diagram shown in figure 6-7. This affinity grouped the customer needs into 10 categories:

1. A spectrum of health care services
2. Physician impact in governance of the system
3. Satisfied patients
4. Regulatory compliance
5. Business flexibility
6. Health care services at a reasonable cost
7. Most clinically effective practices
8. Local care
9. Timely access
10. Minimal change in the current system

Figure 6-7. Affinity Diagram of Customer Needs

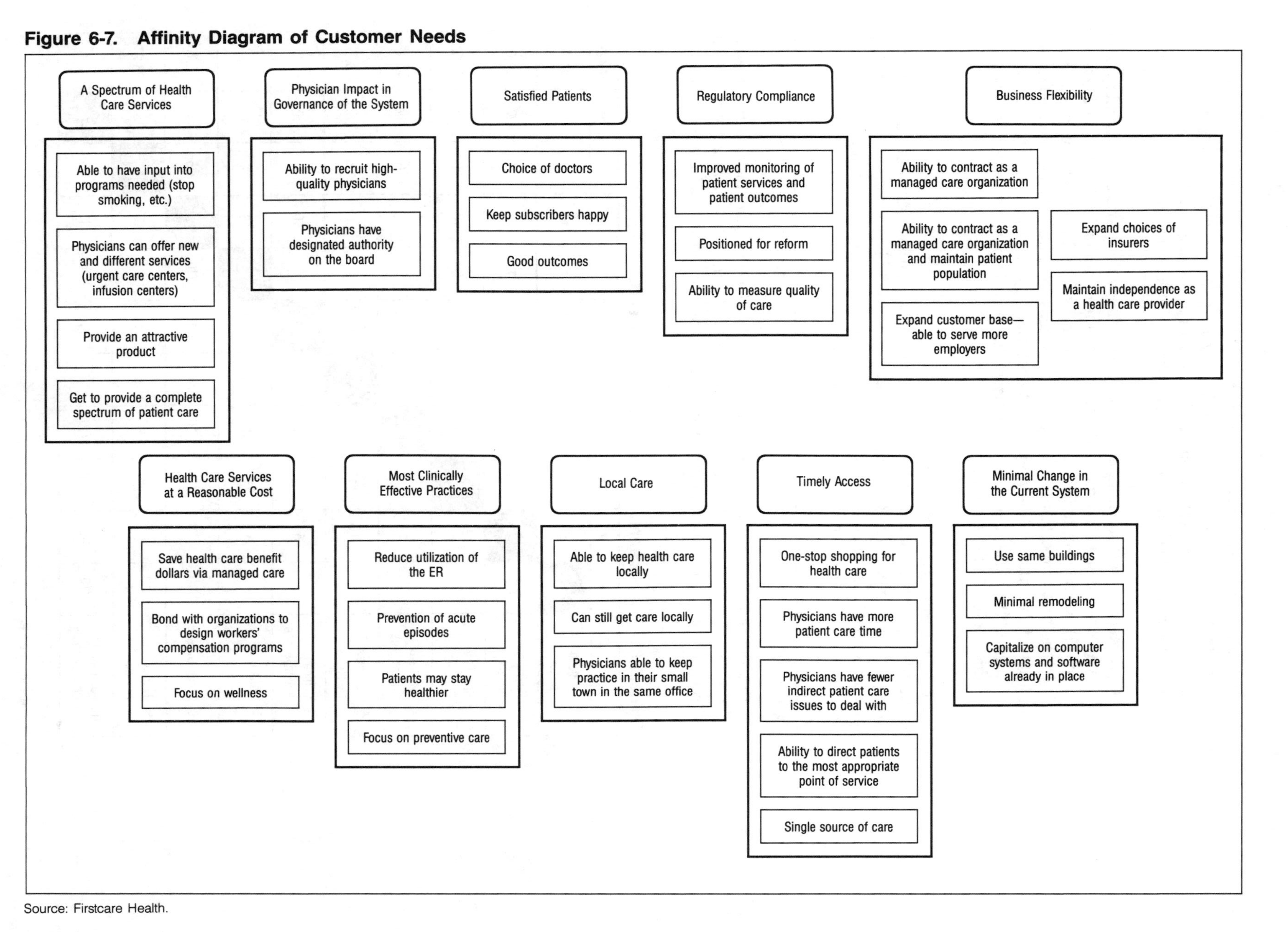

Source: Firstcare Health.

Each category represents an issue that Firstcare Health must address to ensure a successful future. The category titles are even worded in such a way that each one could be a key success factor. But, because Firstcare Health cannot address 10 KSFs at one time, it will have to prioritize the list and identify the highest-impact category titles to develop into KSFs.

- *Worksheet method:* Instead of using an affinity diagram, the leadership team may use a discussion method and a worksheet similar to the one in figure 6-3 (p. 77). In the worksheet method, the team will find a variety of issues listed in the first two columns. Although there may be many issues, the leaders will have to identify a few major ones that the organization must address in the future. Once the team has prioritized the most important issues, it can begin developing KSFs to address them.

Prioritize Issues (If Necessary)

If the affinity or the worksheet method has produced a large number of issues, the top leadership team must narrow the list before developing KSFs. One method for identifying high-impact issues is to use a prioritization matrix, such as the one in figure 6-8. (See appendix B, "Hoshin Toolbox," for prioritization matrix instructions.)

Example

Firstcare Health had identified 10 category titles on its affinity diagram. Each title was an issue that could be developed into a KSF. To narrow the list of issues, the leaders of Firstcare Health compared all possible pairs of issues in terms of their relative importance. For any pair of issues,

Figure 6-8. Prioritization Matrix of Customer Needs

	1	2	3	4	5	6	7	8	9	10	Totals
1. Spectrum of Services		5	1	1	5	1/5	1	10	1	10	34.2*
2. Physician Impact	1/5		1/5	1/5	5	1/5	1	1	1/5	5	13.0
3. Satisfied Patients	1	5		5	10	1	5	10	5	10	52.0*
4. Regulatory Compliance	1	5	1/5		5	1/5	1	10	1/5	10	32.6*
5. Business Flexibility	1/5	1/5	1/10	1/5		1/10	1	1	1/5	5	8.0
6. Clinical Effectiveness	5	5	1	5	10		5	10	1	10	52.0*
7. Reasonable Cost	1	1	1/5	1	1	1/5		10	1	10	25.4*
8. Local Care	1/10	1	1/10	1/10	1	1/10	1/10		1/5	1	3.7
9. Timely Access	1	5	1/5	5	5	1	1	5		5	28.2*
10. Minimal Change	1/10	1/5	1/10	1/10	1/5	1/10	1/10	1	1/5		2.1

*Priority needs

Source: Firstcare Health

the leaders asked themselves, "What is the relative importance of these two issues?" To answer the question, they used the following scale:

- Much more important = 10
- More important = 5
- Equally important = 1
- Less important = 1/5
- Much less important = 1/10

As the leaders compared each pair of issues (for example, spectrum of services compared to physician impact), they assigned numbers in the appropriate rows of the matrix. For instance, spectrum of services was more important than physician impact. Spectrum was assigned a 5 and physician impact was assigned a 1/5. The comparisons continued until all possible pairs were assigned numbers. Row totals indicated that the top six customer needs/issues were as follows:

- Satisfied patients
- Clinical effectiveness
- Spectrum of services
- Regulatory compliance
- Timely access
- Reasonable cost

By narrowing the list to these six issues, the Firstcare Health leadership team could focus development of KSFs on the areas of highest impact.

Note: The prioritization matrix would have worked equally well if Firstcare Health had used the worksheet method of issue identification.

Develop Key Success Factors

The leadership team has narrowed its focus to a small number of issues that are essential to the organization's future success. Through consensus discussion, the team can now develop KSFs to address these issues. (There should be no more than five or six of them.) These KSFs may be recorded on the data collection worksheet.

Example

In its hoshin planning process, Firstcare Health had identified six top-priority customer needs/issues to address in its vision of an ideal clinic without walls. One of those top-priority issues, for example, was clinical effectiveness. The top leadership team decided that a key success factor had to be "Use the most clinically effective practices." Considering each of the six major issues in turn, the Firstcare Health top leadership team specified the following KSFs:

- Provide a spectrum of health care services
- Satisfy patients
- Meet regulatory requirements
- Use the most clinically effective practices
- Provide health care services at a reasonable cost
- Ensure timely access to health care services

Check KSFs against Short List of Customer Needs (Optional)

Key success factors may be checked against the short list of customer needs using a special form of matrix diagram known as a relationship matrix. As shown in figure 6-9, the KSFs go across the top of the matrix and the short list of customer needs go down the side. Using the symbols shown in this figure, the leaders determine the existence

Figure 6-9. Relationship Matrix

Customer Needs	KSF 1	KSF 2	KSF 3	KSF 4	KSF 5
1	⊙	⊙		○	⊙
2		⊙	⊙		⊙
3	○	△		△	⊙
4		⊙	○	⊙	⊙
5		⊙			

The relationship of the KSFs to customer needs:

⊙ Strong relationship ○ Moderate relationship △ Possible relationship

and strength of the relationships between each KSF and each customer need. The leaders look for patterns such as these, which are exemplified in figure 6-9:

- Customer needs that are not covered adequately by the KSFs (customer need 5)
- KSFs that cover a number of customer needs (KSFs 2 and 5)

At this point in the planning process, the planning team can still adjust the KSFs to meet the customer needs.

Example

Firstcare Health decided to check its KSFs against the short list of physician needs. The resulting matrix diagram is shown in figure 6-10. Each of the KSFs had multiple strong relationships to the short list of physician needs. The KSF "Providing a spectrum of health care services" strongly related to four of the customer needs and moderately related to the other two needs.

Conduct a Gap Analysis on Each KSF

So far, the top leadership team has identified the key success factors that will contribute to achieving the vision. The team has checked the KSFs against the short list of customer needs to ensure that no vital customer need will go unattended, no matter which KSF is pursued. From among these KSFs, one or two will actually become the organization's focus–the area for breakthrough change in the hoshin planning process.

The next stage in the focusing effort is to assess where the organization stands on each KSF. In this stage, the top leadership team will give the organization a "report card" based on how well it is currently performing the KSFs. This report card is called a "gap analysis," because it helps the top leadership team identify the biggest gaps between the organization's current performance and its desired performance on the KSFs. To conduct a gap analysis:

1. Develop ways to "grade" each KSF.
2. Collect appropriate data.
3. Attach a performance measure to each KSF.
4. Construct a *radar chart.*

Figure 6-10. Relationship Matrix to Check KSFs against Short List of Customer Needs

	KSF 1	KSF 2	KSF 3	KSF 4	KSF 5	KSF 6
Short List of Physician Needs	**Spectrum of Services**	**Satisfy Patients**	**Meet Regulatory Requirements**	**Clinically Effective Practices**	**Reasonable Cost**	**Timely Access**
Patients stay healthier	⊙	⊙	⊙	⊙	⊙	⊙
Prevent acute episodes	⊙	⊙	⊙	⊙	⊙	⊙
More direct patient care time	○	⊙	○	○	○	⊙
New and different services	⊙	○	△	⊙	△	○
Keep practice in same town	○	⊙		△	△	△
Contract as managed care; maintain patient population	⊙	△	○	○	○	○

Strength of relationships:

⊙ Strong ○ Moderate △ Possible

Source: Firstcare Health

Develop Ways to Grade Each KSF

Each KSF can be graded based on three types of data—customer, competitor, and benchmark:

- *Customer data:* To grade a KSF from the customer point of view, the leadership team will want to refer to historical trends and projections of future customer needs. For example, Firstcare Health would want to judge its spectrum of services KSF based on the opinions of the organization's key customers.
- *Competitor data:* Looking at major competitors helps the leadership team broaden its perspective. For instance, Firstcare Health might give its spectrum of services a high grade based on how well the services satisfy customers. But a comparison of its services to those of an aggressive new competitor in town might result in a lower grade.
- *Benchmark data:* In benchmarking, an organization compares its products, services, and business processes with a gold standard: direct and indirect competitors who are the best in their class or even the best in the world. Firstcare Health might want to research the "full spectrum of service" offerings of a variety of health care organizations.

Collect Appropriate Data

Some customer, competitor, and benchmark data will already be available to the top leadership team. If data for a given KSF are insufficient or unavailable, the leadership team may choose to place the hoshin planning process on temporary hold while it gathers additional information. The team should also make plans to guide future data collection efforts for hoshin planning processes in years to come. As part of the standard hoshin planning process, the team may need to direct efforts to collect new types of data or to reconfigure current data sources. In so doing, they are preparing the organization to have the right data available for future hoshin planning cycles.

Attach a Performance Measure to Each KSF

After considering the various ways of grading each KSF and collecting appropriate data, the top leadership team must develop one performance measure by which it will judge each KSF. These performance measures will appear on the radar chart (discussed below) to remind the leadership team of its grading scale. Firstcare Health chose to grade its spectrum of services KSF by defining a portfolio of services and counting the number of services in that portfolio at any given time.

Construct a Radar Chart

To conduct the gap analysis, the leadership team may use a radar chart, as shown in figure 6-11. The radar chart looks like a wagon wheel, with one "spoke" for each KSF and its associated performance measure. The spoke represents a 1–10 grading scale, with 1 being a low grade and 10 being perfect. The KSFs are assigned a number grade to represent their current status. (See appendix B, "Hoshin Toolbox," for radar chart instructions.)

Figure 6-11. Radar Chart Example—Gap Analysis of Key Success Factors

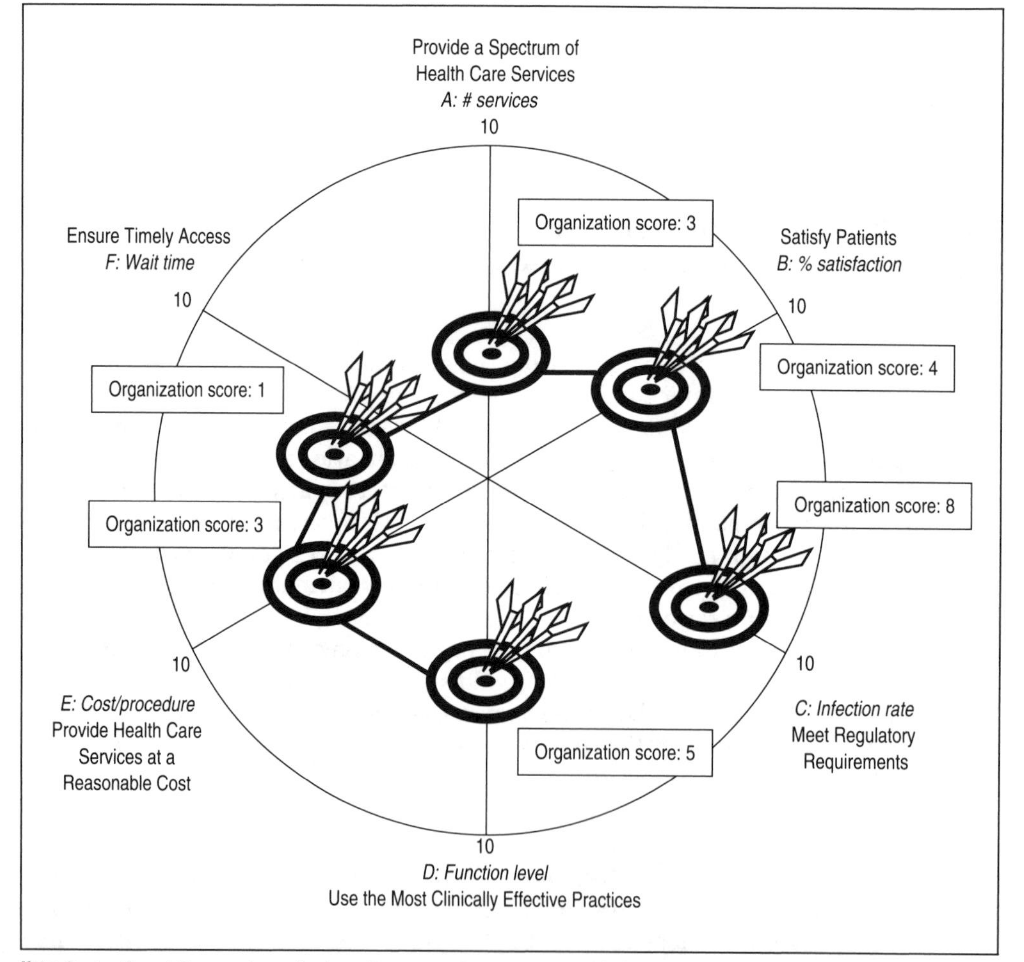

Note: Scales C and F are reciprocal: where lower measurements are good, they are shown as higher ratings.

Source: Firstcare Health.

Example

Once the radar chart is complete, the planning team will have a clear view of the organization's performance on each KSF. The team is especially interested in the KSFs where the gap between current and desired performance is greatest. Firstcare Health noted that its greatest gap was on the ensure timely access KSF. The next largest gaps were on the spectrum of services and reasonable cost KSFs.

See the case studies of Southwest Texas Methodist Hospital and Hewlett-Packard Medical Products Group (chapters 13 and 15, respectively) for examples using the gap analysis.

Select the Focus

The gap analysis may point out the need to improve multiple KSFs. Some improvements may address a single KSF, whereas others may span several KSFs. At this stage in identifying what the organization needs to focus on to achieve its vision, the leadership team chooses one KSF as the organization's focus for the immediate future (that is, the next year). In designating a clear focus, the team is also telling the organization what the focus will *not* be.

The leadership team must go through a three-part process in selecting the focus:

1. Narrow the list of KSFs.
2. Identify the focus.
3. Check the measure.

Narrow the List of KSFs

There are two methods that the top leadership team may find helpful in narrowing the list of KSFs: the interrelationship digraph and a matrix diagram, in particular a relationship matrix. These methods may be used singly or in combination.

- *Interrelationship digraph:* This method can be helpful in narrowing the focus to one KSF from among a variety of viable alternatives. The interrelationship digraph, or ID, as shown in figure 6-12, is a graphic method of showing the cause-and-effect relationships among all of the KSFs. (For instructions on the interrelationship digraph, see appendix B, "Hoshin Toolbox.") Arrows going *out of* a KSF indicate causal or driving forces – that KSF causes things to happen. Arrows coming *into* a KSF indicate outcome or resultant forces – that KSF is an outcome or is driven by other things. Based on the ID analysis, the leadership team may choose to attack a dominant causal force, because making a positive change in that one factor would have a positive ripple effect on many other factors as well.

Example

In the interrelationship digraph of the Firstcare Health KSFs, "Provide a spectrum of health care services" had four arrows going *out of* and one arrow going *into* this KSF. The Firstcare team decided to focus on the spectrum KSF because it was a major driving force in the clinic without walls concept.

- *Relationship matrix:* Another method for narrowing the KSFs is to use a matrix diagram – in particular, a matrix (such as the one in figure 6-10) that shows the relationships between the KSFs and another important variable, such as customer needs. In this matrix, KSFs would be displayed on one axis of the matrix.

Figure 6-12. Interrelationship Digraph Example—Selecting a Focus from the Key Success Factors

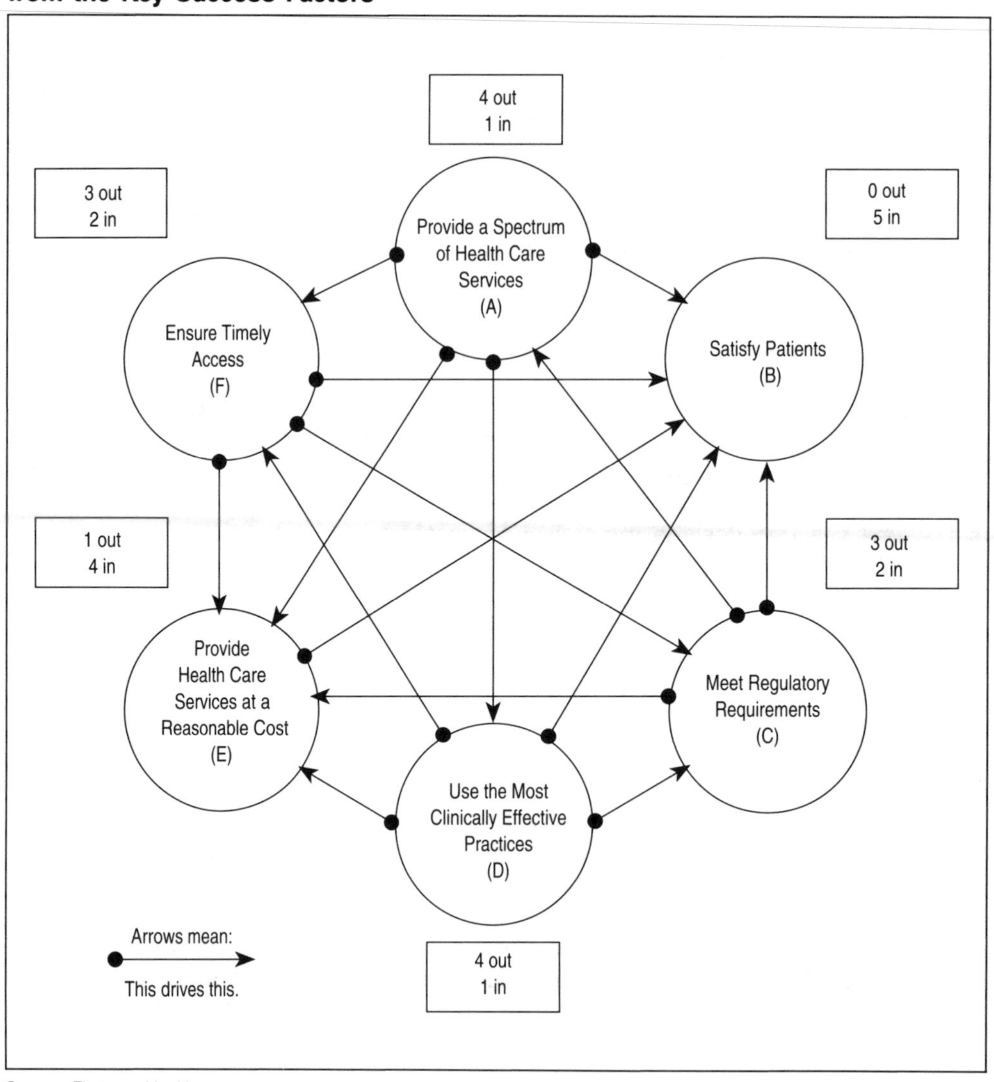

Source: Firstcare Health.

The other axis might be customer needs or vision elements. By using one or more relationship matrixes, the top leadership team should be able to see the potential impact of various focus options on other key factors in the organization.

Example

Firstcare Health noted in its relationship matrix to check KSFs against customer needs (figure 6-10, pp. 87) that KSF 1 ("Provide a spectrum of services") appeared to be strongly related to most of the key customer needs. To check this perception, Firstcare assigned some values to the symbols on the matrix. Traditional values for the symbols are as follows:

–Strong relationship = 9 points
–Moderate relationship = 3 points
–Possible relationship = 1 point

Figure 6-13 was the result of assigning numbers to the symbols in the relationship matrix.

After the leadership team assigned the values to each symbol and added up the totals for each column, these were the results:

KSF	Point Total
1. Provide a spectrum of services	42
2. Satisfy patients	40
3. Meet regulatory requirements	25
4. Use the most clinically effective practices	34
5. Provide health care services at a reasonable cost	26
6. Ensure timely access	34

The KSFs that were most closely related to the key customer needs were KSF 1 and KSF 2. In agreement with the interrelationship digraph analysis, the relationship matrix indicated that "Provide a spectrum of services" was the best candidate for the organization's focus.

Identify the Focus

This is the pivotal point in the hoshin planning process—the time at which it most distinguishes itself from traditional strategic planning. Significantly, this is also the point at which the art of leadership merges with the step-by-step, data-driven decision making that has just occurred.

There is no formula here. The top leadership team must take all previous discussions, tools, and data into account and name the organization's focus. At times, all the tools and data seem to line up and point clearly to one KSF. At other times, the data points appear to conflict or diverge. In either case, leadership judgment prevails. Leaders must find the balance between too much trust and not enough trust in what the data seem to indicate. For example, choosing a KSF as a focus based on the agreement of a matrix diagram and an interrelationship digraph is not as rich a decision as one that takes into account the gap analysis and relative importance of the other KSFs.

Figure 6-13. Relationship Matrix to Narrow KSFs

	KSF 1	KSF 2	KSF 3	KSF 4	KSF 5	KSF 6
Short List of Physician Needs	**Spectrum of Services**	**Satisfy Patients**	**Meet Regulatory Requirements**	**Clinically Effective Practices**	**Reasonable Cost**	**Timely Access**
Patients stay healthier	9	9	9	9	9	9
Prevent acute episodes	9	9	9	9	9	9
More direct patient care time	3	9	3	3	3	9
New and different services	9	3	1	9	1	3
Keep practice in same town	3	9		1	1	1
Contract as managed care; maintain patient population	9	1	3	3	3	3
Totals	42	40	25	34	26	34

Strength of relationships:

⊙ Strong (9) ○ Moderate (3) △ Possible (1)

Source: Firstcare Health.

The leadership team must exercise caution and restraint at this point in the process. There is a tendency to want to bite off too much for the organization to chew–to try to achieve breakthrough improvement in too many KSFs. To test its selection of hoshin priorities, the team can use two guidelines: number and magnitude.

- *Number:* Veterans of the hoshin process advise keeping the number of breakthrough items very small–from one to a very few. As these KSF breakthrough items are deployed throughout the organization, they will multiply geometrically. Left unchecked, they will also overshadow the less glamorous but still vital daily management system. (See chapter 5 for a discussion of daily management.) So it is a good idea to limit the number of hoshin items early in the process.
- *Magnitude:* The magnitude question sounds like this: "Is this focus really a breakthrough, or is it continuous improvement of a more moderate nature, which can be handled by the daily management system?" Breakthrough is defined as significant change in the systems or structures of an organization. Calling an item a hoshin planning "focus" when it is really something that the organization plans to do anyway can create a lot of unnecessary work. The designation of "hoshin" should be reserved for significant changes.

Check the Measures

During the gap analysis, the leadership team developed performance measures for each KSF. Now that the team has selected one KSF as the hoshin focus, it must affirm the measures or develop better ones. At this level, a measure may be fairly broad or global, but it should be quantifiable.

At this point, the leadership planning team is finished with step 1 of the hoshin process. The organization's focus has been selected and is ready to be deployed.

Roles and Responsibilities

During step 1–choose the focus–the primary players are the top leadership team, including the chief executive officer and his or her direct reports. These leaders may call upon the chief planning officer and his or her team for expert assistance.

Top Leadership Team (the Planning Team)

The top leadership team guides the selection of a priority focus. Basing its decision on good information and a solid decision-making process, the team:

- Reviews existing strategic planning material
- Considers a range of options for the focus area
- Selects the focus
- Prepares the focus to be communicated to the rest of the organization

Strategic Planning Staff

Because they are well acquainted with all aspects of the existing strategic plan and the process by which it was generated, the strategic planning staff may be called upon to provide information and clarification to the top leadership team during selection of the focus. The strategic planning staff may conduct market research, collect and analyze data, and provide facilitation and mentorship for the hoshin planning process.

Lessons Learned and Helpful Hints

As mentioned earlier in the chapter, issues that come up during step 1 center around agreeing on a focus and determining the extent of change called for. Leaders also face issues concerning the "process" for determining and communicating the focus. These issues give rise to some common problems such as lack of focus, questions of data integrity, and lack of organizational readiness. The following hints may help address problems commonly encountered during step 1.

Too Many Priorities

The hoshin planning process has a tendency to mushroom and grow. Leadership team members must consciously limit themselves to the breakthrough items that they think the organization can handle while maintaining the healthy functioning and continuous improvement of the organization's processes. The leadership planning team should strive to reserve the designation of "the organization's focus" for a very small number of true breakthrough items.

Integrity of the Data Used in Planning

Hoshin is a data-based process operating in a strategic arena. Although it cannot generate hard data about the future, the hoshin process can point out soft spots in the organization's capacity to collect and analyze good data in the present. For example, if leaders find that they cannot complete a gap analysis without a lot of guessing about their current position relative to their competitors, they should make a note to improve the competitor information data system. By the time the next hoshin planning process rolls around, that data system will be stronger.

Preparation of the Organization

The development of a hoshin plan requires discipline. To keep the process from bogging down, the top leadership team will want to distribute a planning schedule early in the planning process, with milestones and dates. Once all layers of the plan have been developed, they need to be printed and made available to the organization from some central location. It is a good idea to offer training during the first implementation of the hoshin process. A tiered training approach can focus more heavily on philosophy for the executives and more on deployment for the successive layers of management.

CHAPTER SEVEN

Step 2: Align the Organization

The second step in the hoshin process is to align the organization. It has a dual purpose: to develop the plan throughout the organization, and to align resources with the plan.

Expected outcomes from this step are as follows:

- A plan developed in a participative fashion through multiple levels of the organization
- Resources allocated to support the plan

Leadership Issues

In carrying out this step, the leaders are faced with four issues:

1. Maintaining the spirit and intent of the focus
2. Really listening
3. Prioritizing action plans
4. Deciding how far to extend "catchball"

Issue 1: Maintaining the Spirit and Intent of the Focus

The process of aligning the organization tests the clarity of the leaders' understanding and agreement on the focus. As the plan moves from vision to action and from the involvement of a few to the involvement of many, it is easy for the sharpness of the focus to get lost. To maintain focus, all the leaders who selected the focus must be consistent in the way they communicate their reasons for choosing the focus and the vision of success.

Issue 2: Really Listening

Through the catchball feature, those who know what must be done and those who know best how to do it build a hoshin plan jointly. As the plan is defined in increasing detail, leaders must really listen to the patterns of comments from those closest to the work. Subtle nuances and seemingly unrelated observations can lead to a whole new understanding of breakthrough customer service and competitive advantage. Careful, nondefensive listening is the vehicle that allows those patterns to emerge. In addition, top management must resist the temptation to tell others what their means of accomplishing the plan should be. Really listening means collecting—not directing—information.

Issue 3: Prioritizing Action Plans

In step 1, the leaders had to focus on a strategic level. Step 2 requires them to focus tactically. The plan can easily become a "project magnet." Seeing the attention and support that the hoshin plan gets, some people may be tempted to embed their local projects into the plan. Others may fear that lack of involvement in the hoshin plan will reflect badly on their performance. Not all possible projects can or should make it into the final hoshin plan. Through all this, the leaders must keep a clear picture of what must be done and who the necessary players are. This clarity of focus requires rigorous, consistent screening of potential projects.

Issue 4: Deciding How Far to Extend Catchball

In the initial implementation of hoshin planning, leaders may decide to limit the number of layers of catchball. For example, two layers of catchball may suffice in the first year of a hoshin plan, while everyone is learning the appropriate roles and techniques. Later, catchball can extend as many layers as necessary to implement the plan successfully.

This limited catchball must be communicated organizationwide as a rollout strategy. The strategy should be portrayed as an approach to learning about the mechanics of hoshin planning—a pilot test to be expanded over time. Otherwise, limited catchball might be interpreted as a lack of management commitment to full-scale implementation of the hoshin planning process.

Implementation Tasks

Step 2 is about alignment and deployment. The SSM-Ministry Corporation defines deployment as "the process by which the long-term objectives that support the organization's [focus] are communicated and implemented." (See the SSM case study in chapter 12.) During this phase, the plan is cascaded through the organization. It is developed in a participative, collaborative fashion. When *what* has to be done and *how* it will be done are clear to all who are involved in the planning process, the measures of success are set and resources are allocated.

The substeps by which alignment and deployment are accomplished are illustrated in a micro flowchart in figure 7-1. The four tasks are as follows:

1. Develop annual targets.
2. Develop means.
3. "Catchball" the targets and means throughout the organization.
4. Finalize the plan.

Task 1: Develop Annual Targets

The leadership team has selected the organization's focus. At this point in the planning process, the leadership team may not know if the focus is a single-year or a multi-year task. The true time frame of the focus will become clear as the details of the hoshin plan unfold.

Figure 7-1. Micro Flowchart of Step 2

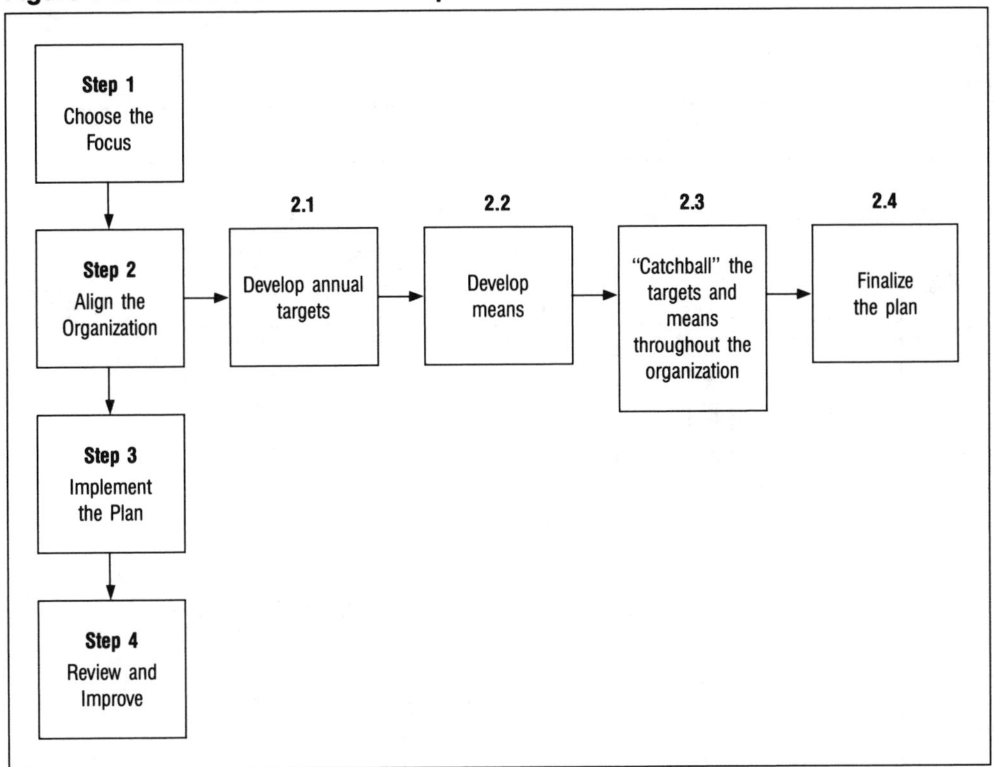

The immediate task of the leadership team is to identify *what* must be accomplished to achieve the plan in the next year. The "whats" that must be accomplished may be called goals, objectives, or targets. For this discussion, they will be referred to as annual targets. The leadership team will go through a three-step process to develop annual targets:

1. Generate a list of targets.
2. Establish a time frame for multiyear targets.
3. Develop measures for each target.

Generate a List of Targets

Just as it did with the KSFs, the leadership team may need to generate a large list of targets and later narrow the list. There are at least two methods to generate annual targets: a combined affinity/matrix method and a barrier analysis.

- *Combined affinity/matrix method:* In this method, the team may use brainstorming or the affinity technique to develop a list of potential annual targets. If the list is much too long to be practical, the team can shorten it using a prioritization matrix, such as the one in figure 7-2. Using weighted criteria such as feasibility, cost, and customer impact, the team selects the highest-rated ideas for further development.
- *Barrier analysis:* This method for generating hoshin annual targets uses the following questions as guides:
  - What are the major barriers to achieving the focus? (Brainstorm a list.)
  - If we had no constraints, what targets could we set to address those barriers?

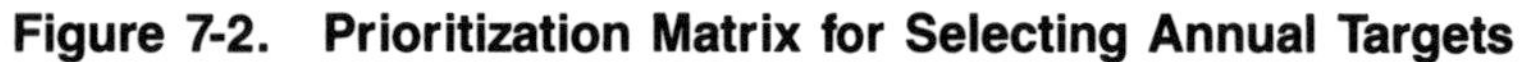

Figure 7-2. Prioritization Matrix for Selecting Annual Targets

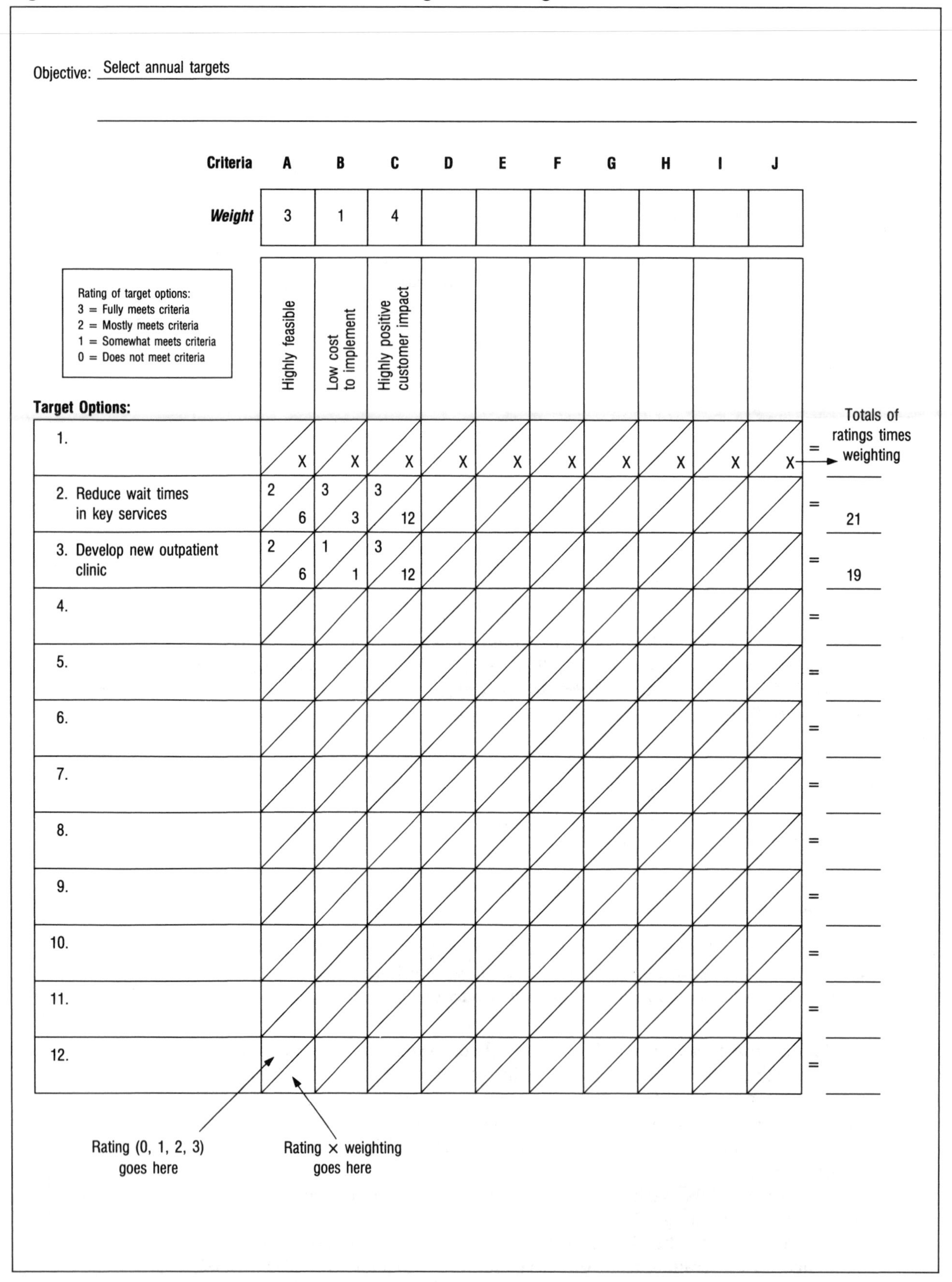

Once the barriers are identified the leadership team can articulate targets to address them. In this case, the target is the positive organizational response to the barrier, as illustrated in the following example.

Example

In the case of Firstcare Health, high cost was a major barrier to achieving the focus of providing a spectrum of services. The top leadership team believed that one target to address the cost barrier would be "to reduce cost of current key services to allow for the development of a broader spectrum of services."

Establish Time Frame for Multiyear Targets

If the organization's focus fits into a one-year time frame, the annual targets describe what must be accomplished to achieve the focus completely. If, however, the focus is a multiyear project, broad annual targets must be developed for each year of the hoshin plan. The planning team may wish to use a chart like the one in figure 7-3 to lay out the annual targets of a multiyear focus.

Develop Measures for Each Target

Once the annual targets are identified, the team must develop measures or indicators of success for each target. In developing measures, the team will want to refer to the various data sources used in step 1, such as customer, competitor, and internal process data. Measures come in two varieties:

- *Outcome measures* indicate whether a result has been achieved. External customer needs (such as patient satisfaction) or measures of health status or functioning may be good sources of outcome measures.
- *In-process measures* indicate whether the process is going well. (Patient complaints in each work unit during a hospital stay is one example). In-process measures may be early warning signals that detect problems before they show up in outcome measures. Internal customers and technical experts within the process are more aware of these than are external customers.

Figure 7-3. Multiyear Hoshin Plan

	Year					
	1				2	3
	Quarter					
	1	2	3	4		
Organization Focus #1 Reduce cost in key services	Service A → (to quarter 3)	Service B → (to quarter 4)	Service C → (to year 2)		Services D, F, E	
	← List here the annual targets to be achieved →					
Organization Focus #2 Provide a spectrum of health care services	Develop measurement system → (to quarter 2)		Develop service A → (to quarter 4)		Develop services B, C	Develop service D

The team will need to select one or two measures for each annual target. (See the case studies in chapters 10 through 15 for examples of measures.)

Example

For its focus ("Provide a spectrum of health care services"), Firstcare Health developed six annual targets. One of those targets is to "develop a system for measuring quality of care across a broader spectrum." Its associated measure is comparison data on utilization versus patient outcomes.

Task 2: Develop Means

Developing or deploying a hoshin plan is a stair-step process, as illustrated in figure 7-4. The hoshin plan is now moving from stair step 1 to stair step 2. The process is defined by a series of *what* and *how* questions. The targets are what must be accomplished; the means are how they will be accomplished.

As figure 7-4 shows, the larger context of the hoshin plan is carried along to the more detailed layers. Level 1's means become level 2's targets, and those who are developing means understand the reason for and importance of their part of the plan. This idea of generating targets and means together—of developing means in the larger context of the targets—is one of the distinguishing features of hoshin planning.

The top leadership team will develop high-level targets and means in a three-step process:

1. Develop potential means.
2. Select and refine the best means.
3. Develop performance measures.

Step 1, developing potential means, requires divergent thinking, once again allowing for breakthrough ideas to occur. Step 2 requires focusing on the minimum number

Figure 7-4. Hoshin Deployment

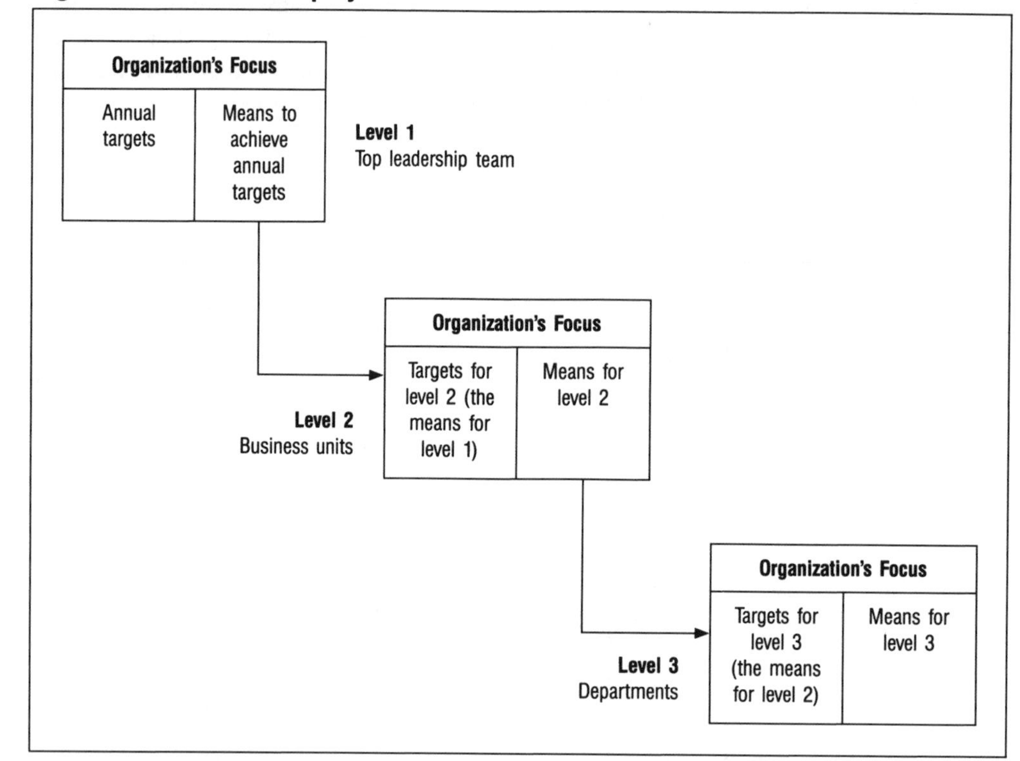

or set of best means. Step 3 ensures that all targets and means are assigned measures to assist in tracking their progress.

Develop Potential Means

Potential means for each target can be developed using the methods described for developing annual targets (brainstorming/affinity diagram, barrier analysis). Another appropriate tool for developing means is the tree diagram. (See appendix B, "Hoshin Toolbox," for instructions. In addition, the SSM-Ministry Corporation case study in chapter 12 contains several examples of the use of tree diagrams to display targets, means, and measures.) Like an outline, the tree diagram is a method of generating and displaying a plan in greater and greater detail. At this stage in the planning process, the leadership team should evaluate, prioritize, and select only the most powerful means to keep them at a minimum.

Example

Firstcare Health used a tree diagram to develop its hoshin plan from the level of the organization's focus (originally the spectrum of services KSF) to the annual targets and beyond. Figure 7-5 shows a top-level, or macro, tree diagram. The "trunk" of the tree, on the far left ("Provide a spectrum

Figure 7-5. Tree Diagram: Organization's Focus and Annual Targets

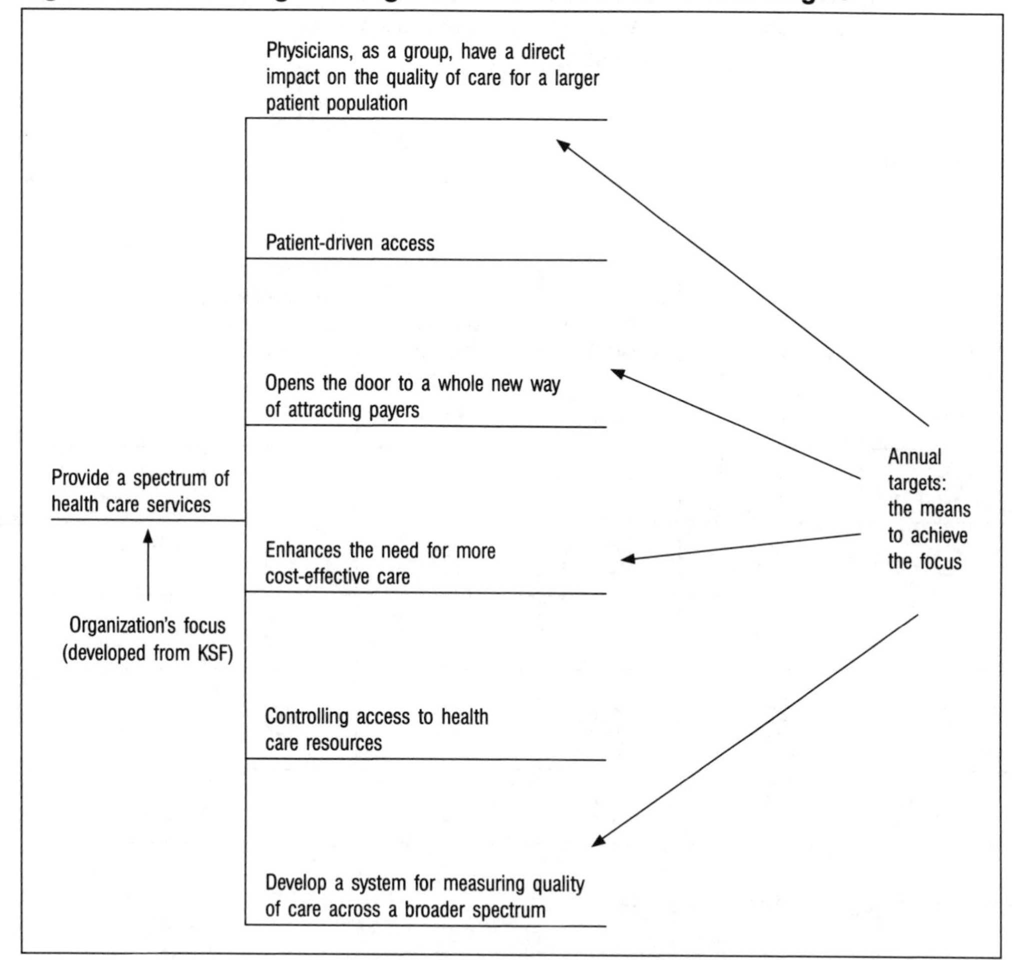

Source: Firstcare Health.

of health care services"), has six main "branches," each representing one annual target. That target is a means to achieve the organization's focus.

Select and Refine the Best Means

Once the means are developed, they may be placed in a target/means matrix, as illustrated in figure 7-6. The target/means matrix has three purposes:

- *Alignment of targets with means:* During development of the means, the matrix keeps the targets visible. This is the essence of alignment.
- *Selection of the best means:* Once the first draft of means has been developed, the matrix is used to check for sufficiency–that is, to see if the sum of the proposed means will really bring about the breakthrough change called for in the target.
- *Refinement of means:* If the means are not sufficient, new means may be developed. Unnecessary means may be eliminated. The plan may be adjusted *before* it proceeds any further.

As shown in figure 7-6, the means to provide a spectrum of health care services are placed in a matrix against six high-level targets, the KSFs, one of which is the organization's focus. Some of the means (for example, 3, 4, and 5) are strongly related to four or five KSFs. Successful completion of these means would have strong, positive ripple effects on all aspects of the organization's vision elements, beyond their obvious impact on the current hoshin plan.

Figure 7-6. Target/Means Matrix

	High-Level Targets (for example, KSFs)					
Means from tree diagram	**Provide spectrum of services (the hoshin focus)**	**Satisfy patients**	**Meet regular requirements**	**Use clinically effective practices**	**Provide health care services at a reasonable cost**	**Ensure timely access**
1. Physicians impact	⊙	⊙	△	⊙	△	△
2. Patient-driven access	⊙	⊙				⊙
3. New way to attract payers	⊙	△	○	⊙	⊙	⊙
4. Enhance need for cost-effective care	⊙	⊙		⊙	⊙	⊙
5. Control access to health care resources	⊙	⊙	○	○	⊙	⊙
6. Develop system for measuring	⊙	△	⊙	○	○	△

Degree of relationship: ⊙ high ○ moderate △ low

Develop Performance Measures

Every target and means developed should have a meaningful performance measure or two attached. A measure is a way to judge the success of the process and/or outcome of targets and means. It indicates relevant units of measurement in a given situation (such as "wait time in minutes" in an outpatient clinic). The measure itself is neutral in that it does not have a specific number attached to it. Once the planning teams set up their measures, they will be able to attach appropriate numerical goals (such as 10 minutes), perhaps after looking at the current capability of their systems or benchmarking other systems.

Task 3: "Catchball" the Targets and Means throughout the Organization

Although the final plan may not be displayed in the target/means format shown in figure 7-6, the process of developing the matrix provides the perfect forum for discussion between the owners of the "whats" (that is, the strategies or targets) and the owners of the "hows" (that is, the tactics, action items, or means). The top leadership targets and means are converted sequentially, first into business unit, then team, then individual targets and means. (See the Southwest Texas Methodist Hospital case study in chapter 13 for a sample catchball worksheet.)

How Are the Targets and Means Expanded?

Like the process of developing high-level means (described earlier under task 2, developing detailed means repeats a three-step process:

1. Develop potential means (using a tree diagram).
2. Select and refine the best means.
3. Assign measures.

Example

Firstcare Health used sequential tree diagrams to expand and detail its means. The means were carried to different levels of detail for different targets, depending on the amount of definition and clarity required. New or breakthrough concepts often require more definition (hence, more layers on the tree diagram) than familiar means. Figure 7-7 shows the expanded tree diagram for Firstcare Health. The sixth branch of the tree ("Develop a system for measuring quality of care across a broader spectrum") is expanded further in figure 7-8.

How Are the Targets and Means Checked?

The plan is checked in two ways. First, any set of means can be checked against higher-level targets using the target/means matrix. (See figure 7-9.) The next step is to troubleshoot the plan in preparation for contingency planning, using a tool called the process decision program chart, or PDPC. (See appendix B, "Hoshin Toolbox," for instructions.) This tool combs through each piece of the plan asking, "What could go wrong?" and developing preventive and contingency plans. The preventive mechanisms are woven into the plan to avoid problems. Contingency or "backup" plans are available to manage problems.

Example

Firstcare Health chose to apply the PDPC to the means from the process decision program chart shown in figure 7-10 (p. 106). For the detailed means labeled "Identify high-utilization services," a

Figure 7-7. Expanded Tree Diagram

- Provide a spectrum of health care services
  - Physicians, as a group, have a direct impact on the quality of care for a larger patient population
    - Physicians have more direct patient care time
    - Improved ability to recruit new medical staff members
    - Physicians will have fewer indirect patient care issues to address
    - Physicians have more designated authority on the board
  - Patient-driven access
    - One-stop shopping for care
    - Choice of doctors
    - Provides to "family" doctor
    - Provides health care locally
    - Maintain stable physician–patient relationship over time
  - Opens the door to a whole new way of attracting payers
    - Ability to contract with third-party payers as a managed care system
    - Ability to provide care locally to employers that have contracted with managed care payers
    - Provide new option in health care services and insurers to local employers
    - Maintain independence as a health care provider
  - Enhances the need for more cost-effective care
    - Focus on wellness and illness prevention
    - Reduce variation in medical management
    - Work with employers to design improved workers' compensation programs
  - Controlling access to health care resources
    - Increased ability to direct patient to most appropriate point of service
    - Reduce duplication in diagnostic testing
    - Single source of care
  - Develop a system for measuring quality of care across a broader spectrum
    - Identify information system needs
    - Develop systems to identify and reduce variation
    - Align high-quality health care providers with the system
    - Generate *meaningful* monitoring reports comparing utilization and patient outcome

Source: Firstcare Health.

Figure 7-8. Detailed Tree Diagram

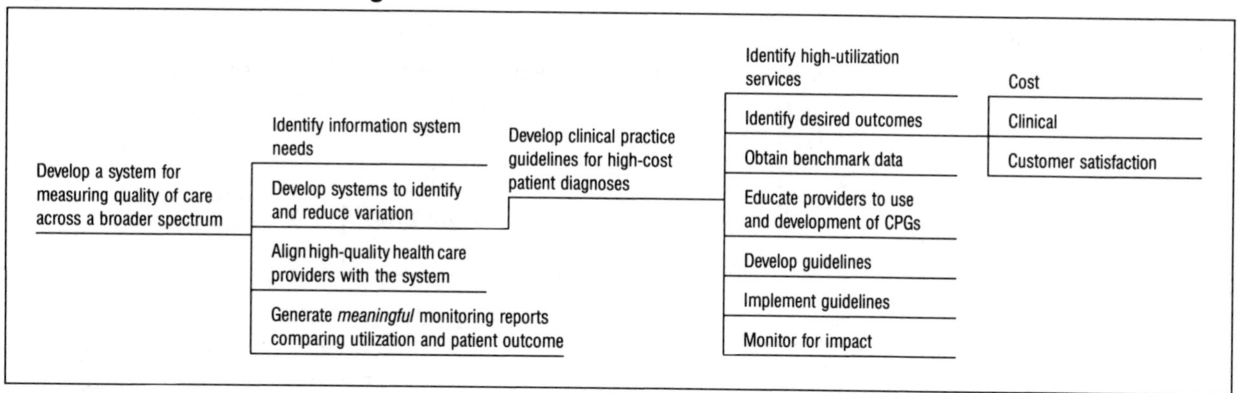

Source: Firstcare Health

Figure 7-9. Target/Means Matrix

Third-Level Means from Detailed Tree (figure 7-8)	KSFs					
	Provide Spectrum	Satisfied Patients	Regular Requirements	Clinically Effective	Reasonable Cost	Timely Access
Identify high-utilization services				○		●
Identify desired outcomes		●	○	●	●	
Obtain benchmark data	△			○		
Educate providers to use and development of CPGs				●	○	
Develop guidelines	○	○		●	○	○
Implement guidelines	○	○		●	○	○
Monitor for impact	○	○		●	●	●

● High relationship ○ Moderate relationship △ Low relationship

Source: Firstcare Health.

potential problem might be that "outpatient data are not available." The countermeasure for that problem would be to develop a system for monitoring the collection of outpatient data. Depending on the timing of this countermeasure, it could be either a preventive or a remedial action.

How Does the Catchball Process Work?

Catchball is a "what-how" discussion and, like the game of catch, it implies a back-and-forth action. If the power of the hoshin process lies in the coupling of target and means development, then the catchball process is the power generator.

The hoshin process is proceeding down the stair steps shown earlier in figure 7-4 (p. 100). At level 1, the owners of the targets might be vice-presidents; the owners of the means might be directors of business units. At level 2, the directors own the targets (which were the means at level 1); department managers own the more detailed means. At each step, the development of a target/means matrix and the process of catchball ensure that:

- The owners of the targets understand them well enough to communicate them to the owners of the means

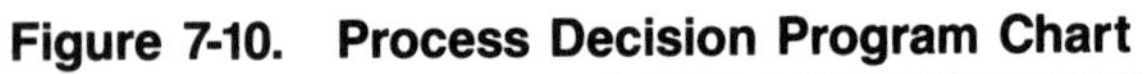

Figure 7-10. Process Decision Program Chart

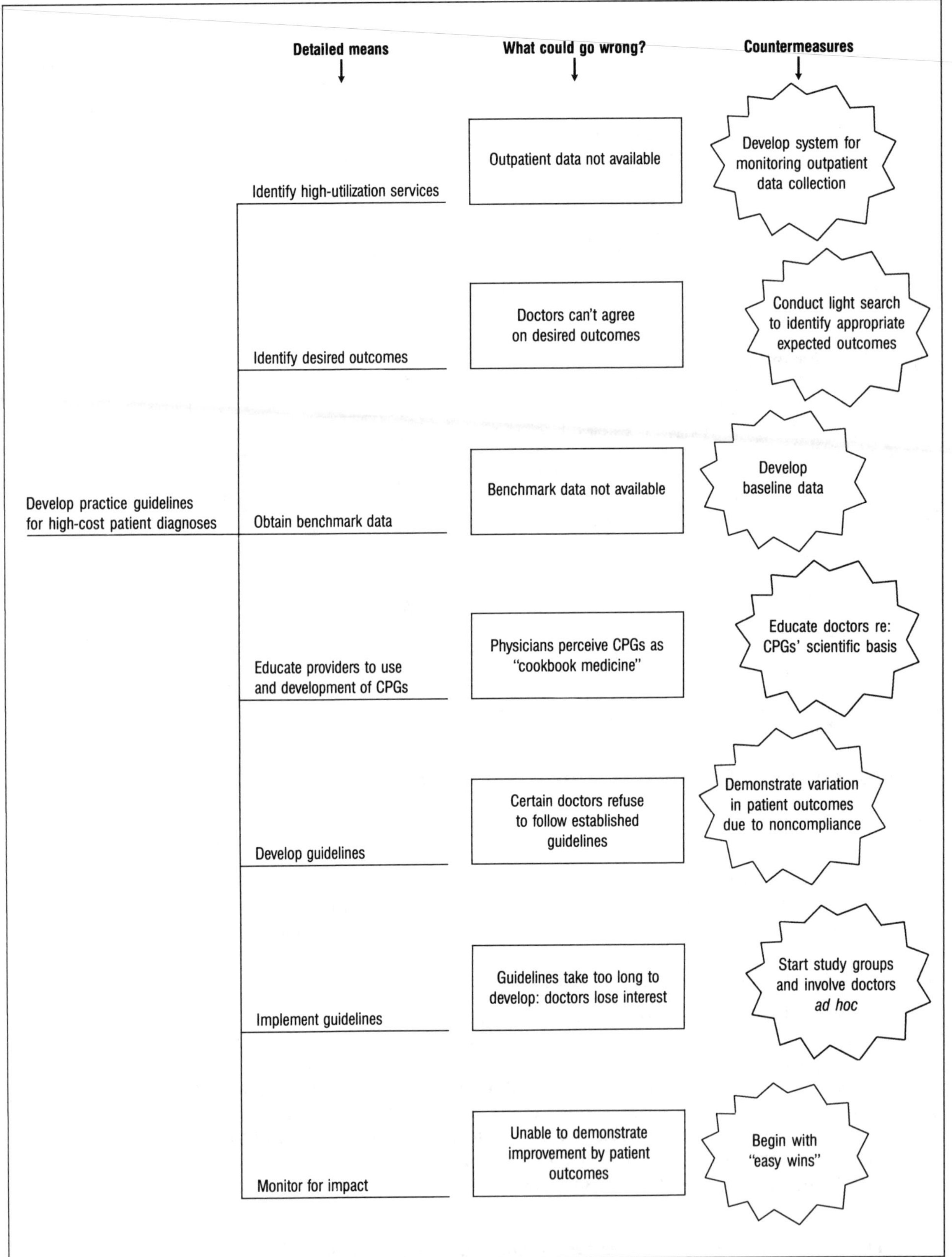

Source: Firstcare Health.

- The owners of the means have a chance to ask questions and clarify what they are being asked to accomplish
- The buy-in and commitment to *both* the targets and the means are being built as the plan itself matures

Catchball loads discussion into the early part of the planning process. It does not mean that the owners of the targets tell the owners of the means how to do their jobs. Rather, by focusing on understanding, it allows the developers of the means to do their jobs more effectively and efficiently and to really own the plan they helped to create.

There are two approaches to means development through catchball: cascading and kick-start.

- *Cascading:* The owners of one level of the plan "throw" their means to the next level of owners and ask, "How can you contribute to achieving this means, which is now your target?" and "How will you measure this contribution?" Through use of tree diagrams and contingency planning and target/means matrixes, this process continues until the plan is developed in sufficient detail. Then the process is reversed, with the plan being reviewed, cross-checked, and coordinated. (At this stage, the owners of a target review all the means associated with that target.) As the plan comes back up the organization, the means are checked for feasibility, duplication, and conflict with other means in the plan.
- *Kick-start:* A variation on the cascading approach is to kick-start the catchball process with a large group meeting of all potential owners of the first two levels of means. The entire group participates in the development of means to support high-level targets. As means are developed in increasing detail, the group may divide into smaller planning teams (subteams) that flesh out means and add potential measures. At intervals throughout the session, the subteams bring their work back to the larger group, and the plan is checked for completeness and consistency. A day or two spent in a kick-start forum may shorten the cascading deployment and communication process by weeks, because all necessary participants are in one room.

One note of caution: Although ownership of the layers of a hoshin plan tends to correlate with organizational layers, *the ownership of the planning item is driven by the nature of the item, not by the organizational chart.* Owners are chosen because they are closest to the work and to the affected customer base, not for political reasons. Figure 7-11 is an example of an ownership matrix diagram showing the means

Figure 7-11. Ownership Matrix

Detailed Means	Owners of Means: Department A	Department B	Department C	Person X	Person Y
Means 1	⊙	○		○	
2	⊙	○		△	△
3	○	⊙			△
4	○		⊙	△	
		⊙	○		
10				⊙	⊙

⊙ Primary responsibility ○ Secondary responsibility △ Keep informed and their appropriate owners. Each means may have multiple owners with varying levels of responsibility, as designated by the symbols on the matrix.

Task 4: Finalize the Plan

The last official act of the planning process is to display the entire plan, including targets, means, who owns each item, and time lines, on a format that will be maintained for the life of the plan. Having a few standard planning formats will keep planners focused on the content rather than on the style of the plan. These formats and the language on them may be modified to fit unique organizational style. Figure 7-12 is a concise format that summarizes important features of the plan on a single page.

Roles and Responsibilities

In step 2 of the hoshin planning process, involvement with the plan expands to include successive layers of management and other members of the organization who will be called upon to develop means.

The CEO

In the process of aligning the organization, the chief executive officer:

- Clarifies upper-level targets to those who will be developing means
- Helps define breakthrough goals
- Listens to means proposed by people closest to the process
- Ensures that good measures accompany the targets and means
- Ensures that resources are made available for carrying out the final plan
- Helps set the planning calendar and stick to it
- Helps break down perceived barriers

Planning Team or Person

The team or person assigned the responsibility for the planning process:

- Helps to set the planning calendar and ensure that it is followed
- Clarifies planning duties and planning items during catchball
- Reviews the entire plan for gaps, overlaps, and conflicts
- Facilitates the flow of vital information

Target and Means Developers

Those who develop targets and means during the catchball process:

- Contribute knowledge and expertise in developing targets, means, and measures
- Ensure that means are tied to the customer
- Create and innovate
- Challenge and question if things do not make sense (for example, if the means do not add up to the target or if the timing seems wrong)
- Test the reasonableness of the means
- Stick to the planning calendar

Figure 7-12. Hoshin Plan Executive Summary

ORGANIZATIONAL FOCUS ______________________________

Targets	Means	Measure of Success	Responsibility (Deployment Channel)		Resources/ Budget	Comments/Priorities	Timeline	Evaluation		
			Owner/ Leader	Team			Qtr 1 2 3 4	Re-viewer	Review Dates	% of Means Achieved
										[: : :]
										[: : :]
										[: : :]
										[: : :]
										[: : :]
										[: : :]
										[: : :]
										[: : :]

Lessons Learned and Helpful Hints

As the plan gets developed, the means and their measures should be tested and refined. The following hints may help during step 2 of hoshin planning, as teams develop means and project the extent of change they will produce.

Ensuring That the Means Bring about the Targets

At the conclusion of the deployment process, the plan should contain the minimum set of means necessary to achieve each target. It is not always easy to predict whether the right means are in place or whether the plan has too many (or too few) means. In addition, problems may arise if means and strategy do not match. For example, the owner of a strategy may believe that what must be accomplished is perfectly clear, but as the strategy is deployed it may become painfully obvious that the intent or extent of the strategy is not clear to those asked to generate the means to achieve it.

Two things can help the plan be deployed correctly and efficiently – in other words, ensure that the sum of the means equals the target:

- *A rigorous catchball process* ensures a healthy dialogue between owners of the targets and owners of the means at any level of the plan. True catchball allows as many iterations as necessary to define, question, and refine the plan. The target/means matrix is a good way to check the plan.
- *Clear specific measures* also ensure clarification of targets and means. Measures are much easier to define at the most detailed levels of the plan. Even so, every effort should be made to attach meaningful measures even to the highest level of the plan – that is, the focus and the annual targets. Measures should monitor performance in two ways:
  –Accomplishment (was this means performed?)
  –Quality (how well was this means performed?)

Defining a "Breakthrough" Change

The definition of a true breakthrough can be troublesome. After all, a breakthrough is something the organization has not been able to do yet. Other than saying, "We'll know it when we see it," a leader may have a hard time giving a clear definition of *breakthrough.* And a clear definition of the target is exactly what is needed to generate appropriate means.

Besides the difficulty inherent in defining *breakthrough,* there is the additional problem of defining the extent of breakthroughs. The questions pertaining to extent are these: How much change does it take to qualify as a true breakthrough? and How much change can our organization handle? One possible method of defining breakthrough clearly is to set a numerical goal in conjunction with a target.

Setting breakthrough goals is both art and science. A goal of 50 percent improvement may be easy to achieve in processes with lots of room for improvement but nearly impossible to achieve in processes that already are virtually perfect. Breakthrough is more a function of the effort it takes to achieve an improvement goal than of the numerical goal itself (such as 50 percent or 5 percent). The following guidelines may be helpful in setting breakthrough goals:

- The goals should have some scientific basis, using data collected from customers, suppliers, competitors, internal processes, the external environment, and benchmarking.

- The question of what constitutes a breakthrough should be carefully thought out. The goal setters need to consider, "Given our system's current capability, is a 20 percent improvement a breakthrough? How about 40 percent? or 5 percent?"

Once the definition of *breakthrough* is agreed upon (including the context for and magnitude of the change required), it must be communicated clearly to everyone involved in the catchball process. In addition, if achieving breakthrough requires definition of new concepts or redefinition of old terms, it is the responsibility of the owners of the targets to pass those definitions along to the owners of the means.

CHAPTER EIGHT

Step 3: Implement the Plan

The third step in the hoshin planning process is to implement the plan. It has a dual purpose: to implement the plan successfully, and to monitor progress of that plan.

Expected outcomes from this step are as follows:

- A plan designed and initiated on schedule
- Relevant information to feed into the review process

Leadership Issues

In implementing the plan, the top leadership team must deal with two issues:

1. Actively guiding the implementation process
2. Emphasizing understanding of both process and results

Issue 1: Actively Guiding the Implementation Process

The hoshin process requires constant, active leadership involvement. There is no such thing as putting the implementation on autopilot. During the implementation phase, leaders demonstrate interest and attention to the progress of the plan without interference or micromanagement. Through supportive inquiries, both casual and formal, leaders model ongoing interest in what they have said is most important to the organization.

Issue 2: Emphasizing Understanding of Both Process and Results

The measurement systems that were put into place during deployment of the plan are exercised fully during the implementation phase. By emphasizing collection and analysis of data, the leaders build the organization's capability to assess and improve while the plan is being carried out.

Leaders mentor others by asking those individuals to update them on progress and to substantiate conclusions with facts. Leaders can make an even more powerful statement about the importance of monitoring by modeling collection and analysis of data on the parts of the plan that they themselves own.

Implementation Tasks

During implementation, the plan flows out like a river across the organization. Each means branches off into smaller and smaller tributaries. Eventually, small teams or even individuals take responsibility for the means and their associated measures. But there must still be a connection between each means and the organization's focus. The name given this connection by AT&T is the "Golden Thread." (See the AT&T case study in chapter 14.)

Two tasks are performed during implementation. These are shown in the micro flowchart of step 3 shown in figure 8-1.

1. Implement the plan.
2. Monitor progress.

Both tasks help keep the means aligned with the focus, and they keep the plan alive all year long. The actual kickoff of a hoshin plan occurs without much fanfare. The real vitalizing force is the monitoring of the plan throughout its life cycle.

Task 1: Implement the Plan

Unlike management by objective (MBO) systems, where emphasis is on the beginning and end points of the plan (setting the objectives and checking the results), hoshin emphasizes *all* phases of the planning process. Implementation is just as active as all the other steps in the process. Once a hoshin planning process has been operating

Figure 8-1. Micro Flowchart of Step 3

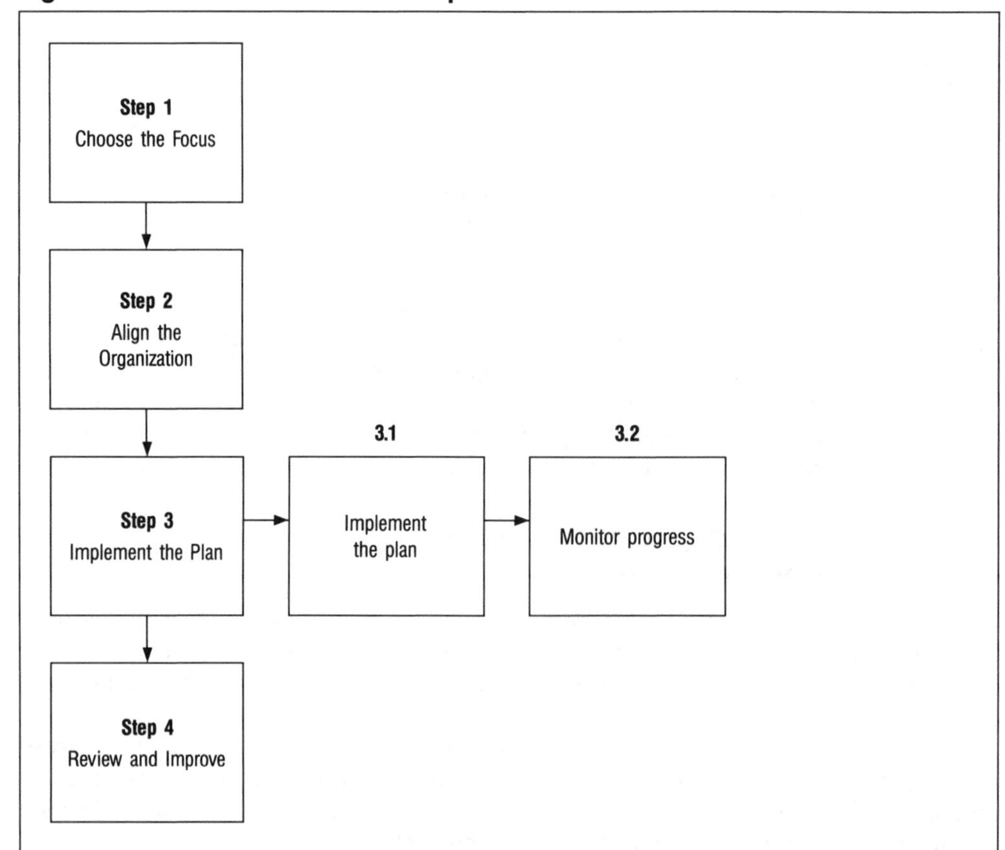

for a few years, implementation and review occur in tandem throughout the life of the plan, as noted in the AT&T case study in chapter 14:

> In the annual cycle, some activities – such as drafting annual objectives, deploying objectives, and conducting annual reviews – occur only once a year. Other activities – such as implementing plans and conducting regular reviews and diagnosis – require monthly or quarterly measurements and adjustments relative to the milestones of the action plans.

Task 2: Monitor Progress

A planning table such as the one shown in figure 7-12 (p. 109) is an effective implementation aid. The simple format summarizes targets and means, who does them, and when they are supposed to be done on a quarterly time line. Hoshin planning emphasizes *process* as well as *results.* Each target and means is tracked *while it is in progress,* as indicated on the planning table time line. Quantitative tracking involves collecting and analyzing data on the measures attached to the target or means. Qualitative tracking involves making notes of comments or patterns that occur during implementation. Both qualitative and quantitative data will be used during the upcoming review cycles.

Hoshin implementation may point out the need for strengthening certain systems and structures within an organization. For example, one capability that hoshin tests is the ability of the organization to collect and share meaningful data across departments. It may be helpful to suggest a standardized, but somewhat flexible, method to help people collect data during implementation to prepare them for data analysis during the review cycles. Figure 8-2 is one such data collection format. The form asks the implementer to:

- Track data on the performance measure
- Observe, list, and prioritize problems encountered
- Evaluate causes to problems
- Enumerate corrective actions taken
- Record learnings

Example

As predicted during troubleshooting of its plan, Firstcare Health noted variability in the availability of outpatient data on high-utilization services. Data collected during the first quarter of implementation pointed out which services were most likely to experience problems with data availability. Before the quarter was over, the team responsible for the affected services had already implemented the countermeasure it had designed during deployment. It put into place targeted systems for monitoring the collection of outpatient data.

Roles and Responsibilities

During implementation, the top leadership team stays in close contact with the process and outcomes of the plan. In so doing, they act as supportive partners with those who are responsible for carrying out the means and they encourage deep understanding of the plan's progress.

The CEO and Management

In the implementation process, the chief executive officer and the management staff:

- Ask people involved in the implementation to show them their data and to discuss the data's implications

- Model the use of data collection methods on the parts of the plan that the individuals own
- Help remove perceived barriers
- Display a bias toward understanding deviations from expectations and implementing corrections and/or preventions based on that understanding

Individuals and Teams

Individuals and teams responsible for parts of the plan are expected to:

- Collect and analyze data
- Gain a deep understanding of the reasons for any deviations from the plan
- Implement countermeasures (corrective and preventive mechanisms) based on a thorough understanding of the plan
- Document data, observations, and countermeasures to use in the review cycle

Lessons Learned and Helpful Hints

This tip comes from an executive who found an effective way to collect and organize data during the implementation phase: "Create a data collection 'graffiti board' in your datebook."

Figure 8-2. Data Collection Format

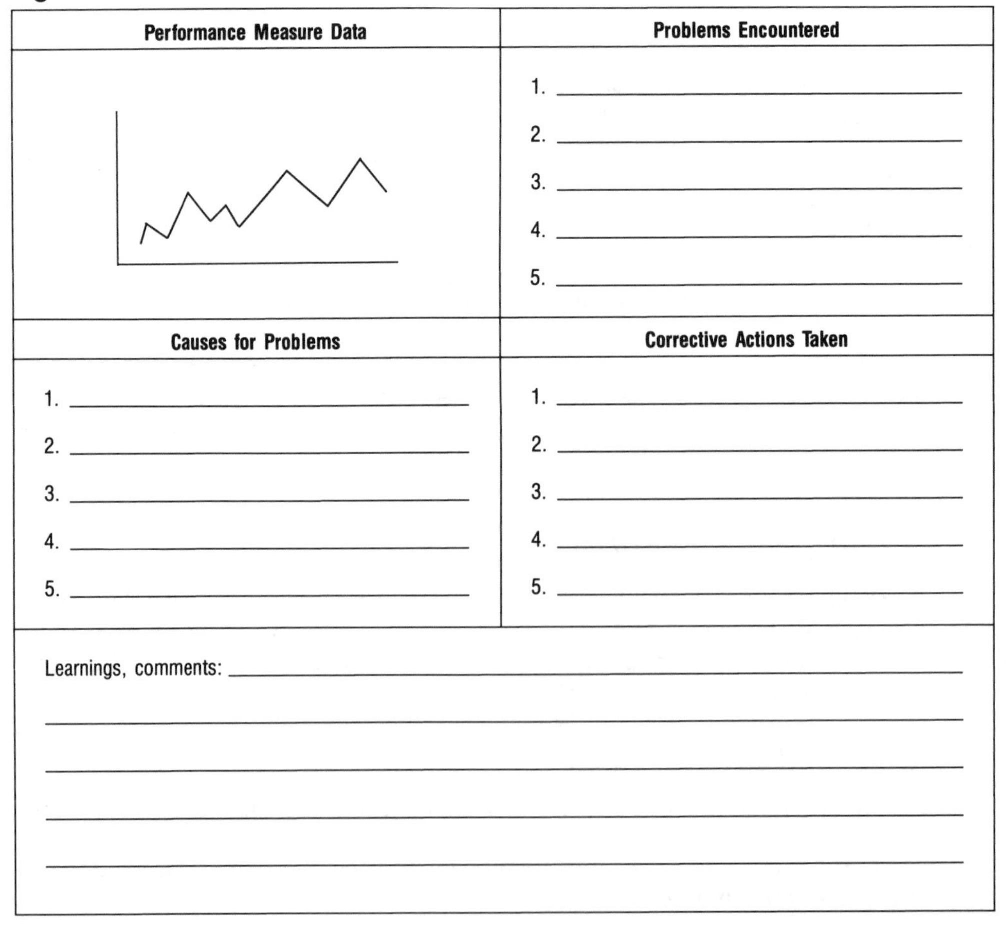

Performance Measure Data	Problems Encountered
	1. ____ 2. ____ 3. ____ 4. ____ 5. ____
Causes for Problems	**Corrective Actions Taken**
1. ____ 2. ____ 3. ____ 4. ____ 5. ____	1. ____ 2. ____ 3. ____ 4. ____ 5. ____
Learnings, comments: ____	

Recording Data in a Datebook

The executive who suggested this tip was never without the 5-inch by 7-inch three-ring binder that held his daily, weekly, and monthly calendars. In the back of the binder, under a tab labeled "Notes," he began to record observations on the progress of various parts of the hoshin plan while visiting different work areas. He also kept track of his own means and measures in that part of the binder. By demonstrating real-time interest in the process of the plan, the executive was modeling the active involvement that characterizes the implementation phase of hoshin planning. He also realized a side benefit from his newfound way of organizing data. Just by having his data and observations current and handy, he reduced from days to hours the time it took to prepare for quarterly reviews.

CHAPTER NINE

Step 4: Review and Improve

The fourth step in the hoshin planning process is to review and improve. This step has a dual purpose: to evaluate both the process and the outcomes of the plan, and to continuously improve the plan and the process of planning.

Expected outcomes from this step are as follows:

- Ongoing diagnosis and correction of problems in the plan itself and problems in the process by which the plan was produced
- Learnings recorded and ready to be used in future planning

Leadership Issues

There are three issues for leaders to deal with in this step:

1. Sticking to a review schedule
2. Creating a climate for effective reviews
3. Holding on to the learnings

Issue 1: Sticking to a Review Schedule

Perhaps the greatest discipline required of leaders in the whole hoshin process is setting a review schedule and sticking to it. Reviews are the lifeblood of the hoshin planning process, but they can easily be overshadowed by the daily pressures of running an organization. It is up to the leaders to demonstrate belief in the importance of reviews by holding them at predetermined intervals.

Issue 2: Creating a Climate for Effective Reviews

Many people see the word *review* as a euphemism for "shoot the messenger, audit, roast" and a host of other meanings they learned to associate with progress checks in the past. Hoshin reviews have a very specific purpose: learning. That purpose can be accomplished only if the proper climate is set and information is shared honestly and completely.

Hoshin reviews invite the sharing of problems as well as successes in an open, fact-based dialogue. Some organizations describe the review climate by saying, "It treats problems like treasures." A "problem" is an unexpected deviation (plus or minus) from the plan. When any problem is highlighted, analyzed, and resolved through a review process, that problem is less likely to make a surprise appearance in the future. If the problem is a positive deviation from plan, learning about it will increase the likelihood that the organization can make that positive deviation happen again. A thorough understanding of the cause-and-effect relationship between the plan and what actually happened increases the organization's sense of control over its destiny and its ability to make good plans happen.

Issue 3: Holding on to the Learnings

Hoshin plans are living, breathing documents. Plans should look dog-eared. Measures should be plotted and discussed. Means may even change midyear, after due deliberation. With the fluid, organic nature of these types of plans, there must be some way of keeping track of both progress and changes. And there must be an organizational memory that lasts more than a quarter or a year – a memory that allows the organization to learn from its mistakes and to profit from its successes.

Documenting learnings may not be everyone's favorite task, but it must be a priority. After the reviews, there must be a system that captures and publishes learnings. There must be a system for ensuring that intended changes to the plan or to the execution of the plan really do take place. It falls to the organization's leaders to design the documents and the methods that will allow them to capture the learning and use it in future plans. Leaders close the learning loop.

Implementation Tasks

The organization has selected its focus and developed plans that include both the means to achieve the focus and the measures that track progress and outcomes of the plan. During the implementation phase, the organization has monitored the plan. As the plan is reviewed, the learnings from all the progress checks are shared, summarized, and prepared for use in future planning cycles. There are two important tasks in this final step in the hoshin process (as shown in the micro flowchart in figure 9-1):

1. Review the plan and make improvements.
2. Review the hoshin planning process and make improvements.

Task 1: Review the Plan and Make Improvements

Hoshin tests the ability of an organization to learn and to act on its learnings. The catalyst for learning is the review system. Like catchball, these reviews are a distinguishing feature of hoshin. In the hoshin culture, great emphasis is placed on conducting constructive reviews:

> It is important to start with the distinction between constructive and destructive reviews. A destructive review is one where the reviewer uses the opportunity to vent frustration, play out personal agendas, exercise inappropriate power of position, or otherwise treat the person being reviewed in a manner that is demeaning or disrespectful. A constructive review is one where the reviewer follows a path of diagnosis, accurately determining the current status of progress and identifying the gaps and weaknesses, leading to feedback that provides a basis for action and that can be tied to a schedule.[1]

Figure 9-1. Micro Flowchart of Step 4

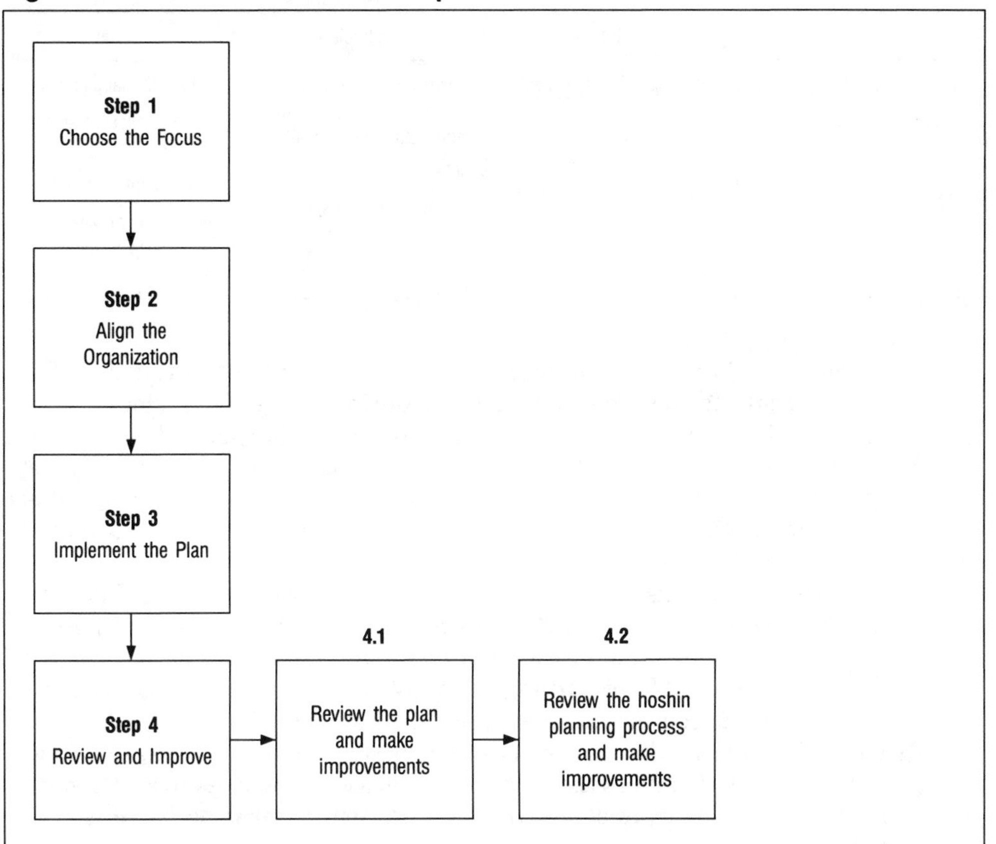

Tips to Maximize Effectiveness of Reviews

Following is a list of tips to make hoshin reviews maximally effective:

1. *Build on existing review cycles.* Rather than creating separate or parallel hoshin review dates, the leaders should schedule reviews to coincide with familiar, ongoing budget or planning reviews. In other words–no new meetings!
2. *Prioritize what is reviewed.* One of the fears expressed about periodic reviews is that managers, especially top managers, will spend inordinate amounts of time reviewing everyone's plan in excruciating detail. The good news for top managers is that they do not have to review everything. The reviews are structured on a bottom-up basis, with each level of review being summarized for the level above it. Reviews are also conducted on an exception basis. If everything went as planned, the review may be quite brief. Finally, reviewers learn over time how to prioritize, so that formal review time is spent on items that benefit from being discussed in a large forum rather than on those that could be handled off-line. A helpful aid in summarizing and prioritizing reviewable material is a standard review table, which is discussed in tip 3 below.
3. *Use a standard review format.* A PDCA-based form such as the one in figure 9-2 keeps the reviewers focused on the content of the review rather than on interpreting or inventing review forms. This review table works for any level of hoshin review and for reviews of daily management items as well. Fill out the table as follows:
   - *Column 1–Plan:* Record the planned target or means exactly as it appears on the plan.

Figure 9-2. Hoshin Review Table

Plan	Do	Check	Act
What was the plan?	What actually happened?	Were there differences (+ or −) between plan and actual outcomes? Why? Show levels of analysis.	What will happen now? Countermeasures in place? Adjustment to plan? Actions to prevent recurrence of negative outcomes?

- *Column 2–Do:* Record what really happened, including supporting data. Note adjustments to the plan that occurred during the review period.
- *Column 3–Check:* Analyze in multiple layers of detail the differences (*both* positive and negative) between what was planned and what actually happened. If appropriate, brainstorm potential causes using a cause-and-effect diagram. (See appendix B, "Hoshin Toolbox," for instructions.) Substantiate true or "root" causes with data.
- *Column 4–Act:* This is the "So now what?" column. Note needed adjustments for the next planning period. Record learnings from the analysis. For first-level learnings, ask, "What did we learn from the misses and the adjustments we made?" For second-level learnings, ask, "What fundamental system changes can we make? How can we avoid problems like these in the future?"

4. *Do not shoot the messenger.* The hoshin review is a dialogue between reviewer and reviewees, with data as the centerpiece. Reviewees must approach the review with the commitment to share true data. Reviewers must desire to hear the truth.
5. *Look for patterns.* Top leaders, who may sit in on several types of reviews during a three-month period, should be looking for repetitive patterns in data. Leaders should encourage reviewees to share anecdotal data, especially customer data, and to be sensitive to trends among the anecdotes.
6. *Ask for data and multiple levels of analysis.* Part of the reviewers' coaching role is to ask (in a nonthreatening manner) for data and for multiple layers of analysis. Reviewers should model the preferred use of data by asking questions such as "Upon what data are you basing your analysis?" and "What charts or graphs can you share with us to illustrate the trends?" When reviewees give a cursory or shallow explanation of deviation from plans, the reviewers have a chance to ask for a deeper analysis. They may even decide to make an appointment to hear the results of the analysis at a later date.
7. *Look for positive as well as negative deviations.* The hoshin review focuses on abnormalities or unpredicted findings. However, a plan that went much better than anticipated calls for just as much analysis as a plan that went poorly. The analysis should focus on understanding three things:
   - What was predicted (planned for)
   - What was done
   - What the cause-and-effect relationship was between what was done and the actual results

   Results are a function of the planning process, the implementation process, and unanticipated factors. Hoshin focuses on a tight coupling between targets and means, improved ability to bring about predicted results, and deep understanding of deviations.
8. *Focus on process as well as results.* Hoshin is a process-oriented planning system. Both the process of planning and the process of implementation are subject

to scrutiny and improvement at each review. Reviewers can model attention to the process by asking questions such as "How can we improve the way we set targets like this in the future?" or "Did your PDPC predict this problem?"

Because hoshin reviews tend to focus on exceptions or deviations from plan, there is a danger that those who followed good planning and implementation processes and achieved predicted results might feel left out! Reviewers need to learn from those who had an "uneventful" review period and to reward them. Appropriate types of rewards are positive comments during the review and notes on the reviewee's performance evaluation.

9. *Create a learning environment.* Tips 4–8 above contribute to the creation of a learning environment in the hoshin review process. Hoshin reviews treat each unanticipated result as a chance to learn. At first this may seem difficult, in that reviewees will want to emphasize good results while downplaying any negatives. Reviewers can display attention to why the deviations occurred. Through their remarks, they can reward efforts to follow good process and to understand, learn from, and prevent deviations. Such a learning environment is based on trust and may take a few review cycles to blend into the culture of the organization.

Structure and Timing of Hoshin Reviews

Figure 9-3 shows the structure and timing of reviews in a hoshin system. The following text examines each level of review and its particular contribution to the hoshin planning cycle. Team, quarterly, and annual reviews are necessary; additional monthly reviews of selected parts of the plan by top management are an option. (**Note:** The PDCA-based review format shown in figure 9-2 is appropriate for all types of hoshin reviews.)

Team Reviews

Team reviews are conducted by those responsible for the action items in the hoshin process. Their frequency is determined by the nature of the items being monitored, probably monthly. The data that feed these reviews may be collected daily or weekly and analyzed monthly. The primary purpose of these reviews is to detect, diagnose, correct, and prevent problems.

Quarterly Reviews by Next Levels of Management

Reviews by the next levels of management occur three to four times a year, compiling the learnings from the team reviews. Target and means owners, managers, and the CEO gather data from various places in the organization to track progress on the hoshin plan. The cross-functional nature of these reviews allows for detection and correction of more systemwide problems than do the team reviews. Adjustments to plans may be made here.

Figure 9-3. Hoshin Reviews

Type of Review	Frequency	Reviewer	Reviewee
Team	Monthly	Middle managers	Supervisors, others
Quarterly	3–4 times/year	Department heads, VPs, CEO	Middle managers
Annual review	1 time/year	CEO, VPs, other top leaders	All those who owned a part of the plan
CEO review	Monthly	CEO, VPs, other top leaders	Selected presenters (for example, strategy owners)

Reviews by Top Management

As figure 9-3 indicates, top management is involved in three types of reviews. Quarterly reviews were discussed in the preceding section. This section discusses two other reviews done by top management—one optional and one necessary.

- *Optional monthly CEO review:* Some organizations choose to put the CEO and the CEO's direct reports in contact with various parts of the hoshin plan on a rolling basis throughout the implementation cycle. Each month, the CEO and the CEO's staff go through a team review with the owners of one of the means. This practice keeps the top management team apprised of the progress and pitfalls of the means owners. The direct contact with the workings of this year's plan helps the executives guide the selection and goal-setting processes on the next year's plan.
- *Necessary annual review:* Sometimes known as the presidential audit, the annual review captures data and learnings from all previous reviews and uses them to feed the next year's hoshin process. Timing of the annual reviews can be tricky. Some organizations actually conduct their annual reviews at the end of the third quarter of hoshin implementation to allow for development of the next year's plan during the fourth quarter.

Task 2: Review the Hoshin Planning Process and Make Improvements

The hoshin planning process itself is subject to improvement. Figure 9-4 suggests an evaluation methodology for assessing the hoshin process and gives suggested scoring criteria. In his book *Hoshin Kanri,* Yoji Akao suggests plotting the results of a hoshin evaluation on a radar chart, such as the one in figure 9-5 (p. 126).[2]

As the evaluation method and radar chart suggest, a hoshin planning process takes several cycles (several years) to perfect. Theory and mechanics that may have seemed unfamiliar and cumbersome at first become second nature to the organization as time passes. Once the hoshin planning process has become somewhat stable (after the first cycle or two), leaders may find it beneficial to summarize in simple "route map" format the annual process and suggested methods or tools they expect to see used.

Boiled down to its essence, hoshin is "(CA)PDCA" with capital letters. Beginning with a "Check" of the previous year's plan, the organization drafts a plan (Plan), carries it out (Do), reviews progress and results (Check), and takes further action according to what was learned in the review (Act). Within the hoshin plan many little PDCA cycles occur simultaneously. Figure 9-6 (p. 127) shows that the hoshin planning system is circular. The end of each cycle feeds the beginning of the next one. Appropriately, the hoshin planning process has been called "self-healing."

Roles and Responsibilities

Strong involvement with the plan and deep understanding of its progress during step 3 (implementation) prepares everyone—from the top leadership team to the owners of the most detailed means—to conduct effective, efficient reviews. The review step is essential to preparing for the next hoshin plan; therefore, executives benefit greatly from the learning that occurs here.

The CEO

During the review and improvement process, the chief executive officer:

- Sticks to review schedules
- Makes the review atmosphere a safe haven for truthful discussion of progress and unexpected results
- Engages reviewees in discussion and dialogue; includes others in the room in the dialogue
- Asks the reviewees for supporting data on the progress of their plans and their analyses of unexpected results
- Recognizes people for following good planning and implementation processes and for getting good results
- Reviews their progress on the parts of the plan that they own

Other Reviewers

Other reviewers involved in this process:

Figure 9-4. Evaluation of Hoshin Planning

Hoshin Planning Concept	Scores * See scoring key below				
	1	2	3	4	5
Overall planning system; hoshin, daily management	1	2	3	4	5
Selection of focus	1	2	3	4	5
Development of annual targets	1	2	3	4	5
Development of means	1	2	3	4	5
Development of measures	1	2	3	4	5
Tracking of progress	1	2	3	4	5
Analysis and review	1	2	3	4	5
Adjustment of plan (this year's)	1	2	3	4	5
Incorporation of learnings into next year's plan	1	2	3	4	5

Scoring Key

Score	Interpretation
1	No knowledge or effort apparent in this concept Good results occur by happenstance
2	Some (spotty) evidence of systematic application of knowledge, effort Use of some tools Few/some good results
3	Organizationwide systematic application of knowledge, effort, data, and tools correlated with results Success in many areas Still obvious areas for improvement
4	Definite correlation between application of knowledge, effort, data, and tools and desired results Success in almost all areas Evidence of innovation Prevention-focused
5	Systematic and effective use of knowledge, data, and tools integrated across the organization Sustained success Anticipating problems World-class performance; role model for others

- Guide reviewees in the collection and analysis of information before the review
- Ask the reviewees for relevant data during the review
- Encourage reviewees to complete all parts of the review form accurately and thoroughly
- Schedule follow-up meetings to coach reviewees who need additional assistance

Reviewees

People who provide information for the review are expected to:

- Collect and analyze data throughout implementation
- Share accurate and complete information during reviews
- Engage in dialogue with reviewers during the review
- Do multiple levels of analysis
- Meet with reviewers for follow-up where additional analysis is needed

Figure 9-5. Hoshin Evaluation Results

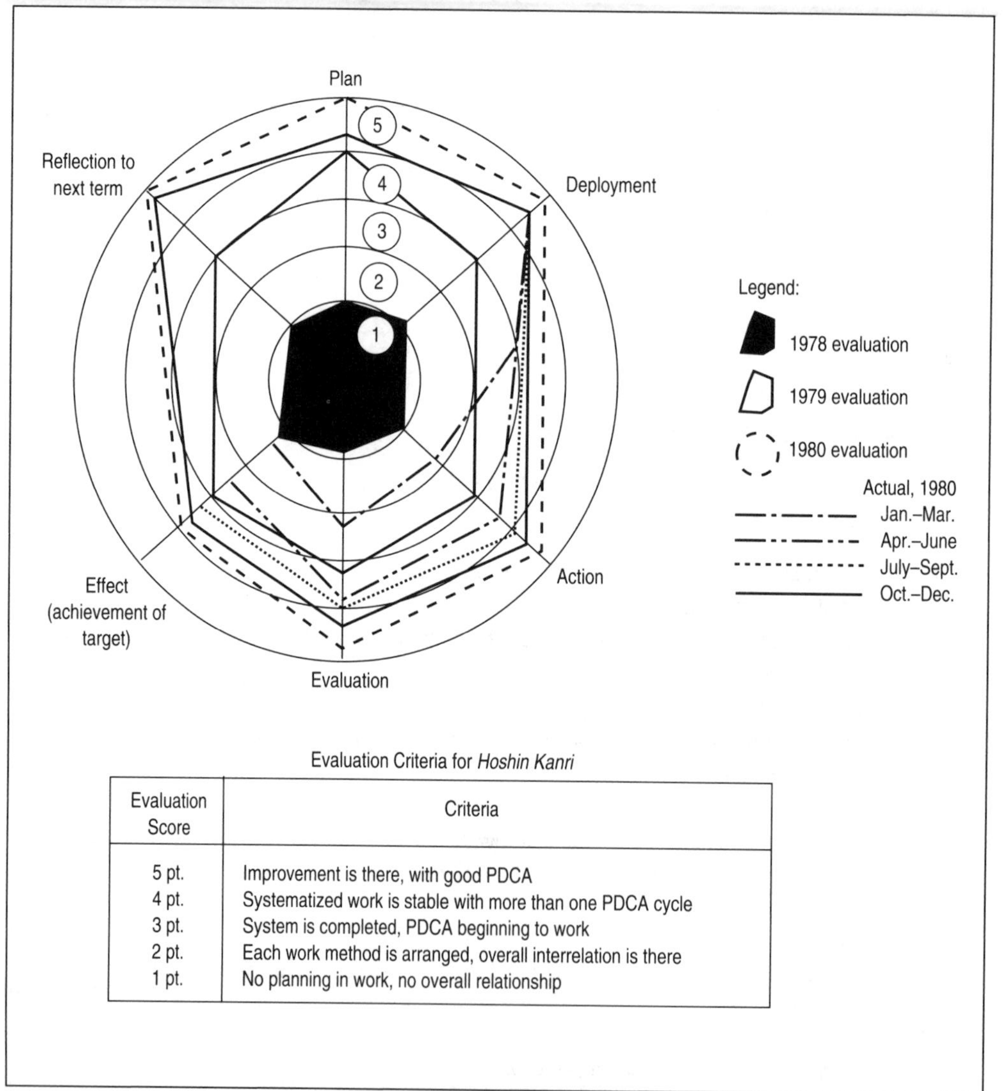

Evaluation Criteria for *Hoshin Kanri*

Evaluation Score	Criteria
5 pt.	Improvement is there, with good PDCA
4 pt.	Systematized work is stable with more than one PDCA cycle
3 pt.	System is completed, PDCA beginning to work
2 pt.	Each work method is arranged, overall interrelation is there
1 pt.	No planning in work, no overall relationship

From *Hoshin Kanri: Policy Deployment for Successful TQM,* by Yoji Akao. English translation copyright ©1991 by Productivity Press, Inc., PO Box 13390, Portland, OR 97213-0390, (800)394-6868. Reprinted by permission.

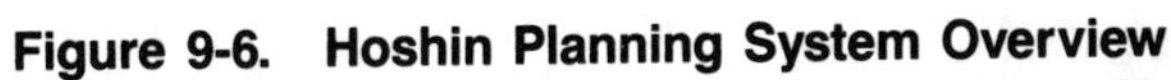

Figure 9-6. Hoshin Planning System Overview

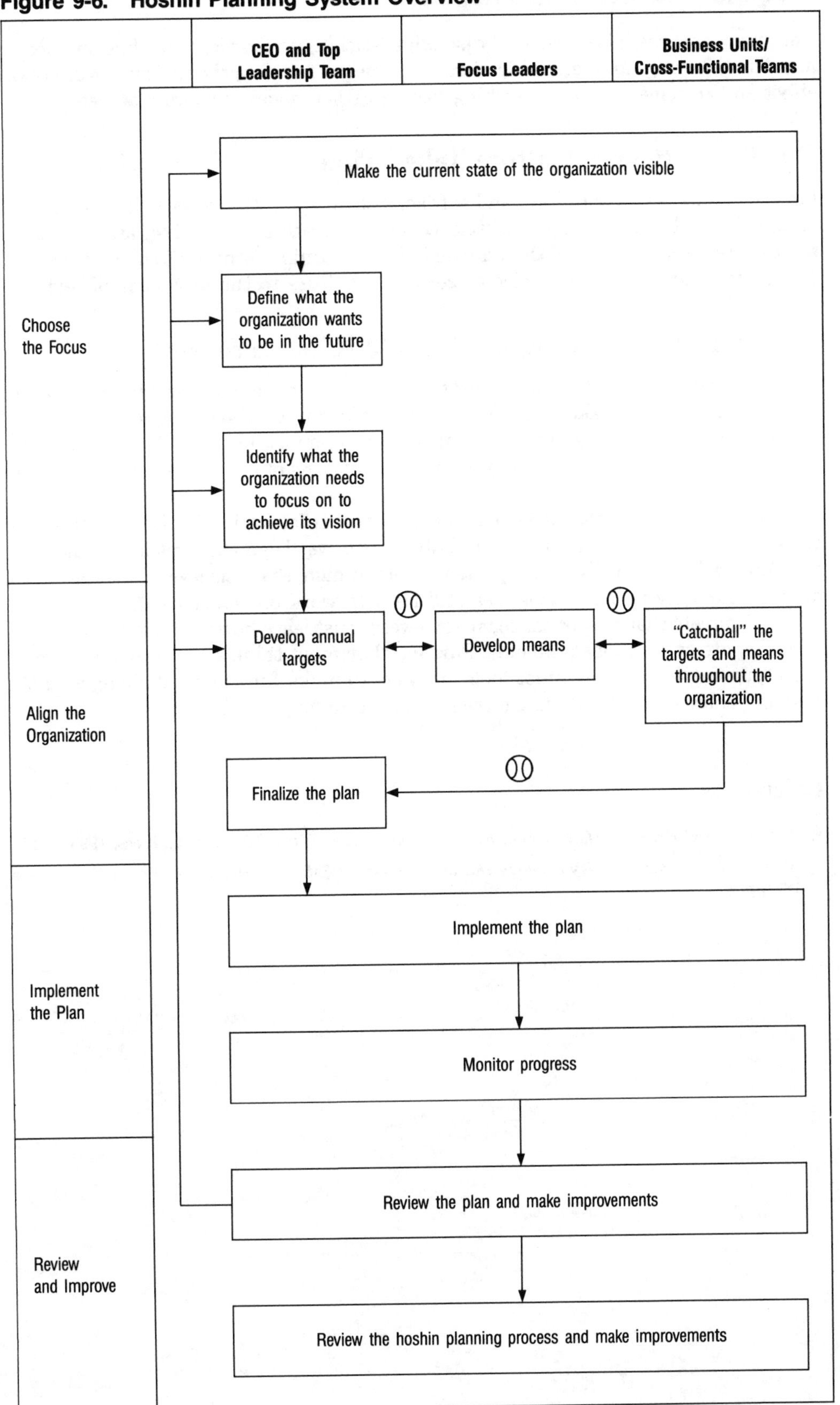

Lessons Learned and Helpful Hints

The review process raises issues of discipline (sticking to a review schedule) and learning. The following hints advise leaders to "keep the faith" as the review culture takes effect and to remember how learning occurs as the review culture matures.

Building a Review Culture Takes Time

Reviews are based on both hard and soft science. Keeping the reviews data-based and process-focused addresses the hard science. Demonstrating that reviews are safe places to share real data and that the emphasis is on learning is part of the soft science. It may take several review cycles to convert a culture to the new style of review.

Review Learnings Progress from "Fix" to "Prevent"

Like building a culture, building an organization that remembers and learns from its successes and failures takes time. The review table in figure 9-3 is a "learning monitor" of sorts for the review system. As people become comfortable with the hoshin review procedure, they get better at filling in the four columns of the review form accurately and completely.

First people learn that it is OK to record true information in the *Do* column of the review form and to discuss it candidly at reviews. Then they get better at using the *Check* column to analyze unexpected results at more than one level. Once the depth-analysis capacity is built, reviewees still need to work on the *Act* column.

To complete that part of the form, reviewees must learn how to think proactively—to anticipate and prevent problems. Further, they must think about ways to do more than "put out fires." They must look for ways to make fundamental changes in the system—changes that may make true breakthroughs possible.

References

1. Collins, B., and Huge, E. *Management by Policy.* Milwaukee, WI: ASQC Quality Press, 1993, p. 105.
2. Akao, Y. *Hoshin Kanri: Policy Deployment for Successful TQM.* Cambridge, MA: Productivity Press, 1991, p. 61.

PART THREE

Case Studies of Hoshin Planning in Action

CHAPTER TEN

Bethesda, Inc.

Dona Hotopp with Gerry Kaminski

Rich in tradition and known for innovation, Bethesda, Inc., was the pioneer in adapting hoshin planning to a health care organization. Bethesda led the way in discovering how this uniquely focused process could work in a nonmanufacturing environment. Long recognized for innovation, the organization has provided the Cincinnati area with the following firsts: a freestanding surgery center, structured alcohol and drug treatment programs, a birthing room program, an outpatient physical rehabilitation unit, employer-focused services such as fitness center management, and industrial health centers, as well as innovations in cancer treatments.

From its beginnings in 1896, Bethesda was built upon a purposeful mission and a sense of commitment to the health of the Cincinnati community. Today Bethesda serves that community as a comprehensive system of hospitals, occupational medicine centers, senior services, and other related health care services.

Bethesda, Inc., is made up of two acute care hospitals, a home health agency, a medical equipment company, a senior services agency, two work capacity centers, and five centers of occupational health. Located in a city that is home to successful companies such as Procter & Gamble, Kroger, and Chiquita Brands, Bethesda provides contract services to medium- to large-sized Cincinnati businesses. Bethesda has recently formed an alliance with Good Samaritan Hospital to create a comprehensive network to better serve the greater metropolitan area.

Bethesda Oak and Bethesda North are the organization's hospitals. Oak Hospital, located downtown, has 434 beds; Bethesda North, at a more suburban location, has 333 beds. The total medical staff of more than 1,300 provides services such as alcohol and drug treatment, cardiac rehabilitation, cardiac catheterization, laser surgery, MRI, and neonatal intensive care. Bethesda, Inc., employs approximately 4,500 people.

In keeping with the tradition of community service, Bethesda's leadership crafted the following purpose early on in their total quality management (TQM) efforts:

> To adopt a leadership philosophy that supports, encourages, and expects all employees to participate in the continuous improvement of service to meet the health care needs of the community[1]

Reasons for Choosing Hoshin Planning

Bethesda defines hoshin planning as "a structured method for planning and implementing major improvements in a few key areas of strategic importance to an organization and its customers."[2] Including customers directly in the definition of hoshin planning is a unique feature of Bethesda's approach. It emphasizes the pivotal role customers play in defining improvements and priorities for the Bethesda system.

In embracing hoshin planning, the leadership at Bethesda determined to:

- Align and focus on key strategic objectives
- Address an urgent financial need
- Enhance cross-functional teamwork and empowerment

Align and Focus on Key Strategic Objectives

Bethesda introduced TQM in early 1989 with the education of senior management and the establishment of the Quality 1 steering committee. The steering committee, led by the CEO and composed of the officers of the medical staff and the senior vice-presidents, adopted a systems approach to quality improvement. The committee recognized the importance of improving the entire system, rather than selected parts of the system.

The steering committee had chosen to implement TQM using the model represented by the GOAL/QPC Wheel (shown in figure 2-3, p. 18). It began by launching six pilot project teams. Later in 1989, another round of project teams began work, TQM materials specific to Bethesda were created, and more managers and staff received methods and tools education. In early 1990, in conjunction with the third set of TQM teams, the steering committee members decided that the time was right to focus the Quality 1 process on strategic objectives. As a result, they introduced hoshin planning.

The committee identified five organizational priorities as important to the entire organization (numbers do not imply prioritization)[3]:

1. Improving the work environment and systems for employees
2. Improving the customer–supplier relationships
3. Improving accuracy
4. Improving timeliness
5. Improving the practice environment and systems for physicians

The first hoshin focus – reducing delays – was based on the priority of improving timeliness.

Address an Urgent Financial Need

Success with the first hoshin focus – timeliness – led the steering committee to try hoshin planning to meet a serious financial situation in 1991–92. An 8 percent reduction in force was necessary late in 1991. Bethesda leadership wanted to hold the productivity gains achieved by the reduction in order to avoid further layoffs. Hoshin planning had worked in reducing delays and was now applied to an urgent business need of improving productivity.[4]

Enhance Cross-Functional Teamwork and Empowerment

One of the initial goals of Bethesda leadership in initiating TQM was to establish cross-functional teamwork and to foster empowerment. Hoshin planning is a process to do both. It requires cross-functional teamwork in all phases of implementation. Direction for all employees, an important factor in true empowerment, is provided through communication of the breakthrough goal, catchball, and hoshin deployment.

Hoshin Implementation

The implementation of the hoshin process at Bethesda has evolved over the years and has been enhanced with each generation of hoshin focus. This case study summarizes the implementation in 1990–91; details hoshin generation, deployment, and review in 1992; and outlines the progress in 1993–94.

1990–1991

Bethesda began its early hoshin planning with training for facilitators and managers in the use of the seven management and planning (7MP) tools within the context of the hoshin process. The Quality 1 steering committee had decided in the spring of 1990 to integrate hoshin planning into the TQM initiative to enhance vertical alignment. Providing training was the first step. Next, the 7MP tools were used at planning retreats at both hospitals. Their power as focused planning methods became apparent.

Choosing the Organization's Focus

In the fall of 1990, the steering committee members applied the tools themselves. They developed a hoshin breakthrough objective for the hospitals to coordinate all the improvement efforts that were under way through teams, task forces, and departmental improvement initiatives. Using the five priority areas in need of improvement that they had previously identified, the committee created an interrelationship digraph.[5] (See appendix B, "Hoshin Toolbox," for an example.) This digraph is the MP tool that identifies the driver, or key cause, among a group of issues. The issue that surfaced as the driver was improving timeliness as a way to affect all the improvement needs. This conclusion was verified by reviewing data from customer research and early quality function deployment (QFD) analysis on customer needs: timeliness was indeed important to meeting key customer needs. So the breakthrough goal deployed in 1990–91 was "to improve timeliness."

Aligning the Organization with the Focus

The deployment process in 1990–91 involved cross-functional coordination and the beginning of catchball (interactive planning discussions) with departments. At both hospitals, cross-functional groups identified delays and stratified them by patient services, technical and professional services, and support services.

Implementing the Plan and Monitoring Progress

After catchball with department managers and staff, department teams addressed the causes of delays using the seven quality control (7QC) tools, such as process flowcharts and fishbone diagrams, and Bethesda's 13-step process improvement model, a systematic way of defining problems, verifying causes, and developing appropriate solutions. Training was provided as needed to a significant number of managers. Delays were reduced, and the organization experienced the power of hoshin planning for focused improvement. This set the stage for 1992 deployment.

Review and Improvement

Departments and teams in all divisions started very enthusiastically and were addressing delays early in 1991 until financial issues became a higher priority for leaders in the hospitals. Because of the external environment, there was a reduction of occupancy, and the steering committee considered the possibility of shifting direction to use TQM to address financial issues. Teams that were making measurable progress in terms of the customer continued their work, and those projects that were not affecting the bottom line were put on hold.

1991: Early Results

The results of the first hoshin experience were encouraging:

1. Reduced delays in many departments in:
   - Patient services
   - Technical services
   - Professional services
   - Support services
2. The organizational experience of the power of hoshin planning for focused improvement

During the first phase of hoshin planning at Bethesda, deployment was concentrated in two hospitals, Oak and North. By the end of 1991, the hoshin effort had resulted in a reduction in delays. As a result of progress made during work on the 1991 hoshin, Bethesda was able to understand the strength of hoshin: how it really does work to focus an organization on what is needed for improvement in line with organizational goals.

1992

The power of hoshin at Bethesda is evidenced by three changes. These are the facility's moving forward with more intensity, setting a more focused goal for further improvement, and utilizing hoshin planning more fully during 1992.

Choosing the Organization's Focus

In 1992, because of external issues and layoffs, the hoshin goal was "to focus on unit optimization so that we more closely match use of resources with patient volume while continuously improving our ability to satisfy our customers." The steering committee determined the 1992 hoshin focus in response to the financial situation of the two hospitals. It was necessary to maintain the productivity gains accomplished through an 8 percent reduction in force at the end of 1991. Hoshin planning was recognized as the method to establish the specific goals, identify the right measures, and achieve the organizationwide alignment needed to hold these gains. To prevent further layoffs, the numerical target was to maintain an 8 percent productivity improvement overall at both hospitals throughout 1992.

Aligning the Organization with the Focus

Deployment began with determining the right measures and providing the data reporting system necessary to track them meaningfully. These activities are briefly described below.

Measures Defined

Leadership applied criteria to determine applicable and practical measures at the department manager level. Some of the criteria used in an extensive study of the issue were as follows:

1. Was the measure understandable?
2. Was information on which the measure was based timely?
3. Was the measure one that managers could control?

Once these criteria were applied, productive hours per adjusted patient day emerged as a key measure because managers had influence over staffing, information could be available on a timely basis, and if productive hours were measured and controlled there would be a positive impact on the total budget. The breakthrough goal was "to focus on unit optimization so that we more closely match use of resources with patient volume while continuously improving our ability to satisfy our customers."

Measurement and Data Reporting Systems Improved

Before divisional deployment was initiated, the organization took six months to improve the measurement and data reporting systems to support the vice-presidents and department managers with consistent, timely, and accurate data. A key insight from the 1990–1991 hoshin planning effort was that lack of appropriate data is a serious hurdle to deployment. Therefore, in 1992 the hospital leadership invested time up front to develop a comprehensive data system to eliminate system barriers.

Key Means Determined

After measures had been determined and the data reporting system developed, the key means of variable staffing was determined by the leadership and used throughout the hospitals. Variable staffing involves directly adjusting staff numbers to fit the changing needs of the hospital. Each division had a target of maintaining 8 percent productivity improvement. Catchball was used with departments to set this initial target. Vice-presidents gave department managers the overall measures, such as adjusted patient days or adjusted admissions. They then empowered departments to develop their own measures (for example, workload units in the lab or patient days in nursing) and plans to achieve the division target and the overall target through the primary means of variable staffing.

Worksheets Developed and Training Provided

The Quality 1 staff developed worksheets on sources of data for each run chart for professional/technical services, support services, and patient services. These measures were also standardized between the hospitals. For example, upon finding that they used different ways of calculating workload units, the laboratories at both hospitals made changes so that they were using the same measures. The development of worksheets and training sessions was key to the successful implementation of variable staffing.

Managers, including the hospital COOs, vice-presidents, and department heads, all received training from the Quality 1 staff and management engineering. Two core facilitators and a number of part-time facilitators assisted in training and just-in-time process improvement coaching. Managers then were able to manually plot their data, better understand the data, and use tools to educate their staff on trends to identify areas for improvement.

Implementing the Plan and Monitoring Progress

After initial training, the vice-presidents met with their department managers to establish department goals and set up the tracking systems. Department measures and biweekly results were rolled up to the division level and then up to the COO. The measures were rolled up and down, allowing the department managers and their vice-presidents to identify problem areas and coach the responsible person on improvement. All levels, including senior management, tracked their own data and displayed run charts in their work area.

A key feature of this hoshin deployment was the consistent use of run charts throughout all departments and divisions and at the hospital level. The four run charts used showed, respectively:

- Productive hours per pay period
- Workload units per pay period
- Productive hours per workload unit measure per pay period
- Total expense per workload unit at the end of each accounting period

Budget and actual data were shown on each run chart. The four run charts were clearly displayed in all areas to make the hoshin planning process visible. (See the example in figure 10-1.)

Implementation and review flowcharts were developed to support hoshin deployment. The flowchart for the director/manager at the end of the pay period indicated input steps for creating the run charts, the biweekly report roll-up from departments, how to plot and calculate total productive hours, and budget deviations; it also indicated when corrective action might be needed. The flowcharts were tools used to standardize the hoshin deployment and provided a mechanism for aligning departments and divisions to meet the hospital target. (See figure 10-2.)

The productivity effort became part of daily work, and the charting of data has continued into 1994. To achieve a closer match between the volume measure and revenue availability, the volume measure was changed from adjusted patient days to adjusted admissions in 1994. A new corporate policy included the measurement strategy, and a pamphlet for new managers on charting measures was integrated into formal management orientation at Oak Hospital.

Review and Improvement

Hoshin review considers results and process. Results of department and division work and results for the organization are part of the review. Hoshin review also encompasses review of the process of deployment, areas for improvement that have been identified at any level, and review of the overall hoshin process itself. In 1992 Bethesda initiated hoshin review at the department level through analysis of results. As an organization, however, it failed to identify "big picture" system barriers or hospitalwide improvement opportunities.

The vice-presidents and the COO reviewed biweekly the results of the hoshin deployment as displayed on the run charts. They made changes quickly to keep the hospitals on track in reaching and exceeding the hoshin goal. The review process also encouraged process improvement. Managers used the run charts to identify department improvement opportunities with their staff. A review form using the plan-do-check-act (PDCA) cycle was used biweekly, monthly, or quarterly to identify changes to the plan or an improvement opportunity. An example is shown in figure 10-3 (p. 139).

To reinforce the integration of process improvement and hoshin deployment, flowcharts were developed for the director/manager at the end of the accounting period as well as the end of the pay period, and for the vice-president at the end of the quarter. The VP's flowchart indicates that an improvement process at the unit or steering committee level should be done at the end of each quarter so that improvement would be made regularly during the year. Figure 10-4 (p. 140) shows an example.

The review process in 1992 was an area for improvement as Bethesda moved into the third generation of hoshin planning. The flowcharts were not as widely used as had been planned. Formal hoshin reviews of process as well as results could have identified major systems in need of improvement and accelerated formal process improvement throughout the hospitals. Therefore, a formal review process was a key need for improvement as the organization moved into 1993–1994.

Figure 10-1. 1992 Biweekly Run Chart: Productive Hours per Workload per Pay Period (Hours/Units)

Cost Center 1670 Department L & D Unit Measure

	1/11	1/25	2/08	2/22	3/07	3/21	4/04	4/18	5/02	5/16	5/30	6/13	6/27	7/11	7/25	8/08	8/22	9/05	9/19	10/03	10/17	10/31	11/14	11/28	12/12	12/26
Budget	11.18	11.18	11.18	11.18	11.18	11.18	11.18	11.18	11.18	11.18	11.18	11.18	11.18	11.18	11.18	11.18	11.18	11.18	11.18	11.18	11.18	11.18	11.18	11.18	11.18	11.18
Actual	10.60	11.06	10.35	10.80	10.27	10.77	9.81	9.82	9.73	9.38	8.37	9.42	9.54	8.72	9.41	10.78	9.76	9.24	9.11	10.14	9.38	8.61	9.97	9.10	9.04	8.66

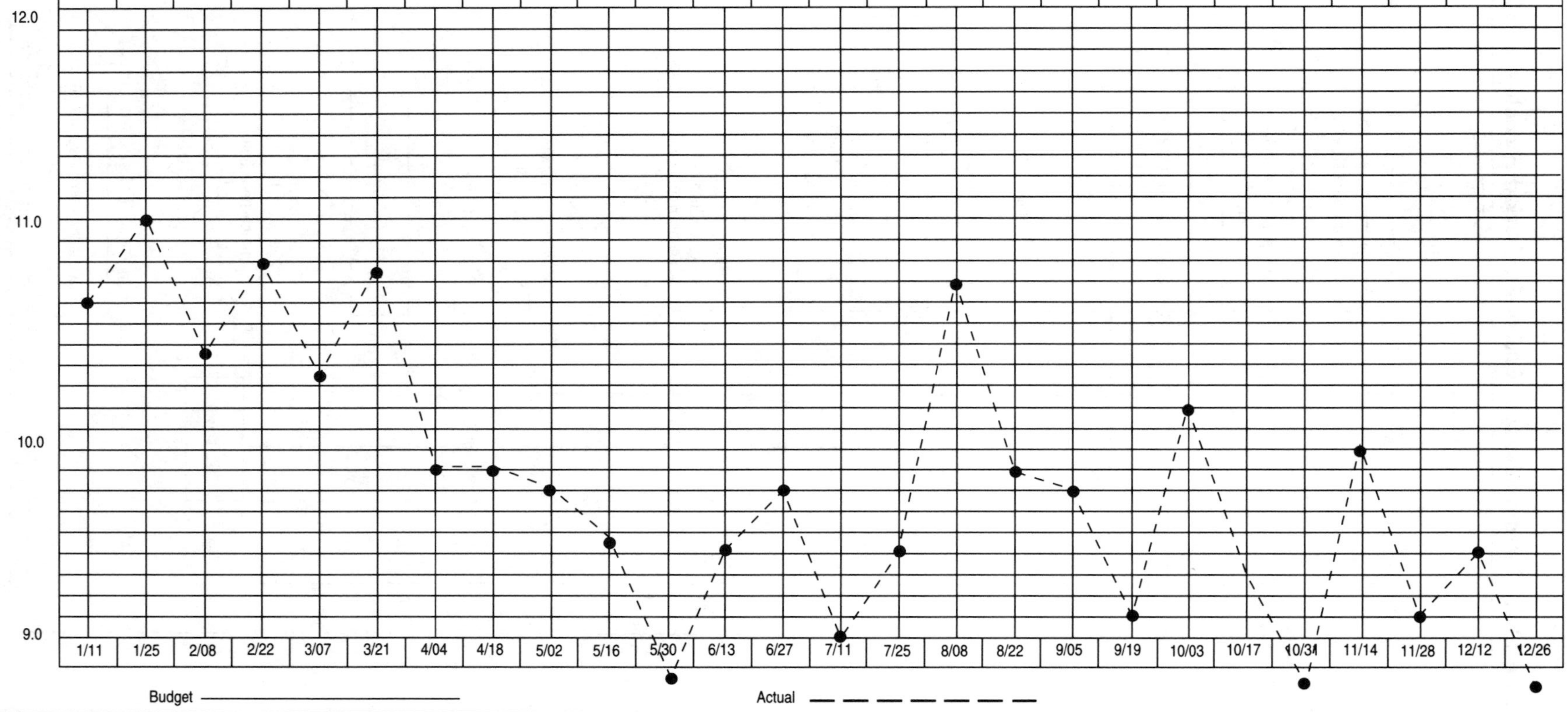

Figure 10-2. Director/Manager End of Pay Period Flowchart

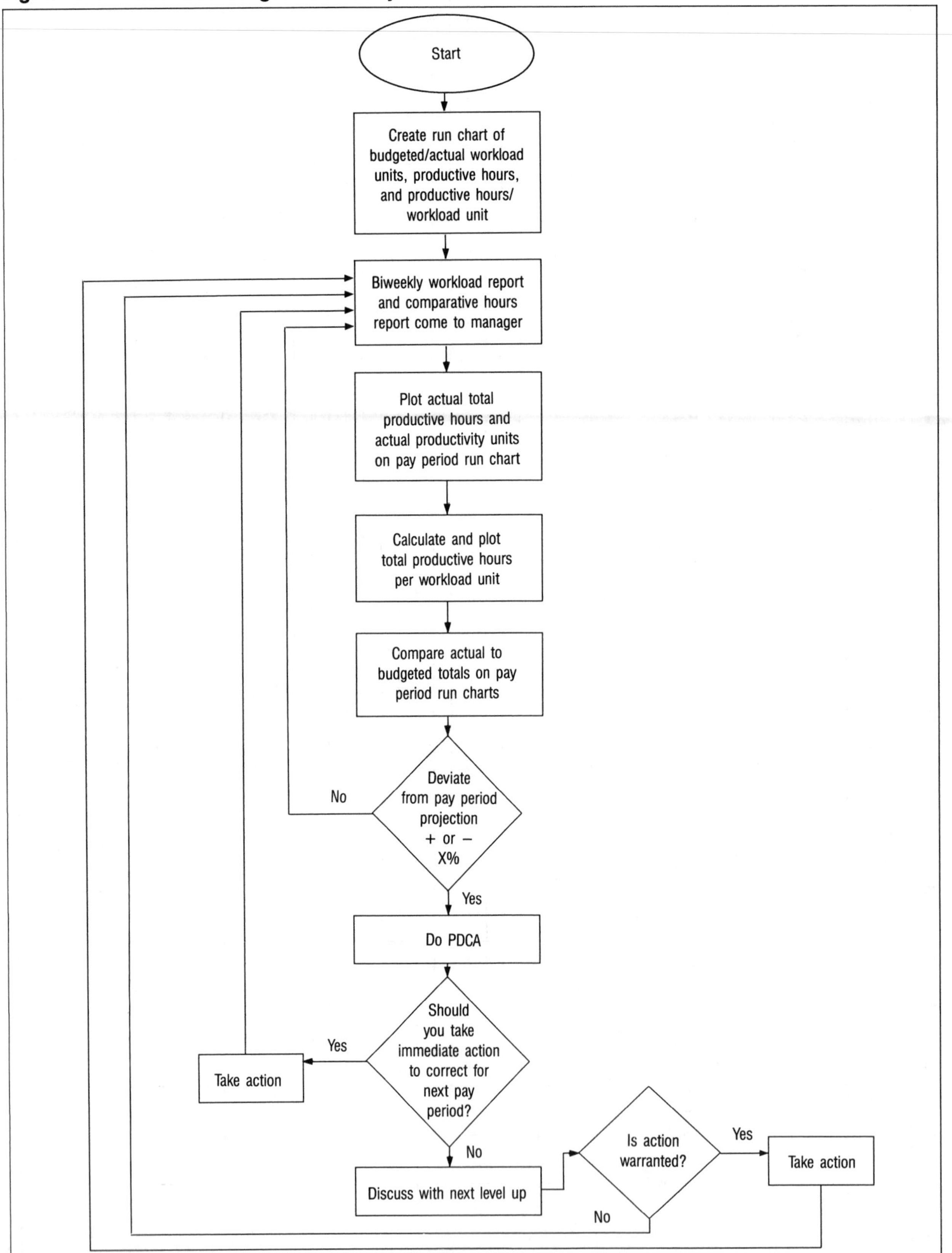

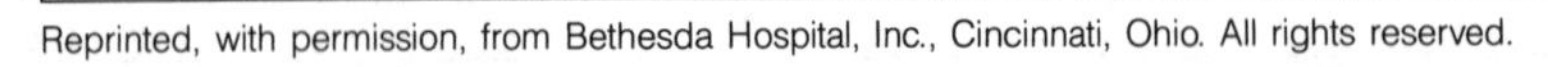

1992: Measures of Success

Bethesda measured the following results of hoshin planning in 1992:

- An 11 percent productivity improvement
- An improved data reporting system
- Reduced waste in productive hours
- Consistent patient satisfaction

The two hospitals exceeded the 8 percent productivity goal by 3 percent to reach an overall improvement of 11 percent. Bethesda's current strong database is a result of the effort to reach this goal. The two hospitals now have standard units of measure, timeliness guidelines, and standardized data forms. Accumulating and analyzing data is a focus for managers, and they are trained to track and use data in decision making with their staff.

Continuously improving patient satisfaction was an element of the hoshin goal. As measured by a Gallup survey, patient satisfaction measures held steady or improved with the new levels of staffing.

1993–1994

After the success of hoshin planning in 1992, the Quality 1 steering committee generated a new focus for 1993–1994.

Figure 10-3. Bethesda Hospitals, Inc., PDCA Form

Individual Completing Form: ______________________

Department/Team: 1614 6 South Oncology Med/Surg.

[x] Monthly review
[ ] Quarterly review
[ ] Other: ________ Date: 2/19/93

P Plan	D Do	C Check	A Act
What did you plan to do?	What did you actually do?	Why did you have to do something different from what you originally planned? Why did this happen? (cause theories) If you used a measure, what were your expected versus actual results? If different, why?	What are you doing about the differences? How are you changing your plan?
Staff according to variable staffing sliding scale plan.	6 South merged with 2 West on 12/19/93, and prior to the move it was necessary to overstaff for several reasons.	Reasons for overstaffing: 1. Double-staffed for moving day 2. Chemotherapy given to patient on 1 West/550. (6 South nurse taken to 1 West for 30–45 minutes. Had to overstaff on next shift to recuperate also on 5 South for another 2 hours giving chemo.)	After the move back to 6 South, we will continue to staff according to variable staffing sliding scale plan. *The PHPPD for the year 1992: actual 6.6, budget 6.6 **The expense/unit for 1992: actual 121, budget 121 ***Total net revenue 1992: actual 100.6%, budget 100.6%

Choosing the Organization's Focus

In 1993–1994, the hoshin focus at Bethesda was "delighting key customers by responding to their highest-priority demands for effective and low-cost health care." The steering committee added these features to hoshin deployment and review:

- Refocusing the hoshin emphasis on key customer demands
- Implementing a formal review process through a hoshin system audit on flowcharts
- Having the entire organization join the hospitals in implementing hoshin planning as home health services, corporate health services, and senior services became involved

Figure 10-4. V.P.—End of Quarter

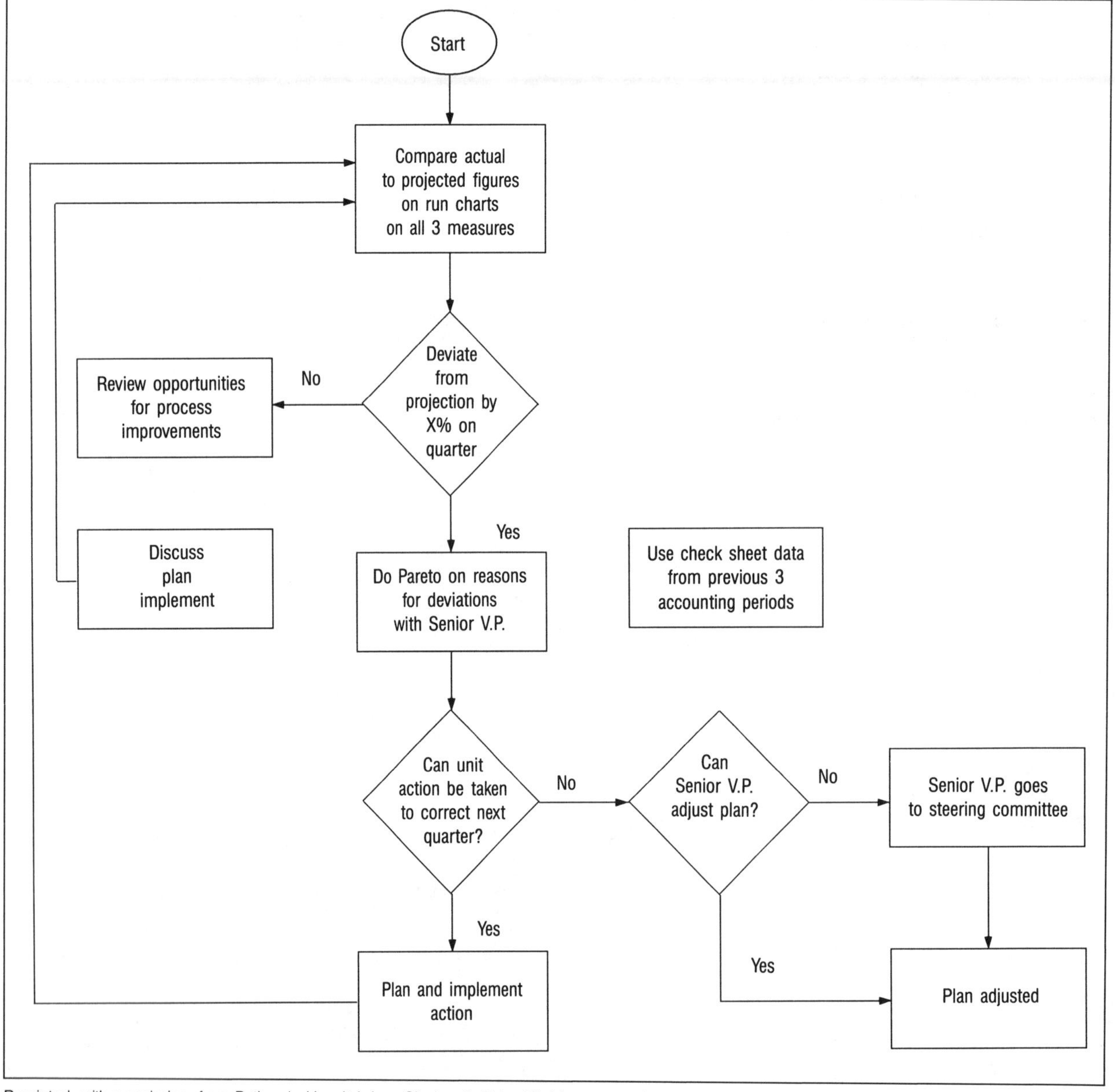

The organization began by identifying key corporate customers. The steering committee assumed responsibility of prioritizing the key customers, identifying and prioritizing their needs, and developing a corporate measurement system. The committee identified large employers and employer cooperatives as the key customers, with the overall demand for low-cost and effective care. It established the hoshin focus of delighting the customer through breakthrough improvements in key quality and cost indicators.

Aligning the Organization with the Focus

Next, the Quality 1 staff facilitated the process to establish the measurement system. Earlier applications of hoshin planning had demonstrated the importance of a valid measurement system. Customer measures for the new hoshin were determined through a complex matrix. Prioritized customer demands were displayed on the horizontal axis, and measures to meet those demands were generated at several levels, from the population level down to very specific measures at the department level. Measurement teams including key employers and insurers as well as Bethesda staff were asked to improve the first draft of measures developed by the leadership team. The Quality 1 staff then collated these data and recommended a set of measures to the steering committee.

The deployment plan for 1993–1994 included these items:

- Determining key process improvement strategies and preliminary targets by the steering committee
- Catchball and finalizing of targets, means, and strategies by all management related to key processes
- PDCA by all management and process improvement teams
- Hoshin system audit (figure 10-5)

Implementing the Plan and Monitoring Progress

As Bethesda began to implement this plan, another priority commanded the steering committee's attention and needed immediate action. The leadership had audited the Quality 1 process and recommitted to making the organization operationally more customer-driven. This commitment and the hoshin focus on the customer led to the realization that the entire organization needed to be more cross-functionally organized to diminish departmental boundaries so as to better serve both the patient and the employer customers. A major innovative restructuring was initiated. The entire system is now being restructured by cross-functional core processes that directly relate to customer needs. This customer-driven structure will allow Bethesda to more effectively meet the health care needs of the community.

The formal hoshin deployment has been postponed for approximately 18 months while redesign and restructuring take place. Departments had taken variable staffing as far as they could in 1992, and major redesign efforts to find new and creative ways to address the staffing issue were necessary. As of 1995, Bethesda plans to resume the hoshin efforts of major process improvement to delight the employer customer.

1993: Results

The results, direct and indirect, of the 1993–1994 hoshin efforts encouraged the reorganization of the system to a more integrated customer-driven structure. A renewed focus on the customer led to new efforts to provide low-cost health services while maintaining and improving quality and outcomes.

A parallel process to the hoshin planning customer focus was the development of clinical paths. The focus of the 1993–1994 hoshin on the employer as key customer highlighted the necessity of increased clinical effectiveness. The means chosen to meet that demand was standardized clinical paths of care. During 1992 Bethesda began piloting clinical paths, and in the spring of 1993 it chose a methodology for faster implementation of clinical paths. Seventeen clinical paths were developed, and the organization is implementing these paths. To take the customer focus into the future, Bethesda also began to construct a case management system combining this approach with clinical paths to create a coordinated care system.

Figure 10-5. 1993–94 Hoshin Implementation Plan

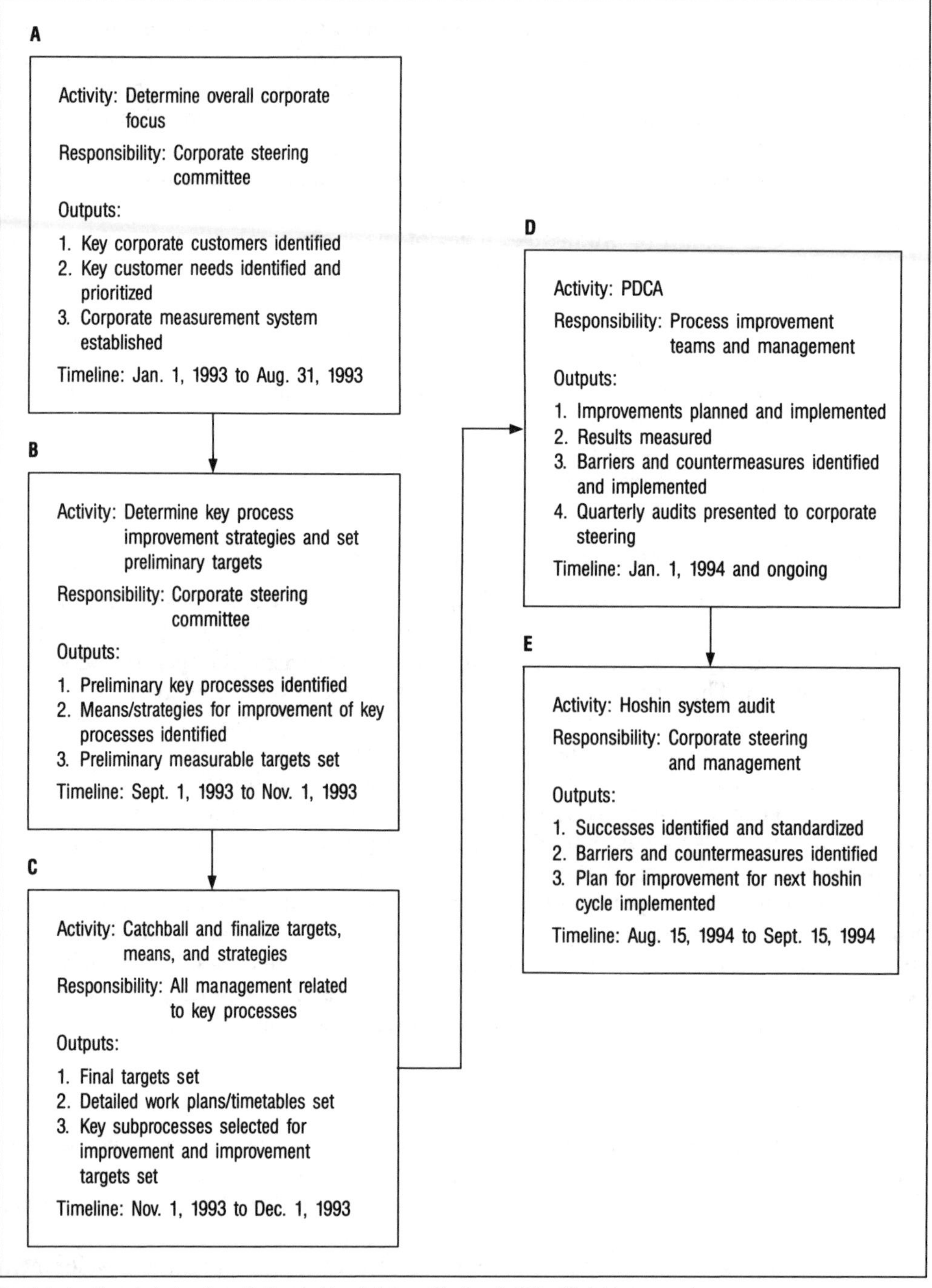

Productivity ratios continued to be monitored in 1994 and appeared to slip somewhat. Although productivity is now a part of daily management, Bethesda's CEO has indicated that the daily management effort may need to be increased. He has explored the issue with the department managers.[6]

Overall Benefits and Results

In addition to the measurable results described above, benefits in the human dimension of change also occurred.

Soft-Side Benefits Achieved

Education, acceptance that TQM can improve business, increased communication, and teamwork are soft-side benefits achieved by Bethesda as a result of hoshin planning. Education of managers at both hospitals in the 7QC tools has helped create buy-in and implementation of hoshin. Through their training in these tools, managers have been empowered to make internal improvements in their own division. Because the education was on a just-in-time basis, the managers are able to utilize their training in a timely manner and to see results from their work.

The 11 percent productivity increase due to hoshin planning efforts has increased acceptance that TQM can be used to improve business results. When Bethesda's hoshin target was directly linked to the budget, hoshin efforts improved the bottom line.

Communication and teamwork among departments, division heads, and the two hospitals have increased dramatically because of concentration on the hoshin target. The common hoshin target and standardization of reports and graphs have worked to ease and improve communication.

Alignment Increased

The focus on an organizational hoshin target has led to increased alignment throughout the Bethesda organization. Such alignment has been identified on three levels: within each hospital, across both hospitals, and throughout departments.

Intrahospital Alignment

Through hoshin planning, for the first time both hospitals had a single focused goal toward which they worked collaboratively. The senior vice-president and COO of Oak Hospital stated that hoshin had a phenomenal impact and that everyone collaborated much more than was previously thought possible.[7] The two hospitals now work as allies, not competitors, and people ask one another for assistance.

Hospitalwide Alignment

The senior vice-president and COO of North Hospital credits the hoshin effort with creating alignment within North Hospital and regenerating and refreshing the hospital's TQM approach. Hoshin focused hospital attention on key improvements and, by having a standardized measurement system in place, helped to advance that alignment. Although management had previously initiated objectives, with hoshin planning "you turn the PDCA cycle, get more understanding of the issues and more employee involvement, and thus you can be more effective."[8]

Departmental Alignment

Departmental managers and systems also are better aligned. Hoshin planning promoted cleanup of reports and establishment of accurate and timely data reporting systems due to the cooperative effort between the information systems division and the financial services division. Department managers were also aligned in creating and selecting these data reporting systems. Increased participation at the department level furthered organizational alignment.

The implementation of variable staffing throughout the organization helped to align the nursing unit with other departments. Nursing services already had variable staffing in place prior to hoshin implementation but, historically, because of staff size, nursing had been scrutinized for productivity. The new hospitalwide integration of accountability for productive hours in all departments was easily accepted and understood by nursing areas.

Customer Focus Enhanced

At Bethesda, hoshin planning has enhanced the focus on both external and internal customers. Customer focus is a major driver of all Quality 1 progress.

External Customers

The first breakthrough goal of improving timeliness was based on an analysis of the needs of patients, physicians, employers, and third-party payers. Whether the teams were working to reduce delays in putting OB patients in exam rooms, admitting patients for hospice home care, or turning around stat IVs, external customers were being better served.

The 1992 hoshin goal of productivity improvement included the phrase "while continuously improving our ability to satisfy our customers." The steering committee and hospital leadership wanted to maintain and improve customer satisfaction while addressing the budget problem. They achieved this objective, but in reality the focus was on the bottom line – becoming more productive. By increasing efficiency and reducing costs, this hoshin focus addressed an important need of the employer as customer.

Internal Customers

Responsiveness to internal customers also improved when the hospital addressed timeliness in specific areas. These areas are shortened response time to nurses' shift change reports and mechanics' work orders.

Key Success Factors

The key to Bethesda's success in achieving its hoshin goal for 1991 and 1992 was the organization's ability to:

- Focus on a real organizational need
- Work successfully in teams
- Make data visible
- Gain senior management support and involvement
- Enhance the organizational grounding in TQM

How these achievements were attained is summarized in the following subsections.

Focusing on a Real Organizational Need

Bethesda leaders agree that focusing the hoshin goal on a real organizational need in 1992 primed Bethesda for success. Everyone in the organization understood the need to maintain productivity gains and how this need tied into the bottom line. Alignment of senior management's needs and concerns with the hoshin goal was a factor for success.

Working Successfully on Teams

Leaders agree that teamwork has been key to Bethesda's success. Everyone was a stakeholder because of tightening economic pressures; thus, the need to monitor productivity was a given and was a priority for all hospital members. Because of the desire to avoid layoffs, everyone worked together to learn more about productivity and to monitor it.

Making Data Visible

The effective use of graphics in displaying data is another reason for hoshin success. Because of the improved data reporting system and high levels of training, run charts and other graphs could be created, understood, and utilized by all levels in the organization. Managers and staff were involved in the manual plotting of points on run charts to facilitate understanding. Members of the nursing staff were aware that nursing managers were analyzing the data and using them to make further improvements.

Gaining Senior Management Support and Involvement

The high level of involvement and support from senior management is seen as a key item in Bethesda's success. Oak Hospital's COO was active in plotting run charts, using TQM tools, and being a good role model. By "getting his hands dirty," he was able to experience barriers that front-line managers dealt with in gathering standardized data and thus was able to understand the significance of hospital systems. The COO cites the importance of other management levels having ownership in the hoshin process. The Quality 1 steering committee members were key to success through educating their managers on quality tools and facilitating the hoshin effort.

Enhancing the Organizational Grounding in TQM

Bethesda had a TQM background before initiating hoshin. The work done on pilot projects, initial efforts at daily management, and substantial training in TQM tools and processes gave the organization the TQM grounding that was necessary for success. For example, TQM education had introduced managers to the 7QC tools prior to hoshin implementation. Just-in-time training for hoshin deployment provided a hands-on experience for them to apply the tools learned.

Problems and Challenges

The challenges faced by Bethesda, Inc., in implementing its hoshin centered on three areas. These were an inappropriate data system, the lack of formal reviews, and organizational priorities (such as restructuring) that interrupted the hoshin timetable.

Inappropriate Data System

During 1991 the hoshin effort was hindered by the lack of effective and timely data and the lack of standardized use of data. Bethesda responded in 1992 by spending six months on selecting effective data, improving data distribution, and standardizing data use in both hospitals. North Hospital's COO acknowledges that no system can perfectly identify what to measure; nonetheless, Bethesda was willing to move ahead using less-than-perfect (but effective) data. Starting with one measure-adjusted patient day the organization had, by the beginning of 1993, moved to adjusted admissions. By the end of the year, the productivity measurement had become a mainstay in the system to adjust operations to volume.

With assistance from the management engineering staff, information and reporting in this area are now standardized and problems of quality and timeliness of data have been resolved. Some units that initially thought variable staffing would be impossible were able to change and adopt the practice once the data became visible.

Lack of Formal Reviews

The lack of formal reviews, especially during 1992, was a deterrent to success that affected the organization's ability to identify and solve problems and remove system barriers. Without formal reviews, departmental improvement opportunities that might have been integrated systemwide were missed. Without formal reviews in 1992, no data were available on the hoshin process that could have documented overall deployment needs. Alignment was achieved, but the power of hoshin planning in revealing key system improvement opportunities was left untapped. The development and initiation of a formal review process has redressed this inadequacy.

Time Out for Restructuring

The restructuring of the Bethesda system in 1994 put formal hoshin planning efforts on hold, but the power of the process to achieve results has been demonstrated over several years. The steering committee plans to reinstate the process once restructuring has been completed.

Roles and Responsibilities

Hoshin planning and implementation has meant new roles and responsibilities for hospital leaders, managers, and staff.

The CEO

The key role of Bethesda's CEO was to initiate the process and to help in selecting the focus, or theme. He supports the implementation in his role as leader of the Quality 1 steering committee. He continues to be involved in monitoring the plans and reviewing results. The CEO ensures that the resources are available for training in the use of the tools for hoshin deployment and for facilitator support for the organizationwide process.

Oak Hospital and North Hospital COOs

The COOs of Oak and North hospitals assert that their roles in hoshin planning were to focus the efforts of the two hospitals. Specifically, they worked to keep the responsibilities of the nursing, technical and professional, and support services departments at both hospitals on track. Once these roles were outlined, the COO role was to lead the hoshin efforts at each hospital. The Oak Hospital COO states that the biggest change in his job since hoshin implementation has been "focusing on nitty-gritty stuff at a high level." Having the COO involved in decisions (for example, what to measure) has helped Bethesda achieve its results.

The Oak Hospital COO also was very visible in his role as hoshin champion, for example, by becoming involved with training in quality tools and maintaining high visibility in his use of these tools. Run charts were posted in his office, and he was involved in the plotting of these charts to facilitate understanding.

The North Hospital COO's job changed when he became involved in a hoshin pilot project to improve surgery. The job changed as he worked more as a team member, was involved in greater communication, and worked toward a shared sense of purpose within the hospital.

Vice-President of TQM and Corporate Education

As head coach of the hoshin effort, the vice-president of TQM and corporate education worked with senior management of both hospitals in the initial design, planning of rollout, and identification of changes that would be necessary to implement hoshin planning. This upfront work was necessary for success, especially with the 1992 goal.

Because her overall goal was to encourage the implementation of TQM across the whole organization, the vice-president focused her time heavily on developing approaches to educate managers in hoshin planning methods and on the goals selected by the hospitals. She coached the steering committee on deployment strategy and led the team of Quality 1 facilitators who worked with the two hospitals. The vice-president's staff developed training in QC and MP tools for all managers.

Clinical Leader

At Bethesda Oak Hospital, the role of the vice-president of patient services has been to work with her division's staff to meet the yearly hoshin goals. She was instrumental in creating employee awareness of *why* they were making the necessary changes, so that they could better understand the importance of their jobs and how the organization was working together toward a common goal.[9]

The vice-president of patient services has also been responsible for coordination between departments. She worked to ensure that all departments work in tandem to meet the division's goal. Catchball was used early on to establish yearly goals for each department. Specifically, the vice-president was responsible for meeting her division's target to keep the organization's productivity at 8 percent. Awareness of how the patient services goals fit into Bethesda's hoshin plan has been effective in helping the vice-president and her staff meet their goals.

Lessons Learned

Reflecting on their years of experience with hoshin planning, the Bethesda leaders found that they have learned some key lessons that they would share with others who are going to begin hoshin planning. These include study of the process, focus on real business goals, and integration with daily management.

Prepare for Using Hoshin

The CEO of Bethesda, Inc., believes that hoshin is an outstanding focus methodology and that it promotes understanding of what is truly important at any particular time. To maximize its value, he advises spending time up front to learn what hoshin is and what it can do. Further, the CEO urges leaders to choose a measurable issue as their theme and to benchmark both before and after deployment.

Align the Focus with Real Goals

The hoshin focus should align with the real and politically correct goals of the organization – "something that senior management is concerned with and is wringing their hands over." Bethesda leaders caution organizations against making the hoshin focus something they *believe* they should pursue but have little heartfelt interest in focusing on. Bethesda's success in meeting its hoshin goal reflects this connection and, furthermore, has been fundamental to the organization's successful threefold goal of meeting the budget, preserving staff employment, and ensuring the organization's future.

Establish Daily Management First

Oak Hospital's COO believes that if a good daily management system with an interlinking measurement system had been in place prior to initiating hoshin planning, the hospitals would have been more capable of maintaining and improving the hoshin effort. The organization defines daily management as a solid understanding of process improvement, well-defined core processes, and well-positioned good measures.

The vice-president of TQM and corporate education believes that an organization can use the hoshin concept of focusing on a few key objectives and measuring key areas early on. However, a good daily management system needs to be in place first so as to successfully deploy hoshin planning.

Apply TQM to Real Work

Another lesson learned by the COOs was that the hospitals were able to use hoshin to transfer the Quality 1 (TQM) effort from a *program* to a working management *process*. In this manner, hoshin was a way to accomplish the "real work" of avoiding another layoff. They have found that there is an obvious need to have systems improvement and that hoshin as a part of TQM is successful partially because it is data-driven. As a data-based process, hoshin allows people to understand data, which leads to buy-in of the data. Familiarity with measures leads to changes in behavior.

Use Understanding of Why Hoshin Is Being Done to Achieve Alignment

To stress how important the role of alignment is to hoshin success, the North Hospital COO related the story of a support services department manager who was very excited about hoshin planning. The manager had always tried to do what was expected of him, but it made a tremendous difference in his motivation to know *why* he was doing it. Knowing the hospital's goals and how important his department's role was in reaching those goals delighted the manager.

Expect Initial Skepticism from Clinical Staff

Clinical leaders should expect initial skepticism from staff members being introduced to hoshin planning. The attitude that "this is no different from what we've been doing" will subside, however, once people see the power of hoshin in focusing on one priority. Leaders should be patient and help staff use the visual graphics that show the advantages of hoshin deployment. A hospital undertaking hoshin might look to nursing for leadership, because nursing has traditionally established annual goals and has established mechanisms for effective deployment and follow-through.

Seize the Opportunity for Major Change

Bethesda's vice-president for TQM and corporate education believes that the changing health care environment may be conducive to clinical and community applications of hoshin planning. Organizational change is a must. The necessity for rapid change in health care overall should be viewed as an occasion to use hoshin planning to create the breakthrough changes that will be expected by future customers.

References

1. Joint Commission on Accreditation of Healthcare Organizations. *Striving Toward Improvement.* Oakbrook Terrace, IL: JCAHO, 1992.
2. Kennedy, M. Using hoshin planning in total quality management: an interview with Gerry Kaminski and Casey Collett. *Journal on Quality Improvement* 20(10):577–81, Oct. 1994.
3. JCAHO, 1994.
4. JCAHO, 1994.
5. Gerry Kaminski, vice-president of TQM and corporate education, Bethesda, Inc. Interview by Dona Hotopp, Jan. 25, 1994. (Also subsequent quotes.)
6. L. Thomas Wilburn, Jr., CEO, Bethesda, Inc. Interview by Dona Hotopp, July 1994.
7. William F. Groneman, senior vice-president and COO, Bethesda Oak Hospital. Interview by Dona Hotopp, Jan. 31, 1994. (Also subsequent quotes.)
8. Jim Connelly, senior vice-president and COO, Bethesda North Hospital. Interview by Dona Hotopp, Mar. 8, 1994. (Also subsequent quotes.)
9. Linda Schaffner, vice-president of patient services, Bethesda, Inc. Interview by Dona Hotopp, Jan. 31, 1994. (Also subsequent quotes.)

CHAPTER ELEVEN

Our Lady of Lourdes Medical Center

Dona Hotopp and Owen McNally

Poverty, infant mortality, school drop-out rates, and drug and alcohol abuse in Camden, New Jersey, all soar high above the state and national averages. Camden has been designated by the state as a New Jersey health professional shortage area, one whose problems go beyond the medical arena. In this setting, Our Lady of Lourdes Medical Center is committed to providing health care and to extending the healing mission of Jesus to the city and to all of southern New Jersey.

Our Lady of Lourdes Medical Center is a catalyst in this community, which is actively fighting the battle to raise the quality of life for its residents. The vision of Lourdes confirms this dedication to high-quality health care and community improvement:

> To be a Franciscan center of holistic healing excellence, a provider of quality patient and family-centered healthcare promotion services, a catalyst and major participant in the revitalization of the City of Camden, a national healthcare leader in community benefit and community activities.

The 375-bed tertiary care medical center hospital opened its doors in 1950 and today serves as the regional center in four areas: cardiac diagnosis and surgery, dialysis and transplantation, perinatal care, and rehabilitation. Lourdes is proud of its school of nursing, its pastoral care department, and the Osborne Family Health Center and Lourdes Wellness Center.

Lourdes maintains an affiliation with the University of Medicine and Dentistry of New Jersey. The medical staff has nearly 400 active members and more than 100 courtesy employees and consultants. Lourdes was a national finalist in the 1992 and 1994 Foster G. McGaw Prize competition, recognizing its achievement in community service and innovation in expanding access to health care.

Reasons for Choosing Hoshin Planning

Our Lady of Lourdes defines its hoshin plan as "a fact-driven, structured process that focuses on improvement opportunities and key system bottlenecks; plans and develops capability-driven breakthrough objectives and action plans; and deploys them to all levels of the medical center."[1] The CEO maintains that the focus on key system bottlenecks is an important part of Our Lady of Lourdes' hoshin plan.[2] Even if it is for a joyous occasion such as having a baby, being in the hospital is a stressful time for both patients and their families. Streamlining and simplifying processes can help eliminate unnecessary stresses.

The leadership at Our Lady of Lourdes Medical Center became interested in hoshin planning for four major reasons:

1. To increase Lourdes' availability to help more people by reducing length of stay (LOS)
2. To move toward a customer focus
3. To implement fully the TQM philosophy
4. To link the strategic plan to operations

Each of these motivators is discussed in the following sections.

Increase Service Availability by Reducing Length of Stay

The most immediate and direct influence on Lourdes' decision to adopt hoshin planning was the bed availability problem that the organization was facing. Lourdes was turning away patients in the early part of 1991. With a shortage of available beds, especially in cardiac services, emergency department personnel were regularly forced to send patients to other hospitals. During this same period, referring physicians could not always admit their patients when needed. The leadership at Lourdes determined that it was imperative to meet the needs of cardiac patients and referring physicians. The leaders, having studied the concepts of hoshin planning and having recognized its potential to focus organizational improvement efforts, initiated hoshin planning to focus on solving this availability problem.

Move toward a Customer Focus

A second motivator for hoshin planning was Our Lady of Lourdes' emphasis on addressing the needs of customers as a consistent operating principle. Customer focus ensures that everyone in the organization understands the real needs of all groups that receive its services. Customer needs then become the center of organizational activity.

From the initial stages of TQM implementation, Lourdes focused on its key customers: patients, physicians, referring physicians, third-party payers, and employees. It analyzed and prioritized the needs of each group and identified 14 important customer needs (as discussed later in the chapter). However, in 1991 an action plan for meeting those needs had not yet been identified. Lourdes' strategic plan had been developed before these customer needs were well defined. Hoshin planning was viewed as a way to take the newly identified needs and wants of customers and merge them with the strategic plan already in place. The hoshin planning process would address both customers and strategy.

Implement the TQM Philosophy

The third major impetus for hoshin planning was the recognized need for full implementation of TQM. Our Lady of Lourdes Medical Center has adopted the GOAL/QPC implementation model for TQM as a holistic approach to organizational improvement. (See the GOAL/QPC Wheel in figure 2-3, p. 18.) This approach includes educating managers on how to use TQM tools in their daily management activities and demonstrating how efficient and effective it can be to use cross-functional management processes to address certain issues. To apply all aspects of its chosen TQM philosophy, leadership began to explore hoshin planning as a way to integrate quality, strategy, and business objectives.

Link the Strategic Plan to Operations

One of the management practices that had been very successful at Lourdes was the use of the strategic plan by department managers as the basis for their annual plans and budgets. In 1991 the strategic plan had seven goals, with multiple objectives for each goal. Managers found it difficult to know which objectives were most important for the coming year. Leadership recognized hoshin planning as a way to help department managers focus on the most important actions to accomplish strategic goals.

Hoshin Implementation

In May 1991 the medical center held a three-day retreat, facilitated by an experienced hoshin planning trainer, to initiate hoshin planning and select a breakthrough focus. The quality steering committee, composed of the CEO and 13 hospital vice-presidents, was joined by the planning department staff, four medical chiefs, and other physicians. These 25 persons possessed both the knowledge to form the plan and the leadership positions to make it happen. This same group held a one-day retreat in August that year to finalize the hoshin targets and establish teams to gather data and determine means to accomplish the targets.

Choosing the Organization's Focus

Leaders at Our Lady of Lourdes prepared for the three-day retreat to choose a focus by reviewing the strategic plan, identifying critical processes, and reassessing the external customer requirements (figure 11-1) identified in earlier stages of TQM implementation. Lourdes had no vision statement at this time, so the strategic plan and mission were used as starting points to develop vision elements.

May 1991: Three-Day Retreat

During the retreat, the leadership team used the seven management and planning (7MP) tools to generate the hoshin breakthrough focus. Using the affinity process to brainstorm and group ideas and an interrelationship digraph to identify issues that "drive" others, the team identified continuous service quality improvement as the key vision element. Using additional tools and relating breakthrough options to the strategic plan and critical processes, the team identified clinical quality improvement as a key breakthrough element. Prioritization matrixes, which clarify and quantify criteria for making decisions, were used to relate clinical improvements to both clinical and

Figure 11-1. Key Customer Demands

Physicians and Referring Physicians	Patient	Payers
• State-of-the-art equipment • Trained and competent staff • Ease of scheduling • Adequate specialty services • Communication on patient progress	• Good outcome results • Staff sensitivity to my needs • Clean and safe atmosphere and surroundings • Better food services	• Regulation and control of the industry • More predictable and competitive prices • One-stop shopping as marketing technique • Control cost through utilization • Faster return to the workplace

nonclinical needs of customers. The leaders were convinced that though these needs are often thought to be mutually exclusive, in reality their integration was imperative for success. As a result of this analysis, they identified increasing effective capacity as a major way to make progress in the clinical area.

Next, the team identified key breakthrough targets for increasing effective capacity. It used a necessity/feasibility grid to analyze options regarding their necessity to the organization and the feasibility of their implementation. These are the three major areas that fell out as being most feasible and necessary:

1. Physician utilization and quality monitoring
2. Expansion of outpatient services on and off campus
3. Effective management for timely discharge

A project team was working on effective discharge management, and plans to build an ambulatory center had been drawn up. Therefore, the breakthrough target that would give the greatest payback for the energy expended was physician utilization and quality monitoring. This breakthrough target was the outcome of the three-day retreat. (See figure 11-2.) The hoshin objective was then stated as follows: "to expand effective capacity by improving quality monitoring and physician utilization."

Aligning the Organization with the Focus

During the summer of 1991, the leadership team held monthly sessions with department heads to present the hoshin breakthrough objective. Catchball, an interactive

Figure 11-2. Choosing the Focus: Hoshin Generation Flow

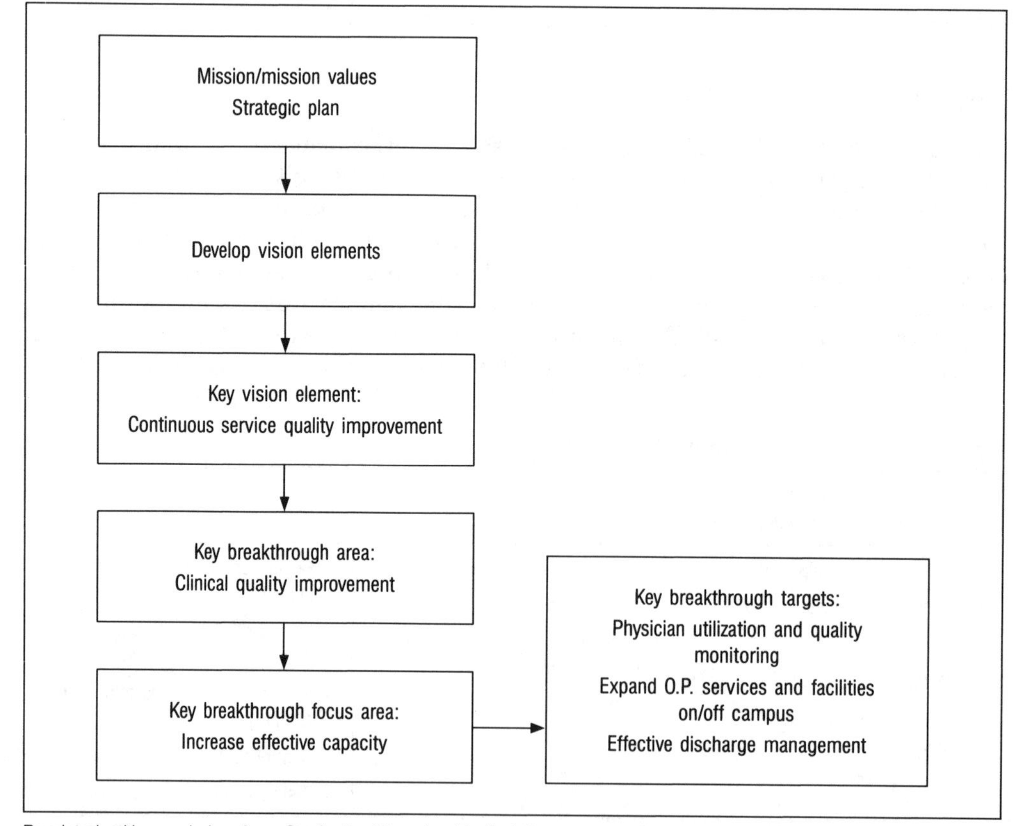

Reprinted, with permission, from Our Lady of Lourdes Medical Center.

back-and-forth communication process between levels, was used to orient and involve department heads. In August 1991 the same 25 medical center leaders met again for a one-day retreat to further develop the hoshin objective.

August 1991: One-Day Retreat

At this retreat, the medical center leaders prioritized four elements as key means for accomplishing the hoshin objective:

- Collection and analysis of quality data
- Reduction of complications affecting LOS
- Standardized practice parameters
- Improved discharge planning

Discharge planning was being addressed by a cross-functional project team, and plans had been made to work on standardizing practice parameters. Therefore, two teams were formed to begin hoshin deployment. The teams were made up of the vice-presidents; the clinical chiefs of cardiology, pathology, and nephrology; and the department heads. One team worked on collection and analysis of quality data, and the other on reduction of complications affecting LOS.

September 1991–February 1992: Hoshin Teamwork

Between September 1991 and February 1992, the two hoshin teams held weekly meetings. They decided to use TQM planning tools to make their goals happen. The teams used one of the 7MP tools, the tree diagram, to break the plan down to assignable tasks.

The first team looked at the data collection processes already in place at Lourdes and tried to identify their capabilities, decide whether any additional data would be necessary, and determine how to design a new system to capture the necessary data and trends. The second team arrived at six major elements affecting LOS:

- Unplanned transfer to special care units
- Adverse drug reactions
- Patient falls
- Failure to act on test results
- Nosocomial infections (infections contracted by patients after hospitalization)
- Equipment issues

By February 1992 the tree diagrams were fairly well developed with each group highlighting the key means for accomplishing the hoshin objective. (See figure 11-3.)

February–May 1992: Data Gathering

The next step involved gathering data to substantiate the assumptions and inferences made. From February to May 1992, the teams collected data in all areas in the existing tree diagram. This led to identification of more than 150 possible hoshin tactics or action items. The exact opposite of what hoshin planning aims to do was happening! Too many action items were suggested, and the group focus was in danger of becoming diluted. Team members became disheartened, believing that the tasks were insurmountable and that, no matter what they did, their efforts would not scratch the surface of what needed to be done.

May–September 1992: Focus and Vision

To compress and align these tactics, Lourdes' CEO met with each vice-president to negotiate a particular focus and responsibility for each division that would positively

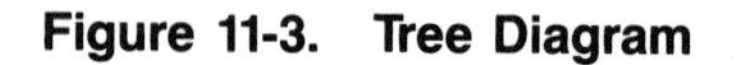

Figure 11-3. Tree Diagram

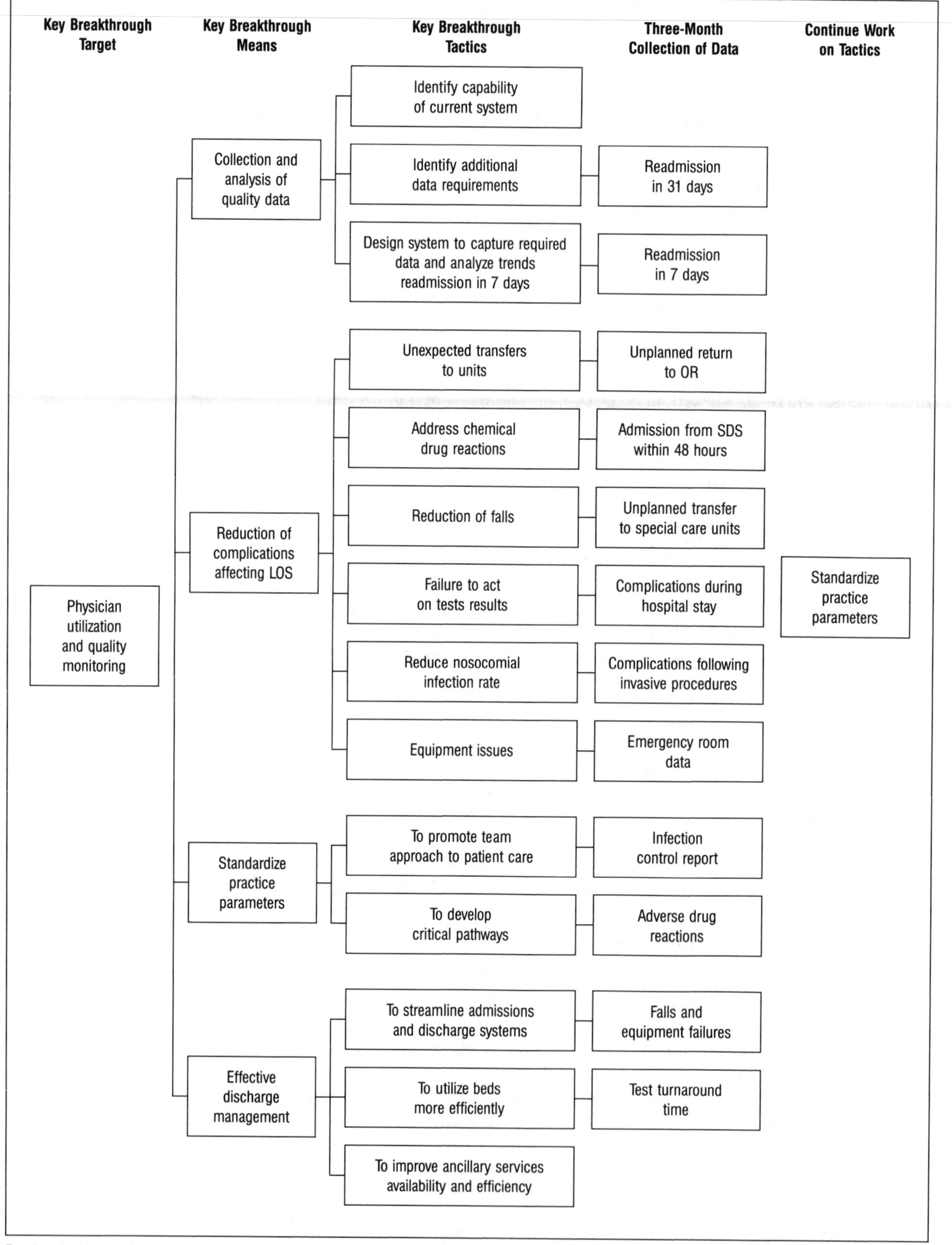
Key Breakthrough Target
Key Breakthrough Means
Key Breakthrough Tactics
Three-Month Collection of Data
Continue Work on Tactics
Physician utilization and quality monitoring
Collection and analysis of quality data
Identify capability of current system
Identify additional data requirements
Readmission in 31 days
Design system to capture required data and analyze trends readmission in 7 days
Readmission in 7 days
Reduction of complications affecting LOS
Unexpected transfers to units
Unplanned return to OR
Address chemical drug reactions
Admission from SDS within 48 hours
Reduction of falls
Unplanned transfer to special care units
Failure to act on tests results
Complications during hospital stay
Reduce nosocomial infection rate
Complications following invasive procedures
Equipment issues
Emergency room data
Standardize practice parameters
To promote team approach to patient care
Infection control report
To develop critical pathways
Adverse drug reactions
Effective discharge management
To streamline admissions and discharge systems
Falls and equipment failures
To utilize beds more efficiently
Test turnaround time
To improve ancillary services availability and efficiency
Standardize practice parameters

affect the organizational hoshin. At the same time, the breakthrough goal (hoshin) statement was enhanced as follows: "to expand effective capacity through reduction of length of stay by improving quality monitoring and physician utilization."

In a parallel activity to developing the focus, leadership at Lourdes developed the organization's vision using catchball with department heads and employees. The hoshin retreats provided data for vision development and the consensus that an articulated vision was needed, generated with the participation of employees, managers, and physician leaders. Affinity charts, tree diagrams, and criteria matrixes provided the catchball tools to gather and display input from all levels of the organization. The TQM steering committee finalized the vision statement in July 1992. Committee members personally communicated the vision and the alignment of the hoshin planning process with the vision to all employees.

In September 1992 a third management retreat was held to regroup and create the focused activity needed to accomplish the hoshin. At this retreat, tactics were grouped and prioritized into twelve organizationwide objectives:

- Identify and reduce adverse drug reactions.
- Optimize patient placement in appropriate nursing unit.
- Reduce incidence of preventable nosocomial infections.
- Increase availability and efficiency of ancillary services.
- Identify capabilities of current quality assurance (QA) data system.
- Implement related tactics affecting LOS, such as critical paths, reduction of lab utilization, and managed care.
- Reduce incidents of falls.
- Reduce failure to act on test results.
- Optimize utilization of equipment.
- Identify additional data requirement.
- Benchmark progress/communicate results.
- Design systems to capture required data and analyze trends.

Implementing the Plan and Monitoring Progress

The vice-presidents and medical chiefs endorsed the twelve organizationwide objectives in the foregoing list. Next they assumed leadership responsibilities as chronicled below.

November–July 1992: Catchball and Hoshin Implementation

Through catchball with their departments and communication with one another, the VPs and clinical chiefs determined:

- Time lines
- Proposed completion dates
- Anticipated outcomes
- Measures for each organizationwide objective

They then developed their division objectives, or "action items." They generated from 3 to 13 division objectives for each organizationwide objective, many with numerical goals. The CEO and the director of TQM coordinated the objectives through division-level communication and coordination of the plan. Tree diagrams and data display tools (such as run charts, Pareto diagrams, matrixes, and bar graphs) were used to develop and monitor the plans. In this way, departments were able to visually trace their actions to the hoshin objective. (See figure 11-4.)

Figure 11-4. Cause-and-Effect (Fishbone) Diagram

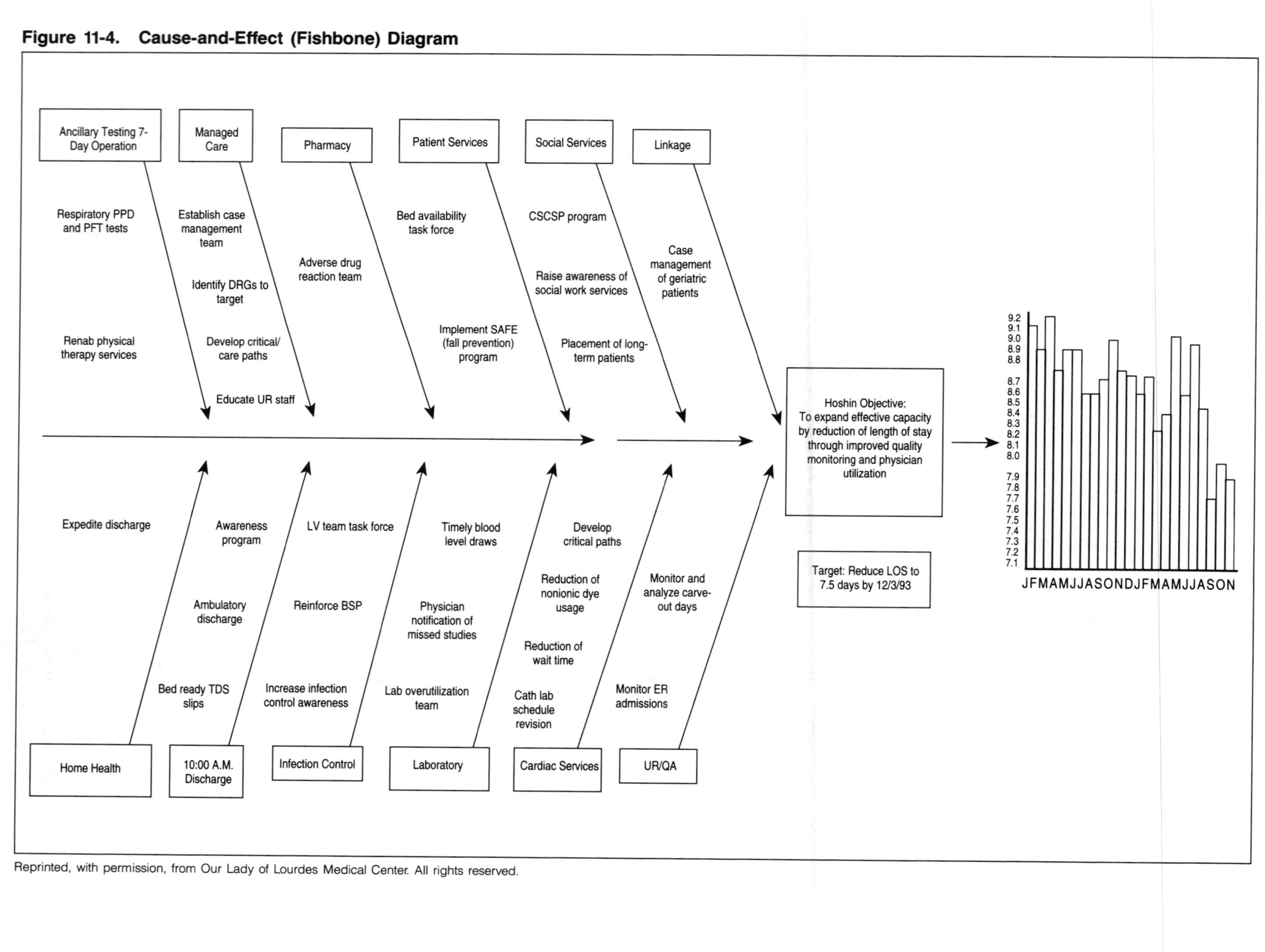

July–December 1993: Implementation and Monitoring

The director of TQM assisted the vice-presidents and medical chiefs by educating the staff in hoshin methods and tools. The TQM steering committee reviewed and improved hoshin deployment at its monthly meetings throughout 1993. In July the committee added a numerical target to the hoshin: to reduce the average length of stay to 7.5 days by December 31, 1993.

Implementation proceeded at various rates of speed. Cardiac services began with a running start, whereas some departments took almost all of 1993 to gather data, generate their means, and clear other agendas in order to actually begin deployment. In many instances, divisions or departments formed cross-functional teams to accomplish their objectives. Work proceeded at the division level throughout 1993.

Review and Improvement

A key method for alignment, coordination, and review was a quarterly hoshin update meeting.

July 1993–March 1994: Review

At the quarterly meetings, the CEO, vice-presidents, and clinical chiefs reviewed progress on three aspects of implementation: quarterly results, the level of involvement of everyone in each department in achieving the results, and visibility through the use of quality tools. For consistency and visibility, in addition to the quality tools, a reporting format was suggested, as shown in figure 11-5. The chart in figure 11-6 was displayed to make the entire deployment process visible and to record overall results.

The review in early 1994 began with an annual review of the entire process for 1993. With their staff, hoshin leaders reviewed results, process, visibility, and plans for 1994 improvements. They brought reviewed data to a hoshin update meeting, and this information was used to create the 1994 hoshin plan. In addition to defining a new hoshin objective, the director of TQM used this opportunity to link the learnings and infrastructure of hoshin planning to improving the overall planning process. Vice-presidents were asked how they could use the hoshin process to deploy more of the strategic plan to fully integrate the hoshin planning process with all the specific strategic objectives of the medical center. Hoshin planning was also integrated into the newly adopted hospitalwide performance improvement plan.

Overall Benefits and Results

Lourdes has enjoyed many benefits from its hoshin planning efforts. Advantages have been in the form of quantifiable results and "soft-side" benefits.

Measures of Success

The hoshin planning process has had a positive effect on the entire medical center. Two divisions in particular have made significant progress and have seen tangible results: cardiac and pathology services.

Organizationwide Results

The most concrete measure of success is the reduction in length of stay, as illustrated in figure 11-7 (p. 162). Lourdes' success for 1993 is measured in three ways:

- *The 1.7-day reduction in length of stay:* In 1992, the average LOS was 9.3 days, which decreased to 8.3 days by March 1993 and was down to 7.6 by the end of 1993.
- *The $3 million savings on a $120 million budget:* All the hoshin teams focused on appropriate utilization of resources. For example, the lab team alone saw annual savings of $60,000 due to reduction of Chem 12 and Chem 20 tests.
- *The issuance of a $500 cash award to each employee as a result of these successes:* The CEO and the president of Lourdes aligned the award with the hoshin and thanked all staff members for showing fiscal responsibility, working well together as a team to provide high-quality care, and accomplishing the total quality improvement initiative.[3]

Another organizationwide hoshin measure is the 10:00 A.M. discharge time. The percentage of patients discharged by 10:00 A.M. increased from 16 percent to 34 percent from 1991 to 1993.

Cardiac Services Results

Lourdes has focused on cardiac services as a key area because of the high volume, complexity of cases, high cost, inability to service referral networks of the cardiologists, and impact on length of stay. Through hoshin planning, cardiac services enjoyed the following results:

- *An overall decrease in LOS,* from 9.48 days in the second quarter of 1992 to 7.06 days in the fourth quarter of 1993. Cardiac services continuously cared for a greater number of cases using fewer total patient days, as displayed in the run chart in figure 11-8 (p. 162).
- *The adoption of three critical pathways in cardiology,* one for cardiac catheterization and two for congestive heart failure (CHF). After the successes of these initial pathways, a critical pathways oversight committee was set up to coordinate the development and implementation of critical pathways hospitalwide. Critical pathways not only streamline services for patients so they have a better idea of what to expect, but also increase efficiency through use of the best methodologies for caring for a particular type of patient. By early 1994, development of five additional pathways had been initiated. During 1994, the development of five additional pathways was initiated, namely chronic obstructionary pulmonary disease, hip fracture with surgical repair, pneumonia, and open-heart surgery with and without catheterization. A case manager process is presently being developed. It is anticipated that the pathways will be used as road maps

Figure 11-5. Hoshin Reporting Format

Indicator	Current Quarter	Prior Quarter	Year to Date	Goal or Benchmark	Statistical Significance	Comments
Hospital-acquired infections	5%	3.5%	4%	3%	<	Increase in bacteremias
Angioplasty success rate	92%	90%	90%	95%	>	QI effort continuing

Figure 11-6. Hoshin Process Flow and Time Line

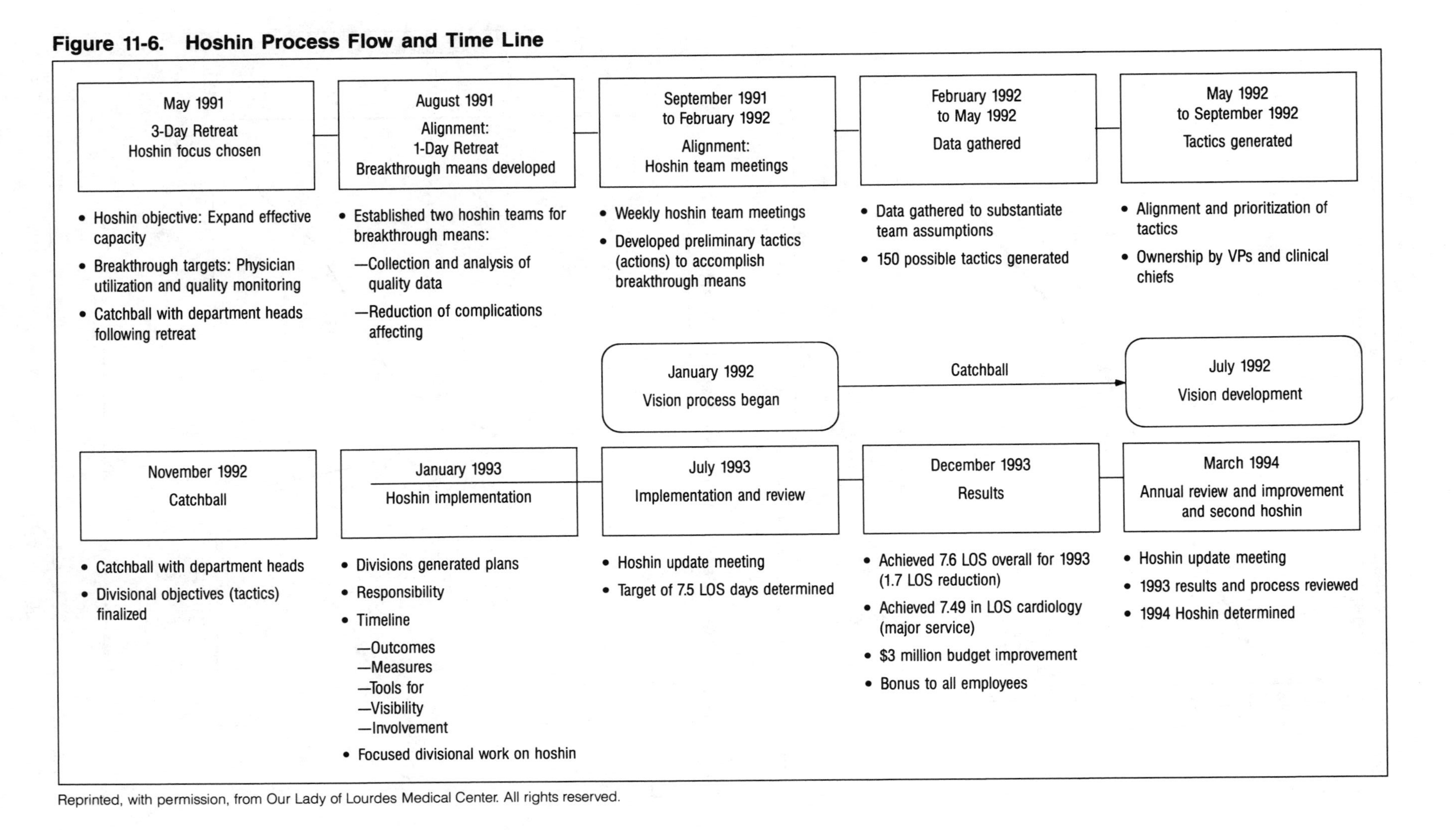

Reprinted, with permission, from Our Lady of Lourdes Medical Center.

Figure 11-7. LOS Reduction

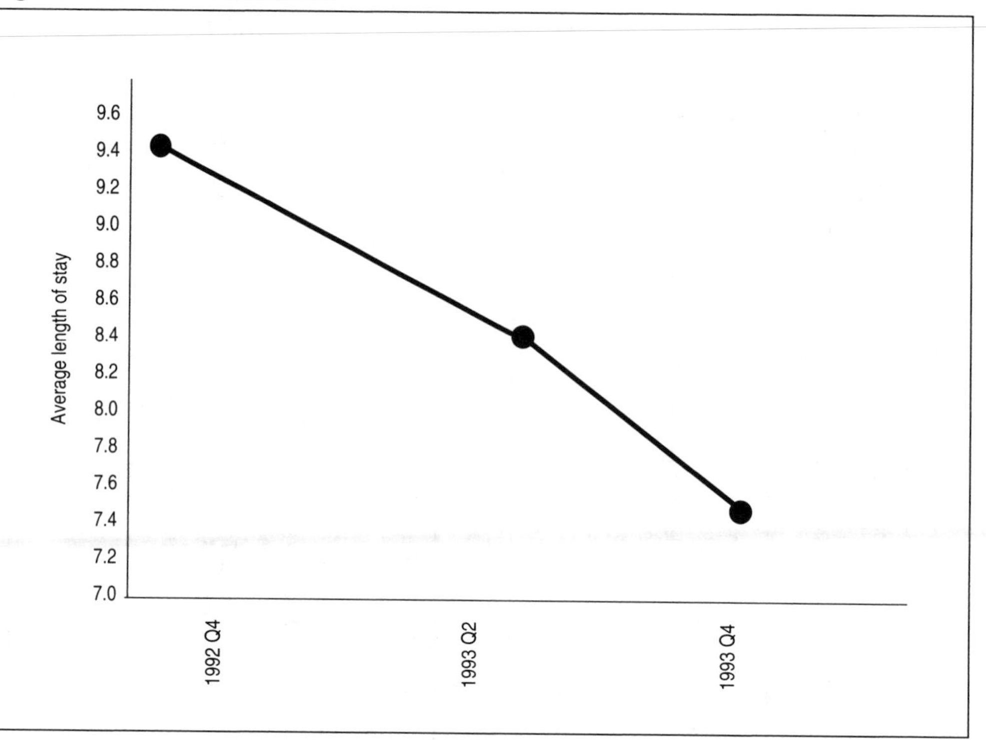

Reprinted, with permission, from Our Lady of Lourdes Medical Center.

Figure 11-8. Cardiac Cases and Patient Days by Quarter

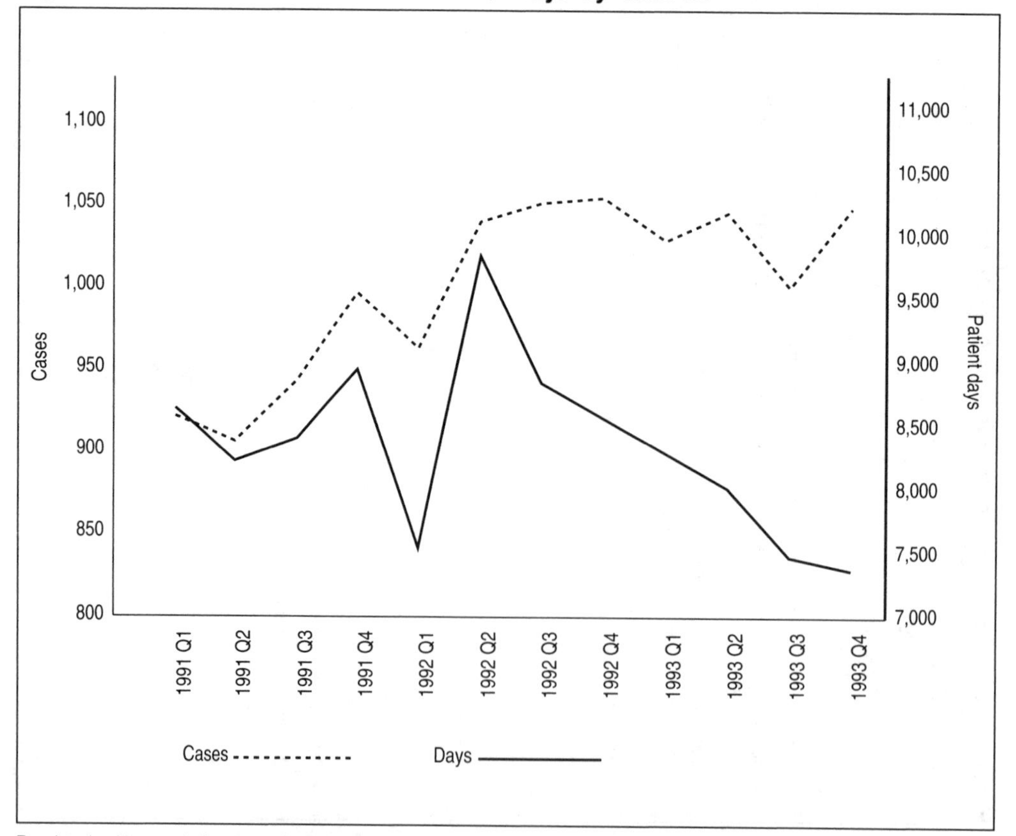

Reprinted, with permission, from Our Lady of Lourdes Medical Center.

for the case manager for quality of care and for resource utilization. Information systems are being developed to ensure that quality monitoring accompanies the case management process by tracking quality indicators such as readmission rates.

- *A decrease in the use of low osmolality contrast agent (LOCA),* from 49.4 percent in the first quarter of 1992 to 16.6 percent in the fourth quarter of 1992, saving $43,500 in 1992–20 percent of the 1991 cost–during a year in which the number of procedures increased. The use of nonionic dye decreased from 49.5 percent in 1992 to between 16 and 17 percent as of November 1993.
- *A decrease in the number of patients having to wait for stress tests,* from 76.2 percent in April 1992 to 20.7 percent by April 1993.

The cardiac services unit continues to monitor these and other projects, while constantly working on standardization of testing and procedures.[4]

Pathology Services Results

Lourdes' pathology division focused on the overutilization of laboratory services, with the following results:

- *A decrease in the number of tests ordered by physicians:* The TQM team charged with addressing the issue of lab overutilization discovered that physicians routinely order either a Chem 12 or a Chem 20 test for inpatients, even though both yield a lot more information than physicians typically use. It is much less expensive to order the specific analyses (for example, potassium or glucose) of a Chem 20. Consequently, with the approval of the laboratory's medical director and the vice-president for medical affairs (both physicians), the team eliminated the routine use of Chem 12 and Chem 20 tests for inpatients.[5] By considering which tests were needed for which diagnoses, a decrease was achieved in the number of hematology and coagulation tests ordered.

  The number of tests ordered decreased an average of 43 percent between April and September 1992 and April and September 1993. The chief of pathology estimated that this saved the hospital nearly $60,000.
- *A reduction in test turnaround time:* Another result of the cross-functional team's work was the establishment of a priority system for ordering tests that worked in conjunction with the 10:00 A.M. discharge effort. If a patient is to be discharged, the lab can now use this system to make sure that the necessary blood count tests are returned in time to ensure a 10:00 A.M. discharge.
- *An increase in physician awareness and involvement:* As a result of the hoshin work, physicians are now more aware of how reducing laboratory utilization helps improve the bottom line at the hospital and how important the laboratory is to accommodating physician demands. The chief of pathology notes that physicians now realize that if they can "lessen the burden on the lab," then the lab can give better responses to more urgent requests from the medical staff.

Additional Team Results

Each division or cross-functional hoshin team measured specific objectives in achieving division plans. A selection of these measures is shown in figure 11-9.

Soft-Side Benefits

Organizationwide, soft-side benefits include the following:

- *Awareness of organizational focus and vision:* Organizations need to have a corporate identity so that employees, no matter what their function is in the

Figure 11-9. Hoshin Team Measure

Cross-Functional Team Objective	Measure	Results—Improvement
Reduce time for ancillary tests	Test turnaround time	27.4% improvement—hematology 14.6% improvement—chemistry
Reduce number of canceled surgeries	Surgeries canceled	14%–9% decrease in cancellations
Reduce lateness in OR	Percent of lateness, first case	64% baseline decreased to 15% average
Reduce number of patient falls	Number of falls	Falls decreased by 28%
Increase concurrent reporting of adverse drug reactions	Development/use of tools, consistent measurement	Macro flowchart of system, matrix chart of barriers completed, cause-and-effect diagram initiated
Decrease number of low birth weight	Percent low birth weight	Decrease from 2.2% to 1.6%
Reduce LOS by active participation of rehab nursing staff	Identify problems, implement improvement	More than 50 problems identified, approaches taken, results collected

Reprinted, with permission, from Our Lady of Lourdes Medical Center.

organization, feel a part of the greater whole. Lourdes' CEO believes that 80 percent of employees realize that the organization is focusing on reducing length of stay and know how their jobs relate to this organizational goal. Through working together toward this common goal, Lourdes is more focused and less disjointed, thus increasing employee morale.

- *Increased communication among staff members:* The chief of pathology stated that, although the focus of the team was overutilization in the laboratory, improved communication among nurses, physicians, and lab workers has helped to promote dialogue and, consequently, has resulted in other organizational improvements.
- *Standardized use of graphics:* With the division's capacity problems made visible through graphics, the chief of cardiology noticed that staff members immediately were able to focus on them. As a result, LOS began to drop even prior to the establishment of team procedures and practices. The consistent use of graphics in hoshin deployment as a cohesive force for all improvement activities helped the teams to grasp the problems and track the results of their work.

The director of TQM explains that, although Lourdes may have improved length of stay using another process, it was the soft-side benefits of focus, communication, and alignment that brought a sense of excitement to the medical center.[6]

Alignment of the Medical Center

After three years of hoshin planning, Our Lady of Lourdes is a more aligned organization. Furthermore, the departmental quality management implementation process has become more aligned with existing structures and systems.

Organizationwide Alignment

- *Task forces and teams* that target such areas as drug interaction, infection control, and discharges from the emergency room are weaving the focus on reducing LOS into their specific team efforts.
- *The physicians,* particularly voluntary physicians, have come on board with the hoshin effort. Not only are they aware of the hoshin objective and work to meet

goals, they are also involved in project teams and show an unprecedented interest in TQM and the management efforts of the medical center. Physicians realize that in the current health care environment their practice behaviors will be measured individually, and they now see the hoshin goal of Lourdes as one that other institutions will want them to meet.

- *The vice-presidents and division heads* have also become more aligned and understand how the hoshin plan works as a vehicle for the vision statement. Each division VP worked on a unit vision statement that supports the hospital vision and leadership statements. As a result, leaders in each division understand not only where their division is headed, but also how their leadership style affects division and organizational goals. The director of TQM believes that by having all members of an organization aligned on a future-oriented goal, the organization can move from a reactive to a proactive stance.

Cross-Departmental Alignment

An example of alignment at work can be seen in the efforts necessary to increase the percentage of patients discharged by 10:00 A.M. To improve upon this percentage, information systems, transportation services, environmental services, social services, administration, home health, nurses, and physicians are working together to educate employees and patients on necessary procedures. Presently the team is focusing its efforts on "changing physician practice patterns."

Customer Focus

Our Lady of Lourdes is constantly working on becoming more customer-centered. The hoshin breakthrough target of increasing effective capacity was derived from a need to serve the customer better. Efforts to achieve the 10:00 A.M. discharge goal have focused primarily on the patient but, indirectly, have improved service to internal customers as well.

Through work done by the pathology team on turnaround time, the physicians are now aware of themselves as laboratory customers. Surveys conducted by the laboratory team have heightened this physician-as-customer focus with an open-ended question, "How can the laboratory better serve your needs?" This has helped the laboratory to better serve physician needs.

Key Success Factors

Our Lady of Lourdes Medical Center has achieved the results described through focus, hard work, ongoing education, and the work of hoshin champions. Key success factors are highlighted by the organization's:

- Grounding in TQM
- Enhanced communication channels
- Willingness to use available resources
- Unity of leadership support
- Shared ownership in the TQM process
- Organizational alignment

Key success factors are addressed by leaders at Lourdes:

The CEO describes organizational readiness, the ability of executives and staff to interact in an open manner, the willingness to use available resources and to move forward without waiting for more sophisticated data, and lack of hesitancy by all involved as key success factors. He notes that, because of these factors, Lourdes was willing to dive right into hoshin planning, without waiting for the "perfect situation."

The director of TQM, in charge of the day-to-day implementation of hoshin, believes that success is attributable to the unified support of leadership – the CEO, steering committee, and operational vice-presidents. He also recognizes the importance of communication through monthly and quarterly sessions and the alignment of information services (IS) and hoshin teams. Information requests by hoshin teams became a high priority for IS. The commitment of those involved – the "stick-to-itiveness" of the organization – is another key success factor.

The staff at Lourdes have taken ownership in the TQM process. Team members have accepted responsibility for maintaining team momentum and for spreading the word about what their teams have accomplished. For some employees, TQM has allowed them, for the first time, to participate in a problem-solving process. There are TQM "champions" at Lourdes who, when the enthusiasm slips or people get discouraged, keep the energy high.

The chief of cardiology asserts that the feeling of ownership gained by involving staff in the *how* of making things happen is a critical element. The chief of pathology acknowledges communication and the adaptation by the medical staff to new practices as key success factors within his division.

Problems and Challenges

Obstacles to implementing hoshin at Lourdes can be divided into two categories. The first is organizational hurdles, or those perpetuated by "what has always gone on." The second is hoshin hurdles, or those specific to hoshin implementation. (See figure 11-10.)

Organizational Hurdles

The organizational problems faced by Lourdes stem from two sources. One is the variation in vice-presidential management styles, and the other is the large number of volunteer physicians on staff.

Figure 11-10. Hurdles in Implementing Hoshin

Hurdles	Countermeasures
1. Difficulty of leadership focus	• Holding a series of management retreats • Utilizing visible exercises and data display • Building on the strategic plan and findings of customer analysts to focus problems
2. Team time commitment	• Recognition of team results • Administrative appreciation of team efforts • Increased staff awareness of how they fit with the strategic plan
3. Need for education	• Director of TQM focuses on education • Keeping education in Lourdes' budget
4. Large number of volunteer physicians	• Up-front TQM and hoshin planning education • Data display, visible graphics • Development of critical pathways

Reprinted, with permission, from Our Lady of Lourdes Medical Center.

- *Variation in vice-presidential management styles:* This variation is countered by monthly meetings with the director of TQM as he works to motivate the VPs to find parameters for their work and new styles of managing their divisions. The director has helped the vice-presidents to realize that although their divisions are independent, all of the vice-presidents and their staff work toward the same hoshin objective. The group has also come to realize that if all parts do not function well independently, they cannot function as a whole.
- *Large number of volunteer physicians on staff:* The structure of Lourdes, which relies on a large volunteer physician community, has posed a hurdle to hoshin implementation. Education on hoshin tools, research and display of data, and the development of critical pathways, however, have given Lourdes the buy-in to hoshin planning needed from volunteer physicians.

Hoshin-Specific Hurdles

The leaders at Our Lady of Lourdes have had to deal with four challenges specific to the hoshin implementation process. These are the need for education, the compilation and synthesis of huge stores of data, team time commitment, and the difficulty of attaining leadership focus.

- *Need for education:* The lack of an adequate teaching staff and the need for ongoing education have been addressed through:
  - Keeping education in the hospital budget
  - Having the director of TQM focus his efforts on the staff education
- *Compilation and synthesis of huge stores of data:* While a large store of data resides in the medical center's information systems, very often teams were not familiar with the kind of data that are stored or did not have individual access to the data. As a result data were often gathered manually that could be accessed electronically. This issue is being addressed as part of 1995 hoshin practice.
- *Team time commitment:* At the beginning, many of the same people were involved in working with multiple project teams. As the number of project teams and hoshin teams has expanded, administration and department heads made efforts to involve different people from all levels on the new teams. To ensure the time commitment required for successful implementation of a hoshin plan, Lourdes focused on recognizing the results of team efforts, that is, letting team members know that hospital leadership appreciated their hoshin efforts. Personal satisfaction on the part of staff and their knowledge of how they fit within the strategic plan eased the pain of demands made on their time.
- *Difficulty of attaining leadership focus:* The CEO describes the focusing effort as a hurdle at Lourdes and recognizes the challenge of "getting your hands around" the hoshin. It has been a problem, he also notes, getting a group of senior executives to agree on what is important. A series of retreats that incorporate visible exercises and data display, build on the completed strategic plan, and promote the quality function deployment (QFD) process have helped bring the problem down to a workable size.[7]

Roles and Responsibilities

The design and implementation of hoshin planning have required changes in the roles and responsibilities of executives, physicians, and staff. Specific changes on the part of the CEO, daily managers, and clinical leaders are summarized below.

The CEO

Lourdes' CEO describes his role in hoshin planning as one of leadership. He acts as a coach, helping the organization maneuver through an unfamiliar process. By maintaining high visibility at meetings, retreats, and in his daily work, he is able to make the organization aware of his commitment to hoshin. As CEO, he is also responsible for convincing the administration that a planning process that encompasses breakthrough thinking and hoshin planning is indeed necessary. He met with each vice-president of the medical center to negotiate specific tactics that each department would assume and has also tied capital budgeting to hoshin implementation.

The CEO's job has changed at Our Lady of Lourdes Medical Center. The responsibility has changed from creating a plan to securing the buy-in, education, and communication necessary for the hoshin plan to succeed. More and more of the CEO's job is to make sure everyone understands what hoshin planning is and to provide the communication needed for everyone in the organization to know where Lourdes is headed.

"Daily Manager" of Hoshin Planning

The director of TQM states that to administer hoshin well would be almost a full-time job. In his day-to-day management of the hoshin planning process at Lourdes, he has found his role to be one of educator of executives and staff in the basics of hoshin planning. In addition, he works with the vice-presidents on their visions and holds monthly meetings with each of them to act as coach, facilitator, and cheerleader. He coordinates the data gathering and review process. The TQM director says that because of hoshin planning his job has changed, in that another level of complexity has been added. He sums up his role as one of adding value through the successful results of his work on hoshin.

Clinical Leaders

The chiefs of cardiology and pathology agree that their role in their divisions' hoshin has been that of day-to-day leader and coach. The cardiology chief's work on critical pathways is directly linked to the hoshin work of the cardiac unit. His responsibilities include determining what information needs to be gathered, working with cardiologists to process data, and providing positive feedback to employees. He has been successful in his role as leader, in part he says, because of the ability of physicians to respond to data. For example, his research and data presentations (analysis and literature) on the number of tests ordered and the cost-effectiveness of using ionic dye allowed physicians to follow the guidelines set up by the team. The policy change was well received.

The chief of pathology's role in his division also includes day-to-day interaction with medical and laboratory staff. He reports that his job has been "an easy task" and that he thoroughly enjoyed the opportunity to work as a team for improvement with the laboratory personnel and the nurses and staff out on the floors.

Lessons Learned

As a result of the hoshin planning study at Our Lady of Lourdes Medical Center, the four leaders can offer an array of advice for an organization about to embark on hoshin planning. Due to space constraints, only five are included here.

Start Early

An organization should "jump into hoshin planning as soon as possible, so all can know where the organization needs to make breakthroughs." Directly after its first quality pilot projects begin, an organization should use hoshin planning to find an organizational focus. Then TQM can be utilized to achieve the results necessary for real transformation. By jumping into hoshin planning early in TQM implementation, the organization can break the barrier of inertia or a poor-quality culture and increase vertical alignment.

Provide Ample Hoshin Education

Prior to involving department managers, provide more education on the hoshin planning process and tools. Education will clarify managers' roles and help them realize that change can happen only with their cooperation.

On the clinical side, focus on early education for physicians on the use of quality tools in hoshin planning. Include proper laboratory utilization guidelines early in the training so that physicians will learn correct procedures and a uniform set of rules and regulations for lab use.

Involve as Many People as Possible

Look for areas within your hospital or division that evidence a particular problem; then develop a team and "attack." Involve as many people in the process as possible, because it is easier to generate buy-in if staff have played a part in developing the projected change. Along with staff empowerment, develop a division focus on specifics. Identifying a specific program and quantifying your current level of production with specific measurements expedites the ability for all to monitor improvement.

Make the Results Visible

It is extremely important to communicate results visibly. For example, post a graphic bulletin board in every department highlighting successes, focus areas, and the work of hoshin teams. Or, hold frequent, high-visibility celebrations. As the director of TQM stresses, "You can't take progress for granted."

Become a Vision-Centered Organization

Hoshin planning at Our Lady of Lourdes Medical Center has been "a method for accomplishing a vision-driven transformation," according to the CEO. As the catalyst for creating a vision, hoshin planning enabled Lourdes to gain employee consensus on the future direction and priorities of the organization. The momentum has changed from operating from the strategic plan to being a vision-centered organization. The director of TQM notes that "prior to hoshin planning, departments may have worked at cross-purposes," but that now "we have a better sense of unity, and the organization is moving forward together. That creates cultural change."

The CEO summarizes his realization of hoshin planning as a driver for improvement: The "real power of TQM starts here [hoshin planning], because it creates something called vertical alignment–the understanding of everyone in the organization of what the organization is working on. Once everyone is focusing on a common goal, there are no limits to what can be achieved."

References

1. Hatala, A., and McNally, O. GOAL/QPC Annual Conference presentation, Nov. 1992.
2. Hatala and McNally.

3. Alexander Hatala, CEO, and Sister Elizabeth Corry, president, Our Lady of Lourdes Medical Center. Letter to employees, Jan. 1994.
4. Jan Weber, MD, chief of cardiology, Our Lady of Lourdes Medical Center. Interview by Dona Hotopp, Jan. 25, 1994. (Also subsequent quotes.)
5. William Harrar, MD, chief of pathology, Our Lady of Lourdes Medical Center. Interview by Dona Hotopp, Jan. 26, 1994. (Also subsequent quotes.)
6. Owen McNally, director of TQM, Our Lady of Lourdes Medical Center. Interview by Dona Hotopp, Jan. 24, 1994. (Also subsequent quotes.)
7. Alex Hatala, CEO, Our Lady of Lourdes Medical Center. Interview by Dona Hotopp, Jan. 24, 1994. (Also subsequent quotes.)

CHAPTER TWELVE

Sisters of the Sorrowful Mother Ministry Corporation

Sister M. Lois Bush and Jon T. Beste

Sisters of the Sorrowful Mother Ministry Corporation (SSM-MC) is the sponsor and corporate umbrella for eight hospitals located in the upper midwestern region of the United States. The net patient services revenue for the system exceeded $310 million in fiscal year 1994. System facilities include the following:

Hospital	*Location*	*Staffed Beds*
Saint Joseph's Hospital	Marshfield, WI	524
Saint Michael's Hospital	Stevens Point, WI	111
Sacred Heart/ Saint Mary's Hospitals, Inc.	Tomahawk and Rhinelander, WI	163
Mercy Medical Center	Oshkosh, WI	236
Saint Elizabeth's Hospital	Wabasha, MN	31
Holy Family Hospital	Estherville, IA	58
Flambeau Medical Center (jointly owned by SSM-MC and Marshfield Clinic)	Park Falls, WI	42
		1,165

The organizational structure of SSM-MC closely follows that of a divisional corporation. The corporate office has responsibility for governance and management of the overall organization, with individual divisions or units having responsibility for their particular operations. In this corporate structure, the individual entities are united in the pursuit of common goals, while retaining sufficient autonomy to address local needs and manage their own operations. Current corporate and hospital bylaws establish SSM-MC as the parent, with the hospitals as subsidiaries.

Consistent with the divisional corporation model, the primary role of SSM-MC is to provide leadership that ensures the long-term viability and growth of the system, its partners, and its affiliates. This leadership role is displayed through four distinct responsibilities:

1. Defining goals, objectives, and strategies
2. Determining and monitoring accountabilities
3. Developing and implementing a corporate growth and integration strategy
4. Providing and coordinating selected services

To maintain a proper balance of central authority and local autonomy, SSM-MC must carry out its responsibilities in a manner that models and promotes a collaborative style.

Reasons for Choosing Hoshin Planning

The Sisters of the Sorrowful Mother have been the primary providers of health care services for more than 100 years and has earned a high degree of community support. Each of SSM-MC's hospitals is the sole inpatient facility in its community, and each has maintained positive relationships with local physicians. For example, the system's largest tertiary care facility, Saint Joseph's Hospital in Marshfield, Wisconsin, is physically located on an integrated campus with the 400-physician Marshfield Clinic.

Despite the system's noteworthy success record, by February 1992 its leadership was becoming increasingly concerned with growing market demands for health care reform. There were important questions about how SSM-MC would meet those demands.

Meeting Market Demands for Health Care Reform

The key question was, "Five to ten years from now, what do we want to look like as a regional health care delivery system?" The answer would ultimately be found within the question itself – a regional health care delivery system. However, the question was less expansive in scope, as it was primarily addressing the future of the hospital system as it was currently perceived.

Until 1991, SSM-MC had utilized traditional planning techniques that were driven primarily by the system's financial requirements and by programs that focused explicitly on the mission and values of the sponsoring corporate member, the Sisters of the Sorrowful Mother. However, previous planning methods often began with certain assumptions that had, in some instances, proved to be limiting factors in creating a truly bold, clear vision for the future. Following are examples of these assumptions:

- The best means of strengthening the system is to strengthen the individual hospitals.
- Growth initiatives ought to be based on facilities and programs, rather than on systems of care.
- Acquisition criteria are a financial matter.
- Collaboration with area physicians and other providers is to be encouraged, although it has been minimally successful to date.

Meeting notes from system planning sessions that occurred during 1992 included the following observations:

- At this time, we lack a definition of what we want to be as a regional health care system.
- System leaders each have a different concept of definitions and preferences regarding emerging alternative health care models and what needs to be done to get there.
- It is unclear whether or how the system should approach the development of linkages between hospitals and physicians across multiple service areas.

Additional comments reflected the need to understand the dynamics of primary and tertiary referral patterns, appropriate physician relationships, implications of managed care, sharing of capital, centralization of services, and geographic barriers.

Essentially, two fundamental questions were being raised:

1. What should be the system's focal point?
2. What means ought to be used to attain that goal?

In the early stages of addressing these deceptively simple questions, SSM-MC realized that outside assistance was needed to ensure an external, unbiased perspective and to learn what had and what had not worked for other health care systems and for non-health care corporations.

Choosing a Focal Point for the System

In January 1991, SSM-MC engaged a national consulting firm to provide guidance on the question of organizational focus. This external industry scan made it apparent that certain management practices were consistently present in highly successful organizations:

- Teams formed the basic work structure.
- Empowerment was widespread.
- Quality management tools were heavily used.
- Changes in assessment criteria were considered openly.
- Benchmarking was done against the best organizations.
- The voice of the customer directed all new products.
- Inspections were eliminated, and emphasis was placed on doing things right the first time.

The scan also revealed that successful organizations introduced only a few changes in any one year, to avoid turning the organization upside down. Whatever changes were to be made, the emphasis was on the process of change and on pushing knowledge and understanding of the plan down through the organization, as well as to outside suppliers and other key stakeholders.

For the next 12 months, SSM-MC's leadership became engrossed in learning all that was being written and said about the future of health care delivery. Then, prior to the start of the new fiscal year, which would begin in October 1993, the leaders determined a clear direction for the system: SSM-MC would focus its efforts on one key initiative that would guide decisions related to all others. It would promote the formation and development of integrated delivery networks (IDNs).

Create Integrated Delivery Networks

This broadly stated organizational focus had immense implications for the future of health care delivery in the markets served by SSM-MC hospitals. It would cause the system to rethink its notion of community and of the meaning of service integration. It would undoubtedly challenge the system to recognize the equally significant – and sometimes conflicting – expectations of other providers in SSM-MC's service areas who would be essential to the successful formation of such networks.

Developing Means to Attain the Goal

Although the first of the two questions had been answered (that of the system's most important focal point), it was not yet clear how this goal would be accomplished. During the next several months, key members of SSM-MC's leadership group, including the system's president and executive vice-president, participated in a variety of workshops and training programs related to quality management and planning techniques.

Hoshin planning appeared to successfully link quality management and planning with the techniques necessary for focusing and mobilizing the entire organization as active participants in the plan's implementation.

At this point, the concept of hoshin planning was not yet fully understood within the system, but it did not take long to recognize its potential. The hoshin planning process provides a framework to:

- Identify options
- Achieve consensus
- Establish key strategies
- Communicate with employees at all levels
- Identify interorganizational linkages
- Mobilize the entire organization
- Empower employees with self-monitoring mechanisms that can be adjusted based on market changes

Furthermore, to the delight of the system's leadership, it appeared that hoshin planning incorporated the full array of the best management practices identified earlier in the review of highly successful organizations.

Hoshin Implementation

Given this detailed description of the system's hoshin, the system's leadership directed the planning sessions toward developing long-term objectives, annual strategies, means and measures – all designed to move the system toward its hoshin. Although the hoshin planning techniques were new to the system, some language used in the former planning model remained the same, such as *long-term objectives* and *strategies.* However, for purposes of hoshin planning, these terms would take on new meaning in the way they were to be clearly and inseparably linked to the system's hoshin. So SSM-MC developed the following glossary of terms for internal planning and communication purposes:

- **Hoshin:** As applied in management practice, the term *hoshin* describes a planning process by which an organization identifies the most important direction it can pursue, which, when successful, will propel the organization forward in fulfillment of the goals expressed in its mission statement.
- **Long-term objectives:** Objectives describe significant, broadly stated actions with greater specificity than the system's hoshin. They identify the major components of the organization's work plan, which, in total, describe more precisely what needs to be accomplished if the hoshin is to be achieved. Generally, objectives are so expansive in nature that they will not be fully accomplished within a single fiscal year. Thus, the qualifier *long-term* is appropriate.
- **Strategies:** Both the system hoshin and the long-term objectives are intended outcomes. However, they provide limited insight as to precisely how to proceed in pursuit of the stated objectives. Therefore, clear strategy statements are necessary. Strategies describe the key critical actions to be taken that will move the organization forward in attaining its stated objectives. Strategies take into account the reality of time and availability of resources. They are considered to be attainable within a defined period (for example, the current fiscal year).
- **Means and measures:** Means are the incremental steps to be taken in support of the associated strategy. They describe what can be done *now.* Means are the building blocks that form the foundation for the next layer of activity necessary to support the attainment of the strategies.

Measures provide a way to determine the completion and relative success of the actions that have been taken. They provide the "check" stage in hoshin deployment. They allow the organization, department, work unit, or individual to know when part of the system's mission has been accomplished.

Organization's Breakthrough Goal

Presently, there is no single health care model that addresses the diverse circumstances and needs of every community. There is, however, little doubt among legislators, payers, and others in health care leadership that significant restructuring must be done to expand access to health services and contain the spiraling cost of care.

Major variables influencing such structural redesign include the geographic proximity of services to patients, the efficient use of resources among the providers for a given population, and the organizational and political preparedness of the providers to make the necessary changes. Ultimately, systemic changes that include a broader approach to community health status planning will be necessary. These changes will be possible only if an efficient delivery model is in place to provide the foundation. The term used to describe such a geographically sensitive, resource-efficient structure is *integrated delivery network*. This network includes the following characteristics:

- It has the capacity to provide (or arrange to provide) to its client population all required health care services – tertiary care, preventive care, home health, and other services – under one administrative structure.
- It is primarily a local or regional concern.
- It has coordinated relationships among its parts that make care more efficient, more effective, and of higher quality than would be provided by separate entities.

Attributes of successful networks include:

- The ability to combine hospitals and physicians under one capitated arrangement
- A full range of "primary" and "specialty" care services
- Clinical integration and management of clinical outcomes
- A common culture (with operating units cooperating and having strategic roles)
- Distributed use of medical technology and information systems
- Joint development of care delivery standards and practice protocols
- Capital for program development and risk sharing
- Financial stability
- Management support systems and services
- Avoidance of service line segmentation and commercialization of health care services

Although the decision had been made that hoshin planning would indeed become *the* planning model for the system, significant education and training were needed across the system prior to fully relying upon the process for deployment of the system's hoshin. Over a period of several months, activities centered on learning the fundamentals of hoshin planning and the use of hoshin-related quality tools. The leaders felt that, if successful, the process would lead to identification of the key long-term objectives necessary to move the entire organization toward its chosen hoshin.

In the transition from traditional strategic planning to hoshin planning, the leaders realized that several of the long-term objectives, operational measurement structures, and provider linkages currently in place could not be changed overnight. Further, it was unclear how the current objectives and programs, especially those that reflected the system's mission and values, would be incorporated into the new planning process.

Therefore, the long-term objectives that would subsequently evolve from the hoshin process would likely need to be augmented with other, nonnegotiable objectives that would preserve the mission and values of the system's sponsor. (See figure 12-1.)

How Hoshin Planning Has Worked

Over a two-day period in March 1993, the system's 45 senior executives met for their annual planning session. They began the unsteady process of incorporating several key quality management tools into the process of establishing long-term objectives and strategies in support of the system's hoshin. These sessions began with this question: "What are all the things the system needs to do across its multiple markets if it is to achieve its hoshin?"

The process of addressing this question included the use of affinity charts, relationship charts, radar (spider) charts, decision matrixes, and other tools. Being new to the process, the participants had to accept a certain amount of ambiguity and trust. Periodically, the hoshin coach who led the group through the process reassured the participants that they were, in fact, still in control of their organizational destiny.

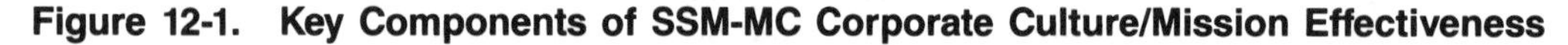

To their dismay, the executives found that the instructions that come with this quality tool kit, like the instructions for assembling a bicycle or a gas grill, do not always apply as shown in the illustrations! Hoshin practitioners should be prepared to modify the rules on occasion, based on both group consensus and common sense, to accommodate the peculiarities of an organization.

Figure 12-1. Key Components of SSM-MC Corporate Culture/Mission Effectiveness

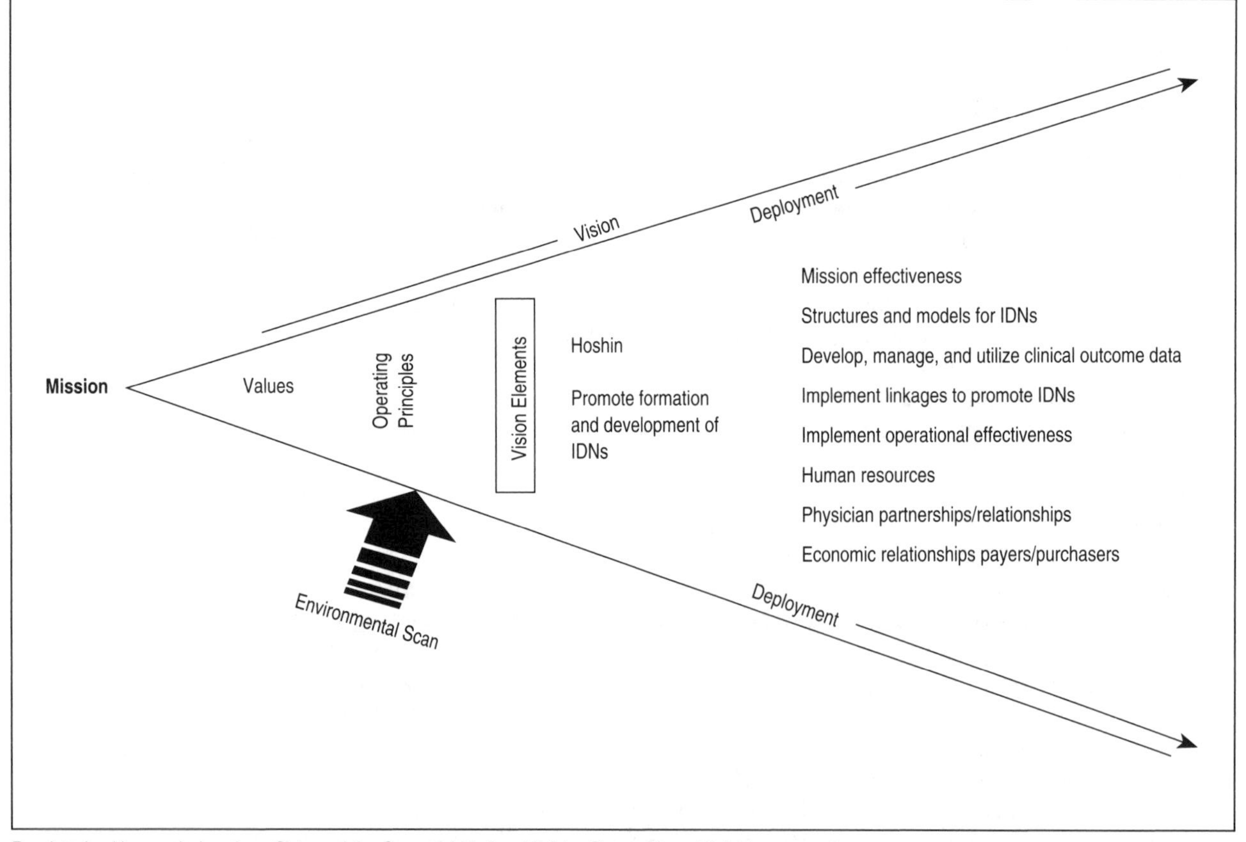

Reprinted, with permission, from Sisters of the Sorrowful Mother Ministry Corporation.

Selection of System Objectives

Following a challenging and enlightening two days of processing, the participants agreed to seven long-term system objectives. Then an eighth objective was added to ensure continued support of the system's commitment to its underlying values. With the hoshin focus on promoting the formation and development of integrated delivery networks, the long-term system objectives are as follows:

1. Develop and promote a coordinated mission effectiveness direction.
2. Develop, manage, and utilize clinical outcome data.
3. Implement linkages to promote IDNs.
4. Implement operational efficiencies.
5. Develop human resources.
6. Establish physician partnerships and relationships.
7. Design necessary structures and models to support IDN development.
8. Develop long-term economic relationships with payers and purchasers.

Development of Strategies and Means and Measures

Following the development and subsequent refinement of these long-term objectives, the question was then asked, "What does the system need to do to accomplish each objective?" This was followed by the use of affinity charts, radar charts, and decision matrixes to identify options and to select the best possible strategies for achieving the named objectives.

Figure 12-2 provides a visual representation of the relationship between the long-term objectives and the system's hoshin. It also depicts the relationship of the resulting systemwide strategies and means and measures that were identified as the best methods for achieving the objectives. The illustration requires careful analysis and discussion. As noted previously, SSM-MC is a health care system consisting of multiple facilities in multiple geographic locations. Therefore, all activities in which the system must be engaged had to be identified in the planning process, even though each activity might not apply uniformly to each of the system's local markets. Accordingly, notice the column headings and notations on figure 12-2. This is the system plan and, for that reason, it includes the full range of necessary actions across the entire system. On a practical level, however, only the first six (A–F) of the eight objectives could be addressed at the local hospital level. The remaining two objectives (design necessary structures and models to support IDN development and develop long-term economic relationships with payers and purchasers) transcend local geographic markets. These are corporate responsibilities. Local hospital teams were not requested to develop specific strategies related to these two objectives.

Prioritization of Objectives

A second major decision had to be made with respect to the remaining six systemwide objectives. Inasmuch as this was the first year for the system in its transition to the hoshin planning model, the leadership team understood that the rate of change needed to be manageable and to occur over an extended period. Full deployment of all six of the remaining objectives across all system institutions could not be effectively managed in the first year of hoshin-based planning. Consequently, by using quality management tools, the leadership group prioritized the six remaining long-term objectives (figure 12-2, objectives A–F), identifying the two that would have the greatest impact in moving the system toward its hoshin. The group consensus was that long-term objectives C and D were of the greatest importance: implement linkages to promote integrated delivery networks and implement operational efficiencies. Figure 12-3 illustrates the relationship of the six objectives (A–F) to the system hoshin and identifies

Figure 12-2. Overview: System Objectives and Strategies (FY 1994)

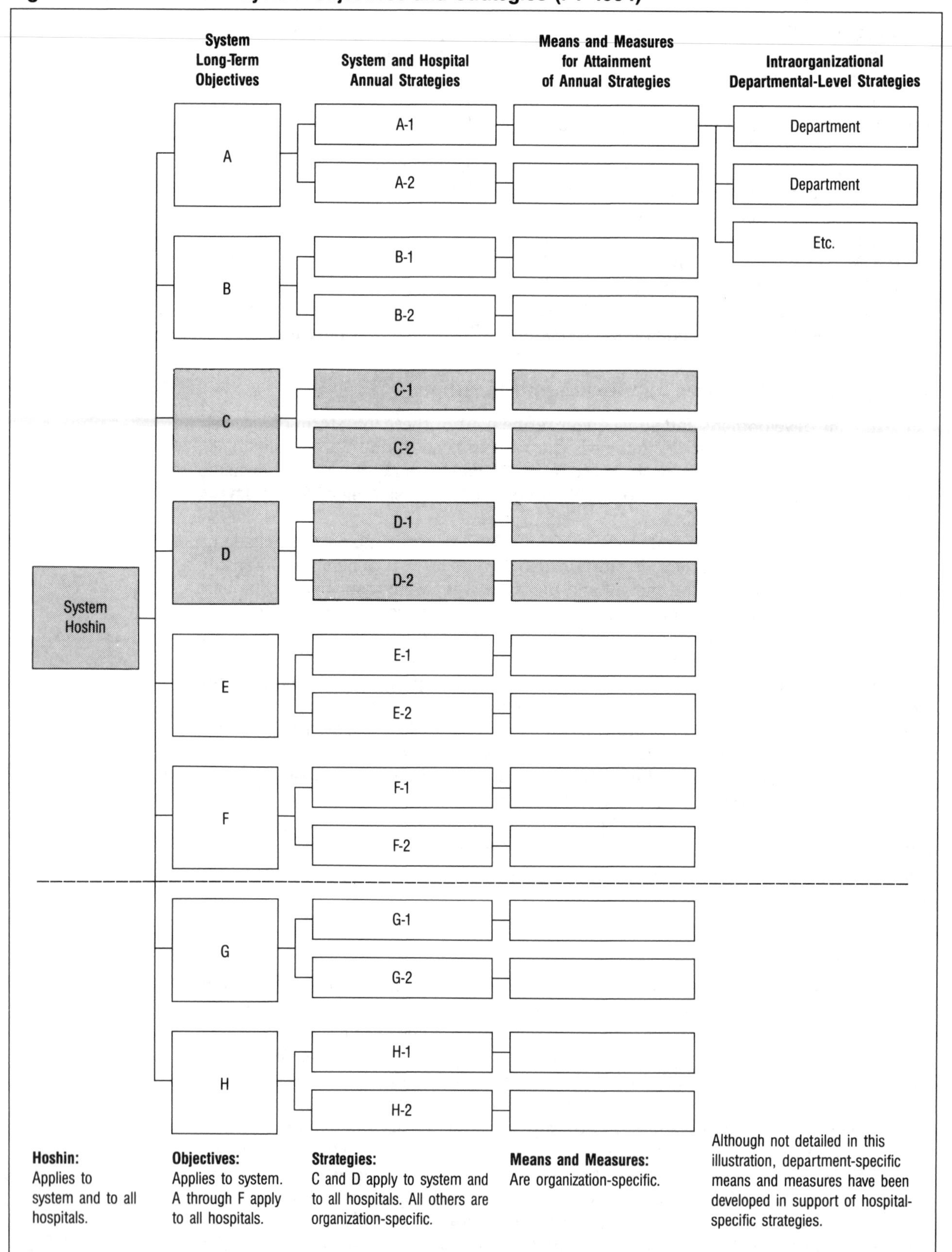

Figure 12-3. Overview of SSM-Ministry Corporation Hoshin Plan

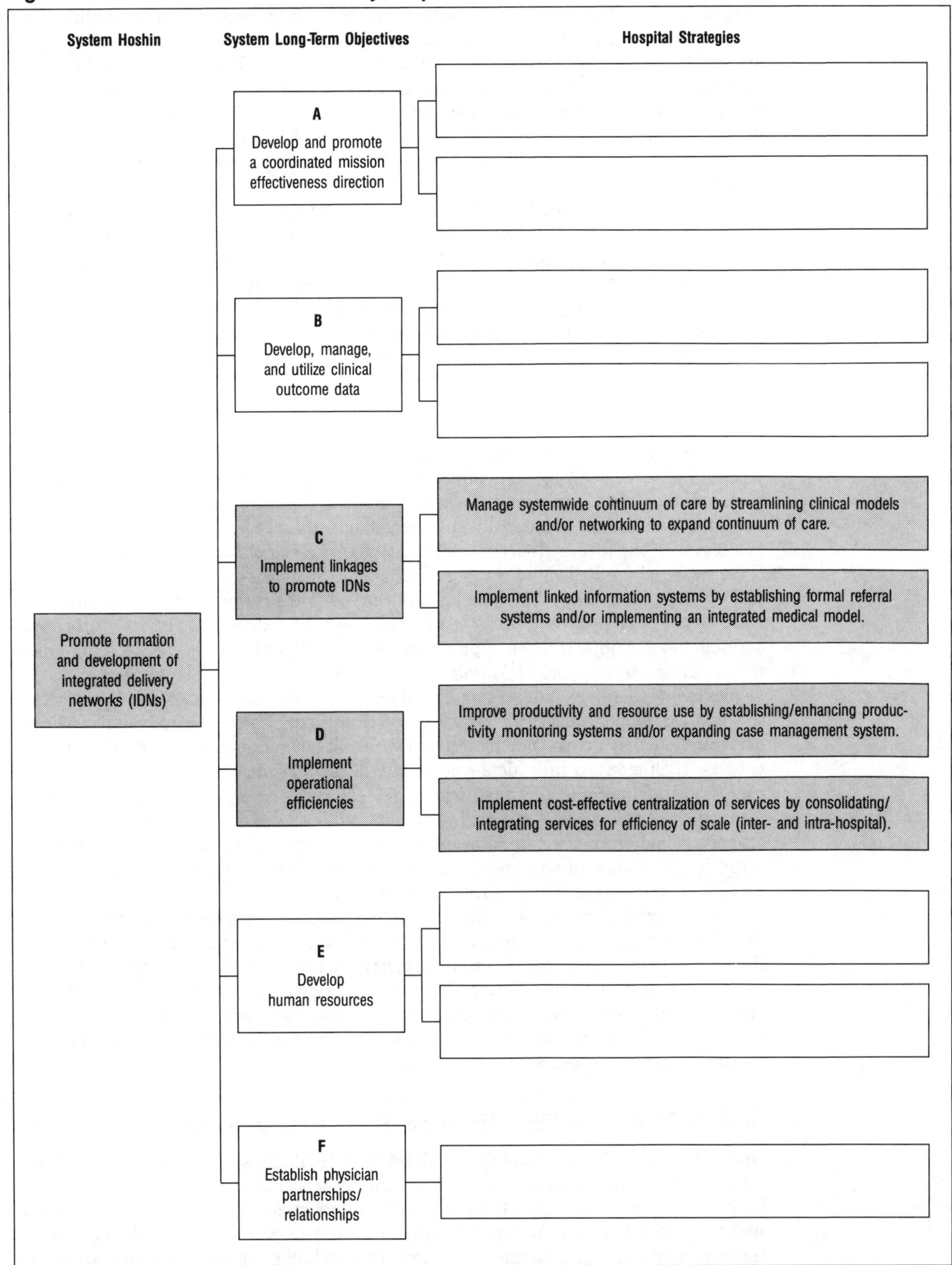
System Hoshin
System Long-Term Objectives
Hospital Strategies
A
Develop and promote a coordinated mission effectiveness direction
B
Develop, manage, and utilize clinical outcome data
C
Implement linkages to promote IDNs
Manage systemwide continuum of care by streamlining clinical models and/or networking to expand continuum of care.
Implement linked information systems by establishing formal referral systems and/or implementing an integrated medical model.
Promote formation and development of integrated delivery networks (IDNs)
D
Implement operational efficiencies
Improve productivity and resource use by establishing/enhancing productivity monitoring systems and/or expanding case management system.
Implement cost-effective centralization of services by consolidating/integrating services for efficiency of scale (inter- and intra-hospital).
E
Develop human resources
F
Establish physician partnerships/relationships

Reprinted, with permission, from Sisters of the Sorrowful Mother Ministry Corporation.

the systemwide strategies that apply uniformly to each of the system hospitals. In communicating this information throughout the management ranks of each hospital, shading was added to the document to visually convey the point that special emphasis was being placed on these two particular objectives. To effectively mobilize the entire organization around these two objectives, it was also necessary that supporting strategies be uniformly pursued across the system. Accordingly, figure 12-3 also illustrates the selected strategies associated with objectives C and D, as identified by the leadership team. Notice that in each instance there are just two strategies per objective.

The decision to limit the systemwide deployment of each objective to just two strategies resulted from one of those glitches not provided for in the hoshin training manual. The team approach to strategy development generated an extensive list of viable ideas. However, nowhere did the hoshin written material advise as to the number of strategies appropriate for effective plan deployment. In the interest of remaining focused and achieving a degree of success in the first year of this new planning process, two "just felt like" the right place to draw the line.

Deployment of the Plan Organizationwide

A key concept in the utilization of hoshin planning is deployment. Deployment is the process by which the long-term objectives that support the organization's hoshin are communicated and implemented throughout the organization. Deployment can be thought of as a series of carefully engineered, inseparably linked plans, each of which is integral to the future structure, stability, and success of the organization. It is the organizational equivalent of an engineering blueprint that conveys a picture of the end product. It focuses individual and collective efforts toward the attainment of the goal. Again referring to figure 12-2, one can begin to realize that the very process of defining system objectives to support the organization's hoshin – and defining hospital strategies to support those objectives – is integral to the deployment process. Deployment, therefore, can be thought of as a repetitive process, at each level within the organization, of collectively defining (or acknowledging) the desired outcomes, then deciding how they are to be achieved and who will be held responsible for the planned actions. Ultimately, a fully deployed plan will include measurements of success for each expected outcome and a periodic check stage to ensure that the plan is moving forward. Through the use of a coding scheme, all levels of activity related to any one organizational objective can be easily linked together. If internal or external events result in the change of any one objective, an effective mechanism is already in place to redirect the efforts of the entire organization.

For deployment purposes within the system, the leadership team arbitrarily decided that each hospital would be requested to establish two specific strategies for each of the four remaining long-term system objectives (A, B, E, and F). (We referred to this as our "rule of two's.") Thereafter, each hospital's management team would identify precise means and measures that would be used to attain each strategy. At each stage, the team used various quality management tools to ensure that a broad, inclusive decision-making process was maintained.

Decision Making on Final Means to Attain the Strategies

Up to this point, involvement in the development of the system's hoshin, the long-term objectives, and the common system strategies was limited to the system's senior leadership group, made up of the executive management group from each facility. Although all the work to this point was crucial to the overall process, deployment of the plan had really just begun. After each hospital management team identified the hospital strategies beyond those related to objectives C and D, it addressed the process of naming the measures and means that would be used to attain the strategies. Because the range of possibilities spanned all departments within each hospital, the process of deciding on the final means required the involvement of the next level of management (department managers) at each institution. The decision-making process once again included the use of quality management tools. Apart from the final outcomes, the very process of involving middle management provided an opportunity for the senior managers to explain the system's hoshin, how it was arrived at, and the role of each operating unit in influencing the system's overall success.

Figure 12-4 is an example of a plan developed by one of the system hospitals, through the point of naming its hospital-specific means and measures. Figures 12-3 and 12-4 illustrate how all six long-term objectives and the strategies related to objectives C and D are carried forward. Strategies associated with objectives A, B, E, and F are hospital-specific. They reflect the best thinking of the hospital management group as to what it realistically believes it is capable of achieving. The far-right column of figure 12-4 reflects the means (the smaller, incremental steps) and the measures that will guide these initiatives.

What Remains to Be Done

Sisters of the Sorrowful Mother is still in the early stages of incorporating hoshin planning concepts; much more work has yet to be accomplished with respect to hoshin deployment. During the first year, the senior management team at each hospital was encouraged to move ahead at its own pace in applying the more advanced deployment techniques. It is important to emphasize that the process of hoshin deployment to the lowest functional levels within any organization is repetitive in nature. Having named the desired outcome for any one subgroup of workers, the same questions need to be repeated: "What primary actions do we need to take to ensure attainment of the desired outcomes?" "What incremental steps and outcome measures will we use to get there?" As these questions are asked at each level throughout the organization, the agreed-upon answers must be put in writing for all to see.

Overall Benefits and Results

The long-term benefits of hoshin planning techniques for SSM-MC are not yet known. However, several short-term benefits are already apparent and have been instrumental in moving the system forward during a period of unprecedented health care reform. Hoshin planning has been effective in making the system's goal of creating integrated delivery networks highly visible within the organization. It also serves as a vehicle for corporate and hospital leadership to engage others in dialogues with respect to the system's vision. People outside SSM-MC have commented that they are attracted to SSM-MC because of its clear vision for the future – made visible in our plans. In addition, the mechanics of the planning process (affinity diagrams, for example) encourage generation of creative ideas that might otherwise be lost. They focus attention on ideas rather than on the individuals participating in the planning process.

Perhaps the greatest benefit of hoshin planning is that it both enhances and expands upon the traditional strategic planning processes already in place in many organizations. Common to most planning processes are activities that result in the formation of multiyear objectives, annual objectives, and strategies – all emanating from the organization's mission or vision statement. Once completed, such information is generally handed down to the operational units with the directive that they are to pursue objectives – with little direction as to how or why. Often not understood or not received favorably by those most critical to attainment of the objectives, such planning processes are rendered inadequate and generally do not produce the intended results.

Figure 12-4. Overview of SSM-Ministry Corporation Hoshin Plan

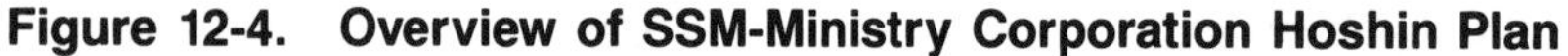

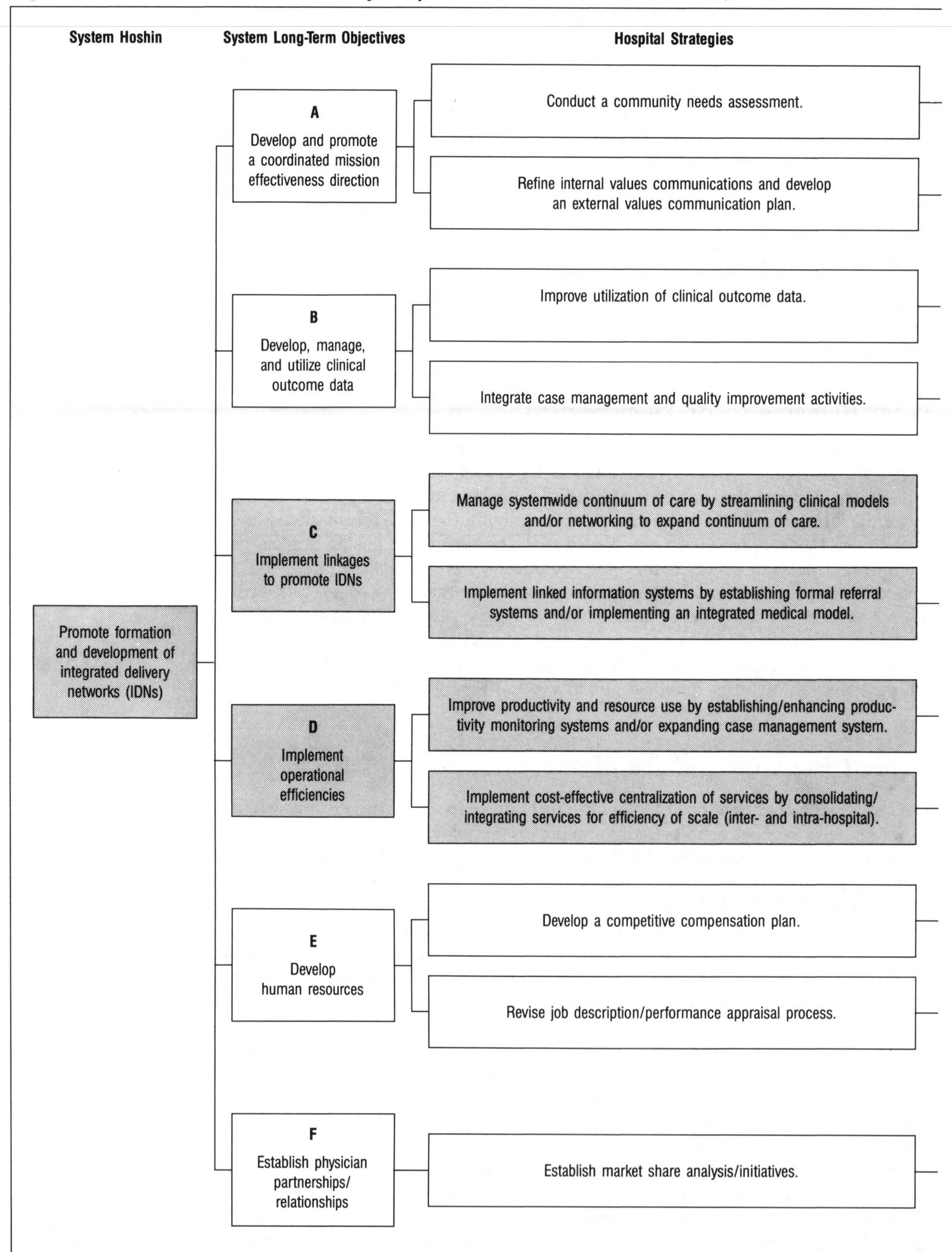
System Hoshin
System Long-Term Objectives
Hospital Strategies
Promote formation and development of integrated delivery networks (IDNs)
A
Develop and promote a coordinated mission effectiveness direction
Conduct a community needs assessment.
Refine internal values communications and develop an external values communication plan.
B
Develop, manage, and utilize clinical outcome data
Improve utilization of clinical outcome data.
Integrate case management and quality improvement activities.
C
Implement linkages to promote IDNs
Manage systemwide continuum of care by streamlining clinical models and/or networking to expand continuum of care.
Implement linked information systems by establishing formal referral systems and/or implementing an integrated medical model.
D
Implement operational efficiencies
Improve productivity and resource use by establishing/enhancing productivity monitoring systems and/or expanding case management system.
Implement cost-effective centralization of services by consolidating/integrating services for efficiency of scale (inter- and intra-hospital).
E
Develop human resources
Develop a competitive compensation plan.
Revise job description/performance appraisal process.
F
Establish physician partnerships/relationships
Establish market share analysis/initiatives.

Hospital-Specific Means and Measures

Participate in the development of the assessment methodology with the system values project team, completed by 9/94.

Develop a FY 1995 community mission effectiveness action plan based on needs assessment findings by 9/94.

Based on outcome from FY 1994 employee opinion survey, develop and implement new internal communications by 9/94.

Establish objectives for externally communicating values program; develop a plan and implement with at least two presentations by 9/94.

Purchase software package to develop a database for analysis and benchmarking of clinical outcomes by 12/93.

Communicate MHAQIP information to medical staff departments to establish clinical CQI dialogue by 6/94.

Establish objectives and policies in the FY 1994 clinical QI plan for integration of case management and QI by 3/94.

Compare case-managed DRG performance to system and regional hospitals' performance utilizing the OHCI database by 9/94.

Assess existing referral patterns with assessment study completed by 3/94.

Identify processes to make referral system functional with plan design completed by 9/94.

Document existing medical record process with flowchart of existing processes completed by 3/94.

Determine medical records user requirements with survey of users completed by 9/94.

Establish valid productivity measurement system with department units of measure established by 3/94.

Refine MIS productivity reporting system and develop revised productivity report format by 4/94.

Develop a plan that defines the criteria for consolidation of departments with plan completed by 1/94.

Identify opportunities for future integration of services by 1/94.

Assess organization's compensation program and prepare a needs assessment report by 3/94.

Prepare a feasibility study evaluating potential compensation strategies and make a recommendation for FY 1995 implementation by 9/94.

Assess job description/performance appraisal needs and prepare a needs assessment report by 3/94.

Prepare a feasibility study evaluating strategies and make a recommendation for FY 1995 implementation by 9/94.

Establish a market share committee composed of senior management staff to analyze data and develop action plans by 12/93.

Hoshin planning differs from other methods in several ways: First, it involves a wider array of managers earlier in the process of setting the key organizational objectives. Consequently, a greater range of options are considered and the end results have a higher level of understanding and buy-in. Second, hoshin planning carries the process forward and downward within the entire organization to the lowest practical work unit. It is, therefore, an effective means for communicating objectives (expectations) to others in the organization. Third, it constructively engages the lowest-level work teams in identifying the means they deem appropriate for attainment of key objectives and the measures to be used as benchmarks in determining their level of success.

Key Success Factors

Although the literal translation of the term *hoshin kanri* is said to be "a bright, shining object"–something that points the way–it is not the proverbial silver bullet that will solve all the problems of an organization suddenly in need of an effective planning process. In fact, in the early stages of training and plan implementation, it will create added uncertainty for even the most experienced planning team. Given this caution, certain success factors should be in place: organizational readiness for hoshin, stakeholders in the process, and a hoshin coach.

Being Prepared for Hoshin Planning

Key to an organization's success in making the transition to hoshin planning is the quality of the planning processes already in place. If an organization is not open to and somewhat experienced with a structured and participative planning model, hoshin planning will require a quantum leap of faith if it is to be even moderately successful. Organizational preparedness is both structural and cultural in nature and should not be underestimated.

Including Everyone with a Stake in the Organization

A second noteworthy success factor is that the process needs to include all key stakeholders in the organization–certainly their interest, if not their active participation, in the planning process itself. For example, it did not take long for SSM-MC's planning team to realize that in the process of developing long-term objectives and annual strategies, they were (implicitly) making decisions that would require a shared vision, mutual understanding, and consensus on key objectives with physicians who, while not employed by the system, are essential to its long-range success.

Using a Hoshin Coach in the Early Stages

A third key success factor is the use of a fully trained and experienced outside coach during the early stages of learning and applying hoshin planning concepts and techniques. Using a hoshin coach will alleviate latent doubts about personal biases and will enhance the learning experience for all participants. Furthermore, an experienced coach will be able to anticipate and thus help avoid pitfalls that can occur during the learning process. Perhaps of greatest importance, an outsider can allow all members of the organization to focus on the substance of the issues being addressed, free of the added task of deciding on the most appropriate techniques to be used at each stage of plan development.

Problems and Challenges

Two main problems were encountered in implementing hoshin at SSM-MC. They had to do with trying to move ahead too quickly and trying to include too many good ideas in the plan.

Lack of Patience

Following the initial introduction and training by a few members of an organization's management team, the tendency may be to jump in and attempt to apply the planning techniques with other members of the management team who have not yet been schooled in the art of hoshin planning. To do so would be to risk rejection. As one such person acknowledged more than a year after such an encounter, "Our group's tendency was not to take it too seriously. We thought it was just one more of those trendy things that would eventually go away." The basic challenge in the transition from more traditional planning models to hoshin planning is that it requires ongoing discussion and needs to occur over an extended period, perhaps several years. It requires a systematic program of exposure, training, and continuous improvement on all aspects of the process, and a phased introduction of the components into daily practice – one piece at a time.

Too Many Good Ideas

The enormous array of meaningful and valuable ideas, objectives, and strategies generated during the brainstorming processes proved problematic. The initial tendency was to incorporate *all* good ideas into the plan, at the expense of the *few* key things that really needed to be done. As noted earlier, the SSM-MC management group found it practical to deploy just two of the organization's eight objectives uniformly across all system hospitals in the first year of hoshin planning. The group recognized that full deployment would require a great deal of energy and that it was important to the success of the process that the expectations be understandable and manageable in the early stages of planning.

Roles and Responsibilities

A fundamental premise of hoshin planning is that the process and the resulting documents be highly visible within the organization. Success of the process equally depends on the visibility and involvement of the organization's executive leadership. Implicit in the decision to use hoshin planning must be a commitment by the senior officers to alter, where necessary, the organization's culture. The process requires the active, candid involvement of employees at all levels of the organization in determining its future. A decision of such magnitude is not possible without the full understanding and unequivocal support of the entire senior management group. Further, executive involvement needs to be more than an intellectual commitment to such change.

As noted earlier, the introduction of hoshin planning at SSM-MC began with its president and executive vice-president who, along with several of the system's hospital presidents, participated in a series of two- to three-day training sessions. Excited about the prospects for the system, they made the decision to use hoshin planning as the planning model for SSM-MC. To date, a minimum of 45 executives within the system have received formal training at off-site training facilities. Approximately 100 middle managers have been trained in group sessions by expert facilitators brought to the local hospitals. One of the key roles of the system's president is to ensure that these training programs are ongoing.

Lessons Learned

Hoshin planning has the potential to become an effective management and leadership tool within SSM-MC. It can focus the attention of an entire organization, and it provides a visible mechanism by which to link the activities of multiple work units in pursuit of a common goal. Some of the critical lessons learned are summarized below.

Take a Positive Attitude toward the Amount of Training Required

In making the transition from a more traditional planning model, SSM-MC's leadership has learned to appreciate the magnitude of training that is required. It has learned to proceed slowly, bringing others along in the process. Learning new skills and techniques does require more work in the short term – not a welcome thought for already overburdened managers. However, the hoshin methodology is also seen as a bright light at the end of the tunnel. If approached positively, it will enable these overburdened managers to plan and manage their workloads more effectively in the future.

Include Testing for Reasonableness in the Process

At various stages during the planning, participants will often become so totally engrossed in the process of planning that some of the solutions will later be found to be impractical or unworkable. Therefore, testing for reasonableness needs to be included as part of the process. Occasionally, the results will not seem quite right. In such instances, they probably are not. Do not hesitate to arbitrarily correct the course when it seems reasonable to do so. Hoshin planning techniques are just that – techniques. They are to be used and adapted to meet the needs of the planners.

Accept the Challenge to Make Improvements

Sisters of the Sorrowful Mother Ministry Corporation is a more focused organization than it was in 1992, when it first encountered hoshin planning. It should be noted, however, that hoshin planning will not focus an organization that may currently be experiencing a degree of success but that lacks the leadership and courage necessary to accept challenge and make improvements. It will not focus an organization that does not want to be focused. Hoshin planning, at its best, will improve and enhance an already successful organization. It serves to extend the limits of more traditional planning processes, pushing the plan to the vertical and horizontal limits of the organization. It gives visibility to the organization's goals, and it provides employees at the lowest work unit level with the opportunity to knowingly and deliberately participate in the overall success of the enterprise.

CHAPTER THIRTEEN

Southwest Texas Methodist Hospital

Lisa Boisvert with Geoffrey Crabtree

It is no surprise that a hospital with a history of being on the front line of change was one of the first hospitals to embark on the *hoshin kanri* journey. The founding flagship hospital for South Texas Medical Center and the first nuclear-age hospital in the United States (built in 1963 to withstand a nuclear attack), Southwest Texas Methodist Hospital in 1992 became one of the pioneers of hoshin in the U.S. health care system.

The hospital is a 573-bed, tertiary care regional referral center based in San Antonio. It is located in the South Texas Medical Center, a 700-acre-plus complex comprising 7 major health care institutions, 2 freestanding research centers, and more than 15 other providers of health education, treatment, and research. Health care is San Antonio's third-largest industry, behind tourism and the military.

Reasons for Choosing Hoshin Planning

Methodist Hospital, like many hospitals that start quality management initiatives, was prompted both by crisis and by some honest reflection on its existing planning process. The main reasons for engaging in quality management were to improve the financial picture, resolve planning problems, and improve communication throughout the organization.

Improve the Financial Picture

The crisis took the form of a little red ink on the bottom line. This marked one of the rare times in recent history that there were any financial concerns. The most obvious cause for concern was that the length of stay (LOS) was decreasing at an accelerating rate, from 6.5 days to 5.3 days over a six-month period. This, among other things, represented a $900,000 loss for the hospital.

Resolve Planning Problems

As part of the self-examination that took place during this time, Methodist leadership acknowledged that their planning process began and ended at the top of the organization. Each year senior executives devised a strategic plan somewhat in isolation and then announced it to the organization. Frequently, the main points of the plan held little relevance to the actual day-to-day realities of the organization. Other planning problems included the following:

- All planning had a short-range focus.
- It was difficult to measure success.
- There was little clarity of language in the planning process.
- The plan was filed without being used.
- It was fragmented.
- The plan was not designed to handle emergencies.
- Resources were not planned for.
- Planning did not involve the input of the total organization.
- The plan was not realistic.

Improve Communication in Both Directions

Perhaps the most costly flaw of the existing planning process was the awkwardness of communicating it to individuals at all levels of the organization, those who would be responsible for implementing the plan's main objectives. Often in the form of a multipaged notebook with lengthy descriptors, the plan never registered as "real" for managers and staff.

Equally frustrating were the challenges to communication from the front line to the administration. The ideas of those outside the executive circle of influence were not solicited in a disciplined fashion. The very people who expedited hospital processes were overlooked in setting the annual goals and objectives for organizing those processes.

Hoshin Implementation

The existing planning team acknowledged the shortcomings in its planning model and sought an alternative. That alternative was hoshin, which Methodist defines with vivid imagery:

> Imagine an organization that knows what customers will want five to ten years from now and exactly what the organization will do to meet and exceed all customer expectations. Imagine a planning system that has integrated PDCA [plan-do-check-act] language and activity based on clear, long-term thinking, a realistic measurement system with a focus on process and results, identification of what's important, alignment of groups, decisions by people who have the necessary information, planning integrated with daily activity, good vertical communication, cross-functional communication, and the buy-in that results.

It is worth noting that nowhere in the paperwork generated within the hospital regarding this planning process is the word *hoshin* used. Department heads and staff refer to the new process simply as "a better way of strategic planning." The director of strategic planning and market research explains that "since catchball makes this type of planning a staff process, we wanted our staff to adopt this form of planning as 'theirs'" and not just a new planning process that comes from Japan.[1]

Getting Started

In 1992, after attending a three-day hoshin planning course at GOAL/QPC, the CEO of Methodist convened his senior management, medical staff leadership, and board of trustees for a planning retreat. With a hoshin planning expert facilitating the retreat, this diverse team set out to understand and accept their organizational mission and vision and to identify those elements necessary for them to meet and exceed their customers' demands.

Since beginning total quality management (TQM) implementation one year earlier, the hospital had earned a heightened understanding of its internal and external customers. One of the most powerful manifestations of that renewed focus on the customer is the redesign of the organizational chart. Figure 13-1 represents a dramatic shift in the hospital's hierarchical paradigm.[2] This new perspective began to redefine the roles of executives, managers, and employees and how they related to one another throughout the emerging makeover of the strategic planning process.

Figure 13-1. Methodist Hospital: Supporting Relationship Chart

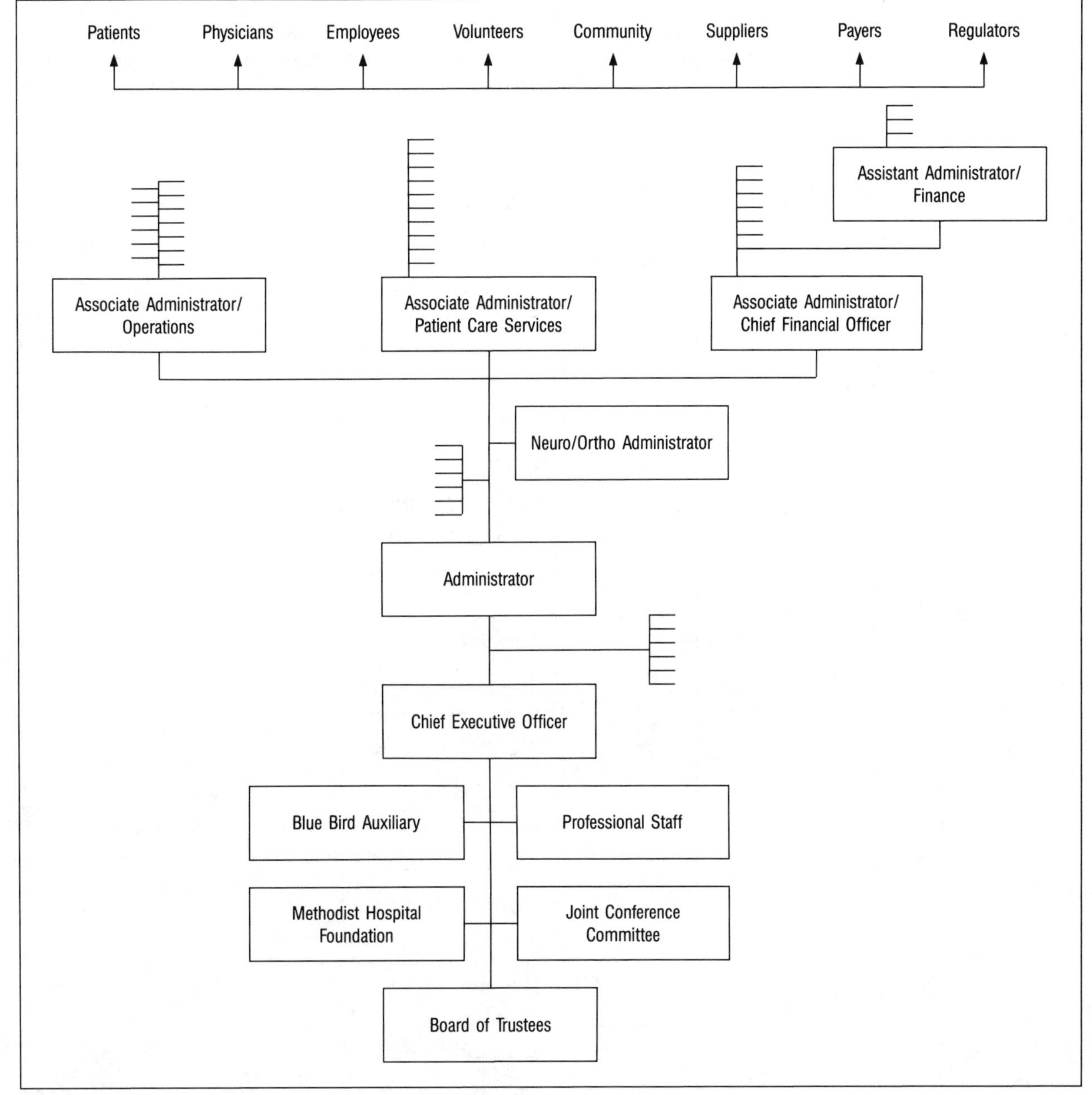

Reprinted, with permission, from Southwest Texas Methodist Hospital.

The CEO notes that, as Methodist began to embrace the new management philosophy represented by TQM and the teachings of W. Edwards Deming, there was some turnover in the leadership of the organization. He adds that "by the time we were ready to experiment with hoshin, we had a set of leaders committed to the new philosophy, [dissatisfied] with traditional planning methods, and willing to give [hoshin] a try."[3] The senior executives were further persuaded to embrace hoshin planning by the clear communication that this was not going to be "the new 'flavor of the month.' There was serious intent to change the infrastructure and the culture in all vital areas."

With the new, forward-thinking planning team at the helm, Methodist embarked on the hoshin planning journey. The overall flow that the group followed is shown in figure 13-2.

Choosing the Organization's Focus

Methodist Hospital's hoshin process was preceded by what seems, at first glance, like traditional strategic planning exercises: customer assessment, environmental scan, financial review, vision and mission development. (See figure 13-3 for Methodist's vision and mission statements.)

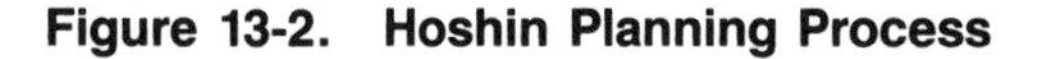

Figure 13-2. Hoshin Planning Process

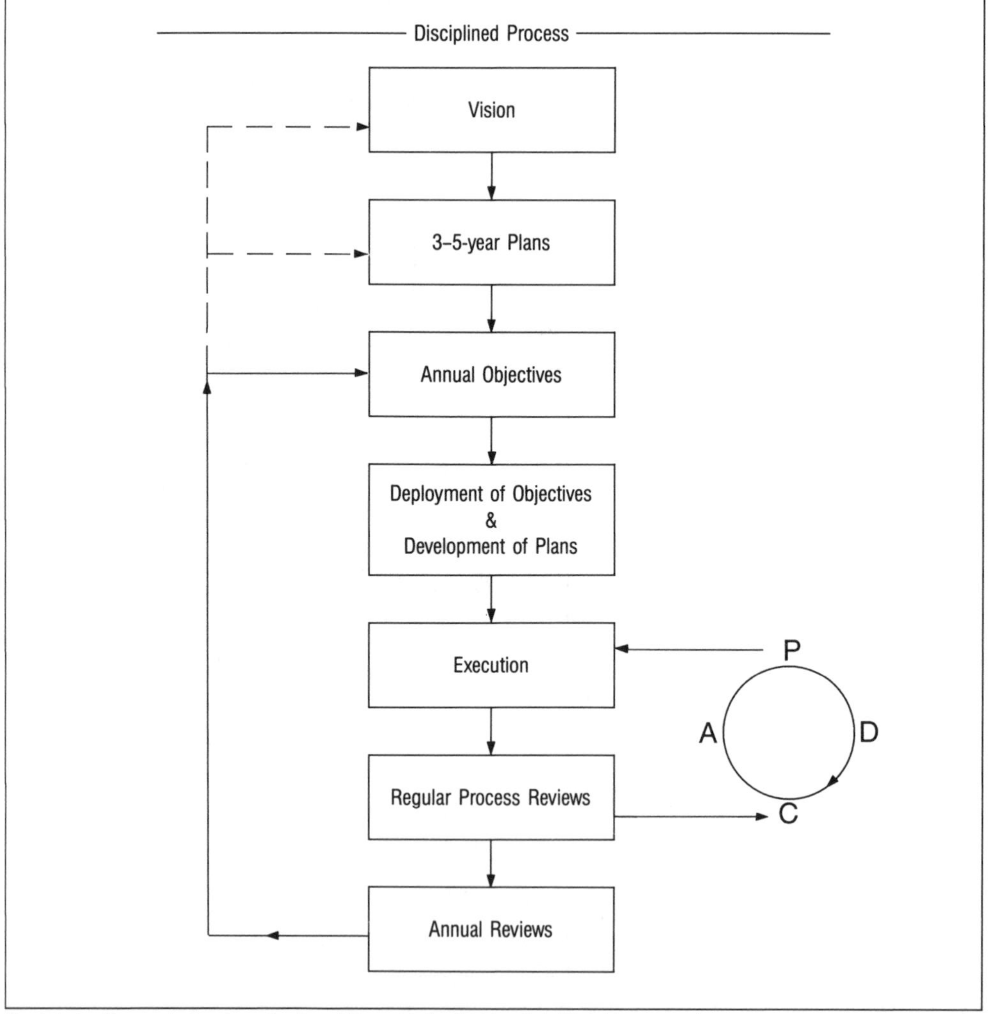

Reprinted, with permission, from Southwest Texas Methodist Hospital. All rights reserved.

The vision was driven by the adoption of total quality management as a culture. The existing mission was put into customer-oriented language. The board of trustees, the executive committee, and hospital staff were asked for feedback on the relevance and wording of the statement. According to the director of strategic planning, "We're still not done. . . . To truly understand your customer requires a lot of effort. The process, by nature, is dynamic. People change their minds about how they want things. To a certain degree we should be flexible with our vision."

Three- to Five-Year Plans

At this stage, Methodist Hospital's process departs from tradition in two essential ways: It is supported by the use of tools for managing verbal data, and it is visible.

Figure 13-3. Methodist Hospital: Vision and Mission Statements

Methodist Hospital Vision Statement

Ultimate Vision:

Patients prefer Methodist Hospital exclusively; the hospital is always full; elective patients insist on admission to Methodist, even if they must wait for a room.

Employees prefer to work at Methodist Hospital exclusively; the hospital is fully staffed; applicants await openings for employment.

Physicians prefer to practice at Methodist Hospital exclusively; physicians consider their relationship with the hospital to be a partnership; physicians insist on admitting their patients to Methodist, even when space is available elsewhere.

Payers (employers, insurers, HMOs, PPOs) prefer to join or create health benefit plans that contain Methodist Hospital as the major preferred provider; discounts are not necessary; new health plans insist on marketing their relationships with Methodist Hospital to the public.

The health care industry cites Methodist Hospital as a model of quality, cost-effectiveness, and value; other health care providers and representatives of government and other industries insist on making site visits here to learn.

Conceptual Basis:

Greatness for Methodist Hospital

We are committed to making Methodist Hospital a great hospital.

A great hospital does more than just accomplish its mission. In addition to healing others, a great hospital has learned how to heal itself.

Operational Basis:

To meet the needs and exceed the expectations of those we serve by working together as a team in a culture dedicated to never-ending improvement.

Methodist Hospital Mission Statement

Individual Basis:

We create healing* experiences.
We cure when we can,
We escort patients to death's door when we must,
But we always create healing experiences.

*The ministry of healing includes the spiritual dimension of the soul, the emotional dimension of the heart, the mental dimension of the mind, and the physical dimension of the body.

Organizational Basis:

The purpose of Methodist Hospital is to provide and constantly improve the delivery of high-quality, innovative health care services in a cost-effective way, while providing an appropriate amount of charitable care to people of the region.

The team used some of the seven management and planning (7MP) tools[4] and others as it developed the key strategic elements that would eventually lead to selection of the annual objectives.

Everyone agrees that the use of tools was an integral part of the hoshin effort from the start. The MP tools not only provided helpful structure to planning discussions, but also made the results of those discussions (plans and actions) readily visible to the whole organization. Also, the tools served as an equalizer of sorts, by making it possible for all employees to participate in planning, which traditionally was only part of management's job. In this way, the language barrier between management and staff was broken down, and everyone can now communicate with the same effectiveness on meaningful matters.

Strategic Initiatives

Using the tools, the executive council/steering committee identified five strategic initiatives in the first year that would evolve into the main pieces of the five-year hoshin plan. The five current initiatives in order of priority are:

1. *Total quality management:* Continue the integration of TQM and continuous quality improvement (CQI) throughout the hospital and its constituencies. Continue to increase the focus on customer-driven strategic planning, resource and expense efficiencies, an aggressive physician's education program, ongoing employee education, and the formalization of quality outcome measurements for all customers.
2. *Hospital and physician relations:* Continue to review and improve systems and processes affecting physician relations with the hospital. Adopt managed care initiatives as the primary strategic goal for fiscal year 1994. Investigate and formalize additional, appropriate, and beneficial collaborative mechanisms, including an assessment of physician recruitment needs, physician-directed process improvements in quality outcomes and measurements, ongoing physician practice assistance, and appropriate communication systems with all stakeholders.
3. *Partnerships and collaboration:* Pursue and implement, where appropriate, collaborative interests and/or formal affiliations with like-minded organizations in San Antonio and the region – to include other health care providers, area businesses, and constituencies.
4. *Outpatient services:* Develop and implement a more formal service line structure for outpatient services. Investigate and implement, collaboratively or otherwise, sub-acute care programs and other types of long-term care programs.
5. *Wellness and prevention:* Identify key wellness incentives and integrate them into a formal wellness and prevention program for Methodist employees. Design and implement an audit and review system to assist in ongoing benefit design improvements. Integrate this project into the managed care strategic initiatives.

Breakthrough Goal

The team selected total quality management for the first-year hoshin, or breakthrough goal. The journey to the selection of this goal included a review of the mission and vision, an affinity diagram[5] to brainstorm main strategic objectives, an interrelationship digraph[6] to identify which objectives were the drivers (figure 13-4), and a radar chart for gap analysis (figure 13-5, p. 194).

These exercises led to the realization that two important elements were missing from the current planning system – a formal method for performing situational analysis and a comprehensive understanding of customer needs and expectations. The retreat team agreed that these elements would be achieved through the successful implementation of TQM.

Figure 13-4. Interrelationship Digraph Exercise and Results

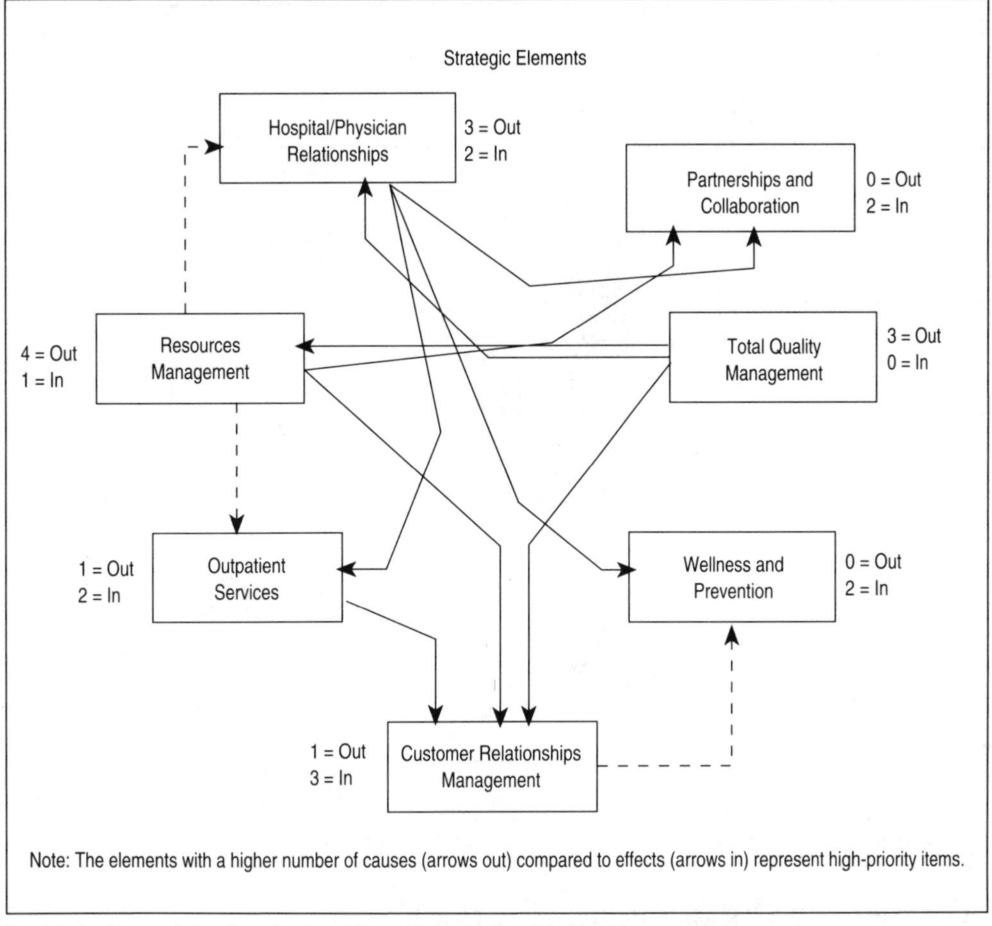

Reprinted, with permission, from Southwest Texas Methodist Hospital.

Selection of TQM as a hoshin is fairly unorthodox. In a presentation delivered by the CEO and the director of strategic planning on their application of hoshin, they contended:

> Some would argue that TQM is not a strategy, it is a culture. We would agree under normal business situations. Our limited situation analysis . . . indicated tough times ahead – specifically in how we deal with rising costs, a changing reimbursement marketplace, and a continuing, overriding desire to exceed quality expectations for all of our customers.
>
> The culture change brought on by systems thinking, which is embodied in the teachings of TQM, became the necessary driver of all of our efforts. It had to, for TQM was not something to be simply turned on like a light.[7]

So the planning team members trusted the process that led them to their conclusions and embraced TQM as their first-year hoshin. This was revisited in year 2.

The administrator of Methodist Hospital shared an interesting insight about the selection of the key drivers in the strategic plan. He notes that, traditionally, a strategic plan would provide one set of priorities, but people's daily focus would be somewhere else. With Methodist's set of hoshin priorities, the chosen drivers are the things people live with every day. The plan is useful because it is relevant to the realities of the organization.[8]

Figure 13-5. Radar Chart: Gap Analysis Exercise and Results

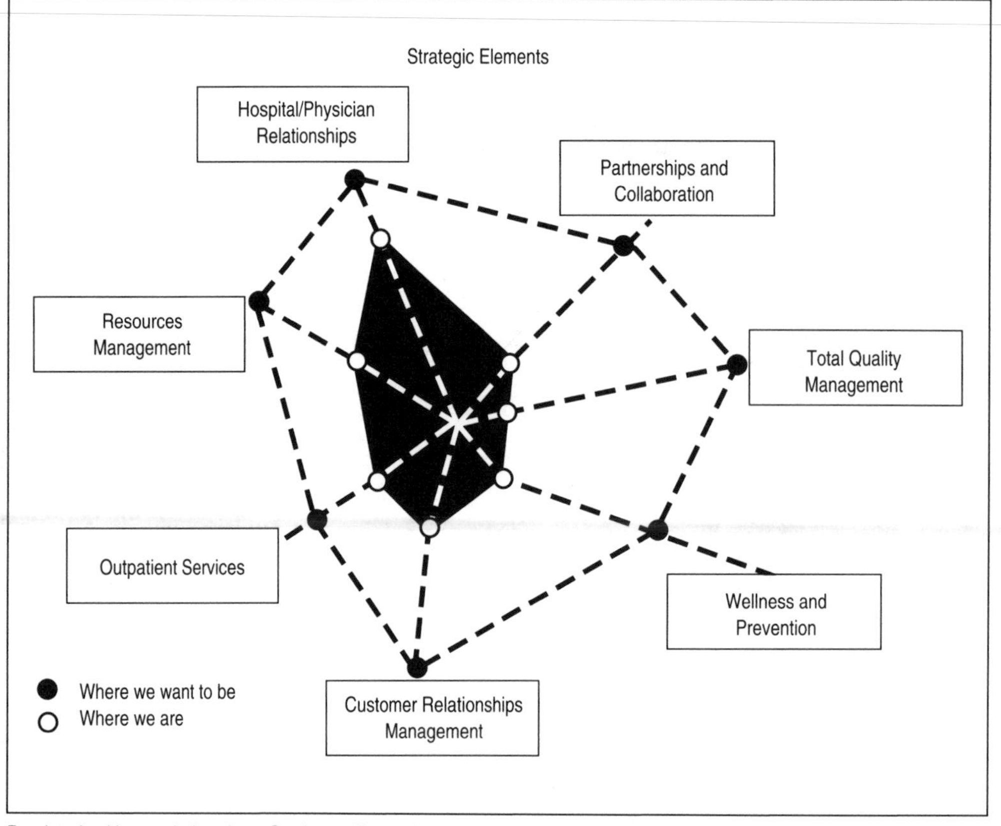

Reprinted, with permission, from Southwest Texas Methodist Hospital.

Aligning the Organization with the Focus

Catchball is the process by which Methodist's management solicited and encouraged input into the main strategic elements of the organization from everyone in the organization – even those not usually included in the circle of planning influence. Methodist launched the catchball process to its employees with the following statement:

> In throwing this ball to you, we are asking all staff members to consider the information in [this] presentation and to provide us with feedback in a number of specific ways that you will find on a response sheet prepared for this purpose. That input will be provided back to management so that we can adapt the plan accordingly.
>
> In October, the plan will be finally deployed throughout the hospital and will contain additional details and instruction regarding its implementation. This deployment will be made easier by the fact that:
>
> 1. The plan has been made better by staff input, and
> 2. The staff will be more familiar with it, having seen it once already.

This is a different approach from the one used previously, wherein plans were decided by top management and simply distributed to those who "needed to know."

Year 1: Catchball

In 1993, year 1 of hoshin implementation, Methodist requested input from the organization with the "Catchball One" questionnaire (identified as exhibit A) shown at the end of this chapter. Sometimes an organization will use the input it receives and then make another cycle of requests for feedback on the changes. The hoshin planning process often includes several cycles of this catchball process.

Methodist made the request for feedback only once in its first year of the new planning process. Reasons for this single pass included time constraints, lack of familiarity on everyone's part with the new planning process, and the fact that in this first iteration the feedback was generally not good. Varied feedback to first-year catchball is to be expected.

Year 2: Catchball

In year 2 (1994), catchball was done for two iterative cycles, with better feedback than was experienced the year before. This indicates some maturity in the organization's planning process and a heightened level of awareness and acceptance of the now fully operational planning method.

Finally, attention was called to the fact that discipline and creativity in designing catchball processes are pivotal to their success. Merely introducing the thought of catchball does not guarantee a response. Methodist added rigor to its process for soliciting input from all employees through the use of a thoughtfully designed response sheet. (See exhibit B, "Barrier Questions and Comments," at the end of this chapter.) The sheet not only provides structure to ensure that the organization receives the information it needs, but it is sufficiently open-ended to allow for flexibility in the feedback.

Year 1: Deployment of the Strategic Plan

Figure 13-6 shows the macro-level picture of the deployment of the 1993 strategic (hoshin) plan. This one page effectively illustrates the feeders to the plan, the main objectives, the key focus, and the main areas of measurement. The adaptability of hoshin for concise, focused communication is one of the features repeatedly touted as positive by Methodist planners.

An example of the detailed and disciplined application of measures typical of the hoshin review process can be seen in exhibit C, "Fiscal Year 1993 Strategic Plan Development Measurements," located at the end of this chapter. Indicators were broken down into these four categories: hospitalwide indicators, training objectives, activities objectives, and expense control objectives, with a schedule of reporting. Notice that the measurement categories correspond directly to the indicator categories set forth in figure 13-6. The selection of indicators is important and thoughtful and is done at the early stages of the planning process.

Year 2: Deployment of the Strategic Plan

In a similar fashion, Methodist completed a macro deployment strategy for the second-year strategic (hoshin) plan (figure 13-7). The new main initiative, hospital and physician relations, is broken down into five high-level targets for achievement in 1994. These targets were then compared to each other in an interrelationship digraph, and managed care was revealed as the driver—the target that, if achieved, would have the greatest impact on the other four.

That driver is then broken down further to show four key smaller goals (targets) that must be achieved to succeed in improving hospital performance in the area of managed care. Then, to the right of each goal will be listed means (tactics) for goal achievement.

This steady reductionism helps break large organizational goals into manageable pieces that can be more easily communicated to the entire hospital. The "bite-sized" pieces of the plan are also more easily contributed to by all staff levels. The detailed

Figure 13-6. FY 1993 Strategic Plan Deployment

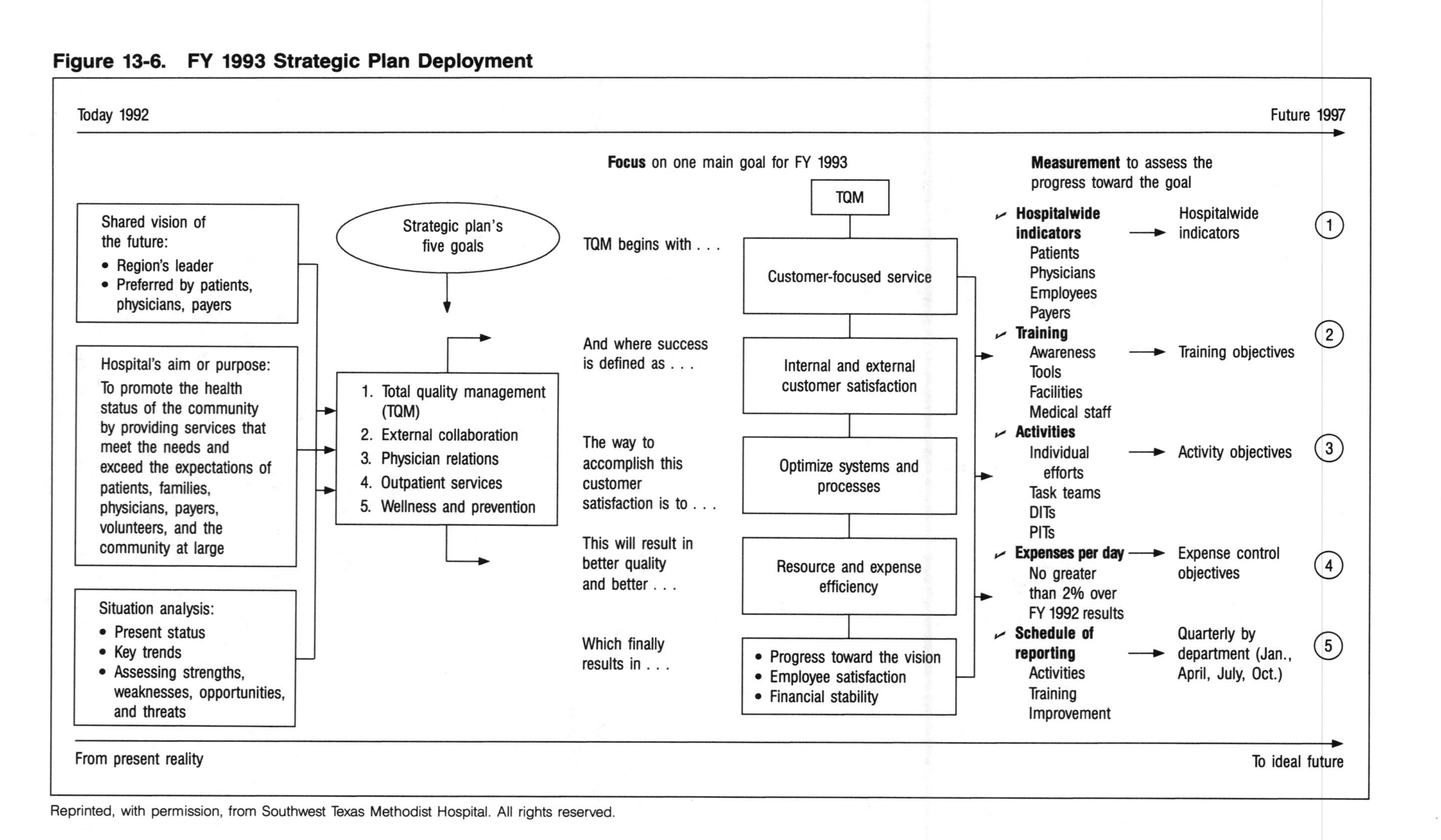

Figure 13-7. FY 1994 Strategic Plan Diagram

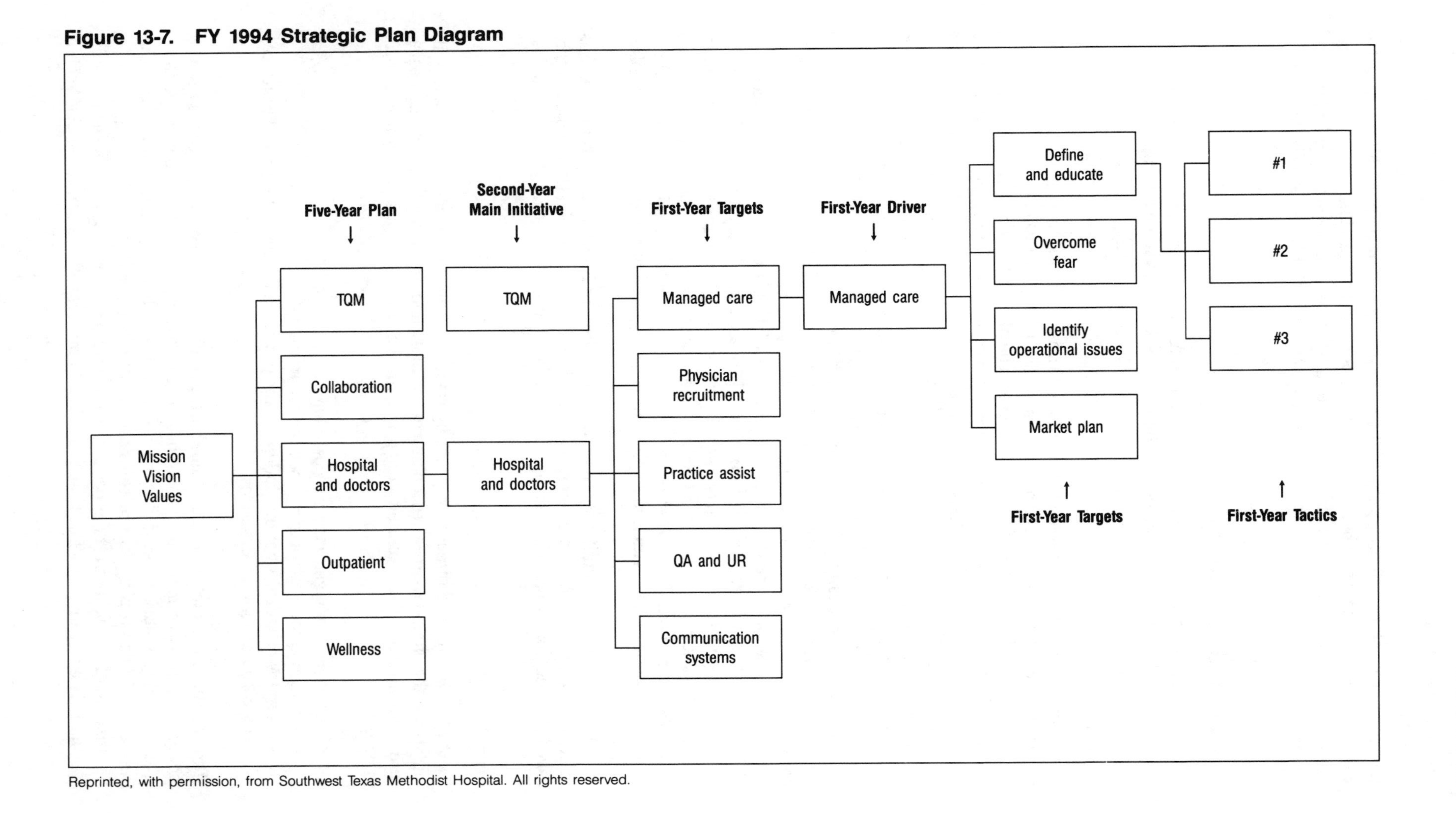

deployment strategy enhances the ability to set relevant measures and to track the targets for improvement. Most important, the consistent whittling away at the larger objectives encouraged Methodist to focus and prioritize its resources. By narrowing in and channeling its efforts in one direction, the hospital increased its probability of achieving success.

Review and Improvement

With the measurement data in hand, the planning team was able to review the success of year 1 as preparation for development of the second-year plan.

Year 2

According to the director of strategic planning, two areas needed to be examined in review of year 1. The team looked at the objectives of year 1 to see whether they had been met, and it reviewed the strategic plan itself to see if the plan still had the same impact. The team used a matrix that set customer demands against the strategies of the plan. (See exhibit D at the end of this chapter.) As a result of that analysis, the team made the previously mentioned change in order of the five originally generated initiatives.

As explained by the director of strategic planning, the number 2 initiative does not automatically become the hoshin after the first initiative has been achieved. The team first has to reexamine the initiatives in light of changing internal and external environments. For example, hospital and physician relations moved from the number 3 position to number 2 in 1994 because of health care reform, increases in managed care, and other environmental changes. The first-year hoshin, total quality management, was continued into the second year, along with this new second-year selection. Notice that it is still represented on figure 13-7 as a key second-year initiative.

The review feature built into the hoshin methodology is an important way to keep the initiatives current and relevant without having to start from scratch and redo the entire plan every year. The process of review is consistent with the spirit of the Shewhart plan-do-check-act cycle, which is explicit in the language and processes of planning at Methodist.[9]

Methodist added validity to its review by including its several customer groups in completion of the matrix referenced in exhibit D. The organization continuously asked, "Is the plan still viable for our customers? Is it still meeting their demands?"

Year 3

As the CEO, COO, and director of planning reviewed 1993 achievements on the hoshin initiatives, they found themselves looking at a rapidly and dramatically changing health care environment. They acknowledged the presence of three major environmental dynamics:

- Increased managed care market share
- An increasingly strong competitor environment
- Many Methodist-loyal but independent physicians now selling their practices to corporate group practices

Many organizations would react by hunkering down and strategizing furiously in the face of such massive environmental upheaval. But Methodist, with its newfound faith in its planning abilities, decided to be bold, face the challenge head-on, and use the flexibility of hoshin planning to the hospital's advantage.

Instead of engaging in the process of setting and reaffirming the five-year hoshin plan as it is entering year 3 of that plan, Methodist has chosen to forgo the hoshin plan temporarily until the crystal ball of the future reveals itself. Specifically, the organization will postpone setting the annual strategic initiatives for six months, place itself downwind of the changing market, and vigilantly watch the changes. It will then set the initiatives when the dynamics of the new market are clearer.

So as not to be caught off guard, the planning team has used existing market and competitive data to identify the three most likely market scenarios. The team then formed three contingency plans based on these scenarios. At the end of six months, it will begin the hoshin process anew and put into place whichever plan is relevant.

Overall Benefits and Results

The $900,000 loss represented in October 1992, prior to implementing hoshin planning, was turned into a $5 million gain within a six-month period. No traditional methods of cost cutting, such as layoffs, were used. Although the CEO credits "some significant gains in expense reduction" (the 1992 hoshin objective) with helping to produce a "fairly healthy" bottom line, he acknowledges that there are many undercurrents to financial results that come from outside the organization, such as managed care advances and demographic changes in the community. Those forces were endemic in the marketplace, of course, and other hospitals in the area were facing similar pressures. "How our organization dealt with these forces was enhanced by our hoshin planning," the CEO commented, though he stopped short of attributing, with any certainty, Methodist's financial turnaround to its hoshin efforts. He offered Deming's famous quote: "The most important things are unknown and unknowable."

Other indicators of success were firmly credited to hoshin, including the following:

- Improved morale
- More efficient use of resources
- Overall expense efficiency
- Less fragmentation
- Greater sense of empowerment for staff not previously included in the planning process

An important positive result of hoshin is the improvement in communication. Enhanced communication among individuals and departments resulted in the hospital's ability to improve processes in a context–the context of how changes in that process might affect other processes in other departments.

The CEO offers the example of a department that revamped a process even though it resulted in costing more money and reducing some indicators of efficiency within that department. But the changes were made because they contributed to some other area and ultimately to the strategic initiative. The leaders did consider the effect of that department's actions on other processes and departments. Instead of penalizing the department for what might look like bad numbers, they now reward this kind of system-oriented behavior. One department's awareness of another has been enhanced.

Key Success Factors

Key factors contributing to Southwest Texas Methodist Hospital's success in its trip so far through hoshin planning include the following:

- Keeping things simple–language and the catchball process, for example
- Recognizing that catchball takes time and being persistent

- Keeping hoshin planning flexible and dynamic and revisiting hoshin objectives regularly as the organizational environment changed
- Making the transition from technical to tactical thinking as more staff became involved in the planning process
- Having a strategic plan—with priority initiatives—on a single sheet of paper, which made a very strong impact on trustees, management, and staff

Problems and Challenges

As with any profound organizational change, some resistance was expected. In fact, the initial planning team chose to move staff quickly away from old paradigms by anticipating questions and challenges and preparing some answers in advance. Exhibit B, at the end of the chapter, shows the actual list of potential questions generated by the planning team and the corresponding comments. In this way, Methodist helps prepare its executive council and, eventually, its department managers for most of the resistance that might arise.

Physician Involvement

One of the concerns that surfaced from year 2 catchball was related to the increased involvement of physicians. Although it was generally accepted that full physician involvement was integral to the achievement of year 2's second hoshin—hospital and physician relations—some viewed the current lack of TQM knowledge among physicians as a potential source of tension in the now finely tuned TQM implementation process.

The CEO's reaction to this bit of catchball fallout was balanced: "These concerns are logical and well placed. However, all persons along the way of this journey are at various points. We have to create a process that is inclusive rather than picking out the people who we feel are educated and working only with them. If we were exclusive, we'd be right back to a self-defeating, oligopolistic mentality."

The key here is that the concerns, although placed in perspective, have been responded to with practicality. In response to this feedback, a target was added under the total quality management hoshin: to implement a physician education program with at least two demonstration projects in participation with the physician/hospital organization and the physician organization.

Education

Education of the staff of a large organization on the power of hoshin and strategic planning in general remains a key challenge. With 1,200 physicians on staff, 3,000 employees, and about a 15 percent attrition rate, the director of strategic planning says, "it's a daunting task to train everyone."

Methodist instituted a two-day training session called "The New Way" and mandated that everyone be involved. The aim was to provide the training in a way that was exciting and made people want to go. The executive council assumed all the responsibility for training this large number of people. By using the whole executive staff, it cut down on the time commitment for each person, but it was still a significant commitment of time. The employees involved agreed that the benefit of having visible participation from executive staff far outweighed the demands on their time.

Empowerment

Empowering individuals at the departmental level to take a greater role in catchball and the development of tactics proved to be another real challenge. Getting people to believe that they have the right and ability to offer input is a constant effort. The education initiative and constantly asking for their opinion are cited as the keys to building employees' confidence in getting involved.

Question 11 in the "barrier questions" document that the hoshin planning team developed (exhibit B) anticipates that people may respond to the changing environment with traditional habits of seeking approval for all improvements. All Methodist staff have been given the authority to use "their best judgment" and to "effect any improvements that are within their area of expertise and responsibility."

In this context, Methodist staff are expected to assess the impact of their actions on others, solicit input, communicate improvements to others, and then to feel "empowered" to make changes without executive approval. This does not mean that wanton changes will be acceptable. The decentralized authority travels with the expectation that everyone will use "good common sense in working with others and sharing one's ideas and improvements."

Change

Methodist has grappled with how to plan within the context of health care reform and the difficulty in developing appropriate breakthrough initiatives in a constantly changing environment. The organization believes that if you're going to be successful in this kind of planning, you have to acknowledge change for what it is – opportunity. Ignoring change will ultimately damage the viability of the organization.

Image

Making sure that the strategic plan language was easily understood at every level was a priority. It was essential to effectively communicate to all staff that hoshin is a lasting way of doing business and not just a gimmick. Successes in this area were achieved through a sound trust in the process, a commitment from Methodist leadership to model the new principles and behavior, and the ability to keep the hoshin process simple and accessible.

Roles and Responsibilities

The manager of the pharmacy department could have been speaking for all department heads when he said, "The reason I've been able to continue commitment on my part and in my department is that there's been continued commitment from the top."[10]

The CEO

The chief executive officer plays an essential and positive role in the successful application of hoshin planning at Southwest Texas Methodist Hospital. Throughout the interviews conducted for this case study, Methodist staff consistently reflected on the leadership role that the CEO fulfilled throughout this process. The sustained commitment on his part to decentralize planning authority and to provide the support, resources, and tools to allow people to fully participate enhanced the quality of the contributions and raised the level of empowerment among staff.

The CEO did not delegate TQM or hoshin planning. He is a fully contributing member of the executive council, which also serves as the TQM steering committee. In short, he is personally championing the new management style and modeling the changes in his own behavior.

Director of Strategic Planning

It is the CEO's example and the steady, knowledgeable guidance of the hospital's director of strategic planning that have provided the ballast for the sails in this process. The director calls his role the "manufacturer" of the CEO's vision. Having someone whose job it is to keep the process on track and to ensure discipline and consistency is vital to the successful manifestation of the vision.

Lessons Learned

Methodist's hoshin experience has taught its leadership many things. The two most important lessons offer encouragement to others considering hoshin planning: First, get input from everyone involved; and, second, have faith in the process.

Get Input from Everyone Involved

For hoshin planning to work, leaders must trust that people are going to give good input to the strategic planning process. The old philosophy that "I've got a good plan and I don't want it messed up by asking people what they think about it" is an outdated and unproductive one. Leaders must not only say that they will listen to the input of the organization, they must create an atmosphere that truly welcomes and uses input. Leaders must make it "safe" for those usually outside the sphere of influence to contribute.

Have Faith in the Process

Although initially hoshin seems process-intensive and demands high usage of resources, it is essential that the organization commit to at least one full cycle of hoshin and not judge it prematurely. Just as with organizational training, which costs money and does not always demonstrate immediate quantifiable results, so it is with hoshin. The message is, stick with it and give it a chance.

The director of strategic planning put it eloquently when he said, "The wonderment and the workability of this kind of planning is that it's customer-focused. It uses PDCA. It is cross-functional in its implementation. It is top-down and bottom-up planning. How else could you, would you want to, strategically plan for the future of our local health care system? Anything else is just playing at planning."

Exhibit A

June 3, 1993
Management Council
Revision June 8, 1993

Southwest Texas Methodist Hospital
Fiscal Year 1994 Strategic Plan

"Catchball One" Questionnaire

Catchball:

The Japanese coined the term *catchball* to mean the communication feedback process that is intended to involve all staff members of an organization. The idea is for management to distribute the strategic plan elements that are most important, explain those plans and the rationale behind them, and focus everyone's attention on the key strategy or the internal "driver" for the year.

In throwing the ball to you, we are asking all staff members to consider the information in the presentation and to provide us with feedback in a number of specific ways that you will find on the response sheet prepared for this purpose. This input will be provided back to management so we can adapt the plan accordingly.

The final strategic plan will be deployed throughout the hospital in October after one more catchball session. This deployment will be made easier by the fact that (1) the plan has been made better by staff input and (2) the staff will be more familiar with it, having seen it twice.

Instructions:

Please review the Strategic Plan Catchball One presentation with your staff. After general discussion, review the worksheet with your staff and brainstorm answers for each question. Please record your observations of these staff discussions after each question. It is not necessary for each staff member to fill out this worksheet. However, it is very important that all staff members participate in this discussion and that their comments are recorded on the Catchball One worksheet.

We would like to have these worksheets completed and sent directly to the Department of Strategic Planning and Market Research no later than June 25, 1993.

Thank you in advance for your help and support of this project.

Catchball One Worksheet

1. What are the reactions to the overall fiscal year 1994 strategic plan?

2. What are the reactions to the proposed first-year targets of the FY 1994 strategic plan?

3. List several ways your department/unit can assist in the fulfillment of the FY 1994 targets of the strategic plan?

4. What are the reactions to the 1994 strategic plan's main strategic initiatives: total quality management and hospital and physician relations?

5. Total quality management remains the key internal strategic initiative, with the continuing target of resource and expense efficiencies. List additional areas of improvement to target in 1994. Hospitalwide? Your department/unit?

6. What ways can your department/unit support hospital and physician relations and managed care strategic initiatives?

7. Are there any concerns about the overall strategic plan and this year's major emphasis?

8. Are there other hospitalwide strategies we should adopt for 1994?

9. Is there a more efficient, understandable way to present the strategic plan? If so, what is it?

Exhibit B

Barrier Questions and Comments

1. What do you want us to cut?

We want you to cut out resource consumption that represents waste, redundancy, inefficiency, and rework, so that your customers will be served better. Management can't really tell people what to cut because management can't possibly know. The people actually doing the work and serving their customers know best what constitutes areas of waste, redundancy, and inefficiency.

2. Where are we going to get the time?

It's never going to be easy to find time to do everything that we need to do. We have that problem now. Managing our time, therefore, becomes a matter of prioritization. As progress is made, there will be additional time created by the elimination of time-consuming activities that represented the waste, redundancy, inefficiency, and rework that is being eliminated.

3. How can I begin when my staff has not been trained yet in the TQM tools and principles?

We do believe that training is important, and we have announced a schedule of additional training that you can receive. But we shouldn't be waiting for the training or anything else to get started. We believe that people want to do a good job, are most knowledgeable about what improvements could be made, and can be challenged immediately to begin putting their knowledge to work. When you think about it, we've always had a responsibility to do our best work, make improvements that serve the customer better, conserve resources, and work cooperatively with one another toward those objectives. Let's not use lack of training as an excuse to do nothing. In one sense, we will never be completely "trained" and will always work to learn and apply the TQM principles and tools better and better in the future.

4. I need more people in my department—so how can I possibly cut anything?

In this question, we've jumped to a conclusion and proposed a solution without study or justification. The old philosophy supported this kind of thinking in the following manner:

a. We're not lazy and we're all working hard to get the job done.
b. Despite our best efforts, we still fall short of getting everything done that we need to do.
c. Therefore, improvement can occur only if we add more people (throw more money at the problem).

In the new philosophy, we accept *a* and *b* above, but we do not reach the conclusion of *c* because we know the results of our work are functions of the people, policies, and procedures followed; materials and supplies used; equipment; and environment. To conclude that the only solution is to add more people is to assume that these other factors are in perfect harmony and that no improvement is possible other than adding personnel to do more of the same.

5. If improvements cause someone to lose his or her job, what happens to that person?

In our mission, vision, and value statement published in January of this year, we made it clear that anyone whose job is eliminated because of improvements in serving our customers will not lose employment as a result. Although circumstances can vary widely, our first choice would be to retrain the person for another position within the hospital. The second choice is to assist the person in finding a job elsewhere. We think it is important for everyone to understand the hospital's intent in this regard.

6. There just aren't any improvements to be made in my area, so what do you want me to do?

TQM principles and operations research convince us that there is a lot of room for improvement in every single area. Anyone who can't perceive areas of improvement either isn't looking or hasn't been trained to look.

7. We could cut expenses if only we could get better support from other departments.

That may be true, but the approach that will result in real improvement will be one of cooperation among departments that are involved in the same processes. These cooperative efforts must be aimed at optimizing the whole system and not just one department at the expense of another. We are not going to tolerate one department's simply shifting its responsibilities to another department in order to cut their expenses. It is possible that one department may operate at a loss to itself in order to optimize the functioning of the whole system. We want to encourage that as much as possible. But such a determination will be made in the full view and knowledge of all departments concerned with a given process. We need to break down barriers between departments and work together toward optimizing the whole system.

8. This won't work if the physicians don't—or won't—get involved.

We agree that physicians are critically important to all aspects of the hospital's operation. We also agree that physician involvement is absolutely critical in many instances. We do recognize that there are many processes that will not require physician involvement or have physician impact. The PDCA cycle calls for us to identify our customers, flowchart the existing process so that we know its boundaries, and brainstorm improvements based on that knowledge. When the customers include the physicians and the flowchart of the process shows physician impact and involvement, then we absolutely must involve them in a meaningful way in improving that process. We have found physicians to be both interested and cooperative when involved in a meaningful way.

9. What if we find improvements that serve our customers better and yet they cost more money?

We understand that our overall emphasis and direction for the coming year has to be on net expense reduction. In improving processes overall, we are convinced that there will be enough cost savings (through reduction of waste, rework, etc.) to be able to fund improvements that cost more. So our overall aim has to be to find enough improvements in a given area not only to fund the portions that will cost more, but to result in a net reduction overall.

10. What if an improvement requires a significant capital expense?

We have a capital budgeting mechanism that will have to be followed. Depending on the size of the expenditure, it may have to be planned in a future month or even year. Its prioritization will depend on its importance and its net effect overall. We should not hesitate to identify improvements that require even significant capital expenditures. We should recognize, however, that there are lots of improvements that we can effect that will not require significant capital expenditures, and those are likely to receive a higher priority for implementation than others.

11. What approvals do we need to implement improvements?

The new management philosophy tells us that we need to empower the staff to effect any improvements that are within their area of expertise and responsibility. Obviously, people have to use their best judgment. Where people think they have a very firm grasp of the issues and a very high confidence level that their improvement will work and not cause problems upstream or downstream from the improvement, they should go ahead. Where people believe an improvement will work but recognize that they have limited knowledge of the possible impacts, they need to work out this idea with those involved through their supervisors prior to implementation. Essentially, it's a matter of assessing the probability of success or failure against the probability of the improvement's causing other problems. We do believe and insist, however, that staff members use their judgment in informing their coworkers and their supervisors about their improvements so that input from others is possible. Informing others also makes sense from the standpoint that if the improvement really does work for one person, it ought to be shared and used by others doing the same job. That's also necessary from the standpoint of changing policies, procedures, or practices so that we are operating consistently. In summary, our message is one of empowerment versus the need to get authoritarian approval to make any move, but this message is balanced by the use of good common sense in working with others and sharing one's ideas and improvements.

12. What incentives do we have (are there any incentives) to really improve processes?

The new philosophy does not espouse the use of games, prizes, slogans, gimmicks, or competition among units. These are all called "extrinsic" motivators that imply that people are interested in making a contribution only if they get some extra or outside reward for doing so. We don't believe that that is the case at all. We believe that people are intrinsically motivated by their own self-esteem, their ability to make a contribution, and their ability to meet and exceed the needs and expectations of those they serve. We do believe that people's contributions should be recognized and appreciated. We do believe that when people continuously make improvements and contributions, their value should be recognized in terms of receiving greater responsibilities and being afforded promotional and developmental opportunities, as well as in their periodic salary review.

13. Will administration back us if improvements have a negative impact on our physicians?

Our physicians constitute one major category of our customers. By definition, a change that has a negative impact on our customers cannot be considered an "improvement." It is true that any meaningful relationship requires some give and take between the participants. Physicians, like everyone else, tend to react negatively to a change that comes as a surprise to them, that they had no input into, and that they do not understand the reason for. It is incumbent on us to involve the system overall. When that occurs, administration does not have to back anyone in opposition to someone else. The parties work together to make the changes that make the most sense to everyone.

14. How much improvement do you want? What is our quota?

In terms of matching expenses and revenues, the projections suggest that a $6.6 million swing in expenses will be necessary in fiscal year 1992–1993 if we are to achieve a zero percent operating margin. That is not a quota. It is simply a fact based on the projection. We do not intend to take that figure, or any figure, and parcel it out to the various departments and units as quotas for reduction. That kind of thinking is simplistic and counterproductive. It is clear that the $6.6 million figure is a substantial one that will require significant efforts from everybody. The kind of effort that we are calling for in this year's strategic plan is intended to be an ongoing effort that never really has an ending point. Why would we ever stop trying to improve things, improve customer service, and become more efficient in the use of our resources? We expect to go by that $6.6 million figure sometime in the next year and continue on toward $10, $12, and $15 million in savings. But we don't want people focusing on a set quota or number for their unit or department. That is the old way, and if we persist in doing that, we will stop making improvements when we hit our number or make our quota. The point is not to stop when we have "done our part" but to continuously improve without regard to limits.

15. Why can't we cut expenses like everyone else and like we did a few years ago?

We realize that there are a few people who would prefer to have the old methodology used. The advantages of the old methodology are that it was quick, it was viewed as a one-time exercise that was performed and then set aside, and it allowed us to escape responsibility for our actions because the quota was imposed on us by "the administration." In the new philosophy, we have grown beyond that thinking. We have grown up and matured as responsible adults. We believe that people are responsible, that they do have intimate knowledge about their work and are in the best position to make the changes that improve processes and serve the customer better, while reducing net resource consumption.

16. What do our customers have to do with cutting expenses?

Customer focus is essential to identifying what our objectives are in the work that we are performing. Once we understand what our customers want and need, we are able to identify areas of activity that are unnecessary or that don't serve those needs well. By knowing customers' wants and needs, we are able to know whether a change that reduces expenses really affects customer service in a negative way. Customer focus enables us to cut the fat and not the muscle.

17. I really can't do anything without approval from my supervisor. So how can my individual effort really work?

See number 11. Supervisors have a tough job and have to balance empowering their staff to work and make changes on their own while ensuring that significant deterioration in service doesn't occur as a result of changes that don't work. Transformation to the new philosophy must start with the individual. Individual effort and improvements must be allowed to occur. In the new philosophy, supervisors are being taught that their roles are those of coach and counselor, support builder, and roadblock remover. In the old philosophy, they were directors, planners, counselors, overseers, and approval authorities. This journey from the old philosophy to the new philosophy is a long, never-ending one. All of us are at different points, and it is incumbent on us to be sensitive to where others are in the journey. We expect that many staff employees will find that they have gone further than their supervisor. In those cases, the staff employees must actually help the supervisor along. We expect to help each other.

18. What happens if this doesn't work?

It is always possible that the most well-intended efforts may fall short. We have a high level of confidence in the people who work at Methodist Hospital. The concepts, principles, and tools of total quality management have really begun to be espoused, appreciated, and practiced. But if we do fall short and a "fire breaks out," we will certainly have to put out the fire. We won't idly stand by and let it burn, but this will be a last resort and it will simply be an acknowledgment that the economic realities required arbitrary action. We are responsible for having a contingency plan for such a worst-case scenario but we do not intend to include layoffs in that contingency plan.

19. No matter how you look at it, if we cut expenses our patients will suffer and our physicians will be angry.

This is old-philosophy reasoning and thinking. To believe this, one has to assert that not a single penny gets spent on waste, rework, unnecessary redundancy, and other inefficiencies. We know that that simply is not the case. It is definitely harder work to understand our processes and find improvements that actually improve quality and service while reducing expenses. That is our charge and that is what we must do.

20. If expenses are the issue, why are we spending so much money on things like a new children's hospital, the 10th floor, and so on?

Some activities are understood only with a long-term view of the future. The hospital's mission is to promote the health status of the community through the services and programs that we provide. As the health care industry continues to change, we will be faced with more and more difficult decisions that require a long-term view of how best to serve the community in collaboration with other hospitals that have the same mission. If you have questions regarding any of these efforts, please let us know. It is our intent to be as forthcoming as possible about any activities that we conduct.

21. We see the financial statement each month, and it shows we are making money. What, then, is the problem?

We have been disclosing our monthly financial statements through management council minutes for all hospital departments for some time now. We have every reason to want all staff members to be adequately informed about the month-to-month financial status of the hospital. With the completion of the south tower, we have finished more than five years of being in an expansion mode. Now that those expanded facilities and services have been largely assimilated, we are able to make accurate projections relative to the financial performance of the hospital in the next one to three years. It is clear from that analysis that if our expenses continue to rise at historical rates of increase, the accompanying revenues would be insufficient to make ends meet. The fact that we have made this assessment and are disclosing all of this prior to its occurring only means that we are fulfilling our responsibilities.

22. Why can't we first cut expenses in the departments that have nothing to do with patient care?

Understanding the hospital as a system belies the statement that there are departments and activities that "have nothing to do with patient care." Even those departments and activities that are not as directly related to patient care activities as others have important functions to perform in terms of the overall system. All parts of the system are going to be required to participate and show improvement in their operations and services to their customers, but we see no reason to single out one kind of department or service as being more or less valuable and important than any other.

23. What can we do about waste that is caused by regulatory requirements from outside agencies?

We realize that there are regulatory requirements imposed on hospitals that are counterproductive, have nothing to do with adding value to patient care, and add a significant amount of time and expense to the services we provide. We can approach these issues in several ways. First, we should really examine those regulations and requirements to find out if we have missed something important. Second, we can examine the intent behind the regulation and see if there is a more innovative way to achieve the aim of the regulation while still reducing the waste and inefficiency caused by our current procedure for complying with the regulation. Third, we can attempt to get the regulation changed or rescinded.

Exhibit C (Southwest Texas)

Fiscal Year 1993 Strategic Plan Development Measurements

Hospitalwide Indicators

1. Patients are delighted about Methodist Hospital when:
   a. The expected clinical outcome is achieved
   b. Nurses are responsive, skilled, caring, informative, and knowledgeable
   c. Requests (call button) are responded to promptly and with sensitivity
   d. Accommodation needs are met and exceeded
   e. Admission procedures are understandable, quick, and efficient
   f. Discharge procedures are understandable, quick, and efficient
   g. Billing and collection procedures are understandable, accurate, and efficient
   h. The value of services received exceeds expectations

2. Physicians are delighted about practicing at Methodist Hospital when:
   a. Available time is maximized
   b. Scheduling needs are met
   c. Hospital staff are responsive, informative, concerned, accessible, and knowledgeable
   d. Reports are timely
   e. High-quality consultants are available
   f. State-of-the-art equipment and facilities are available
   g. The expected clinical outcome is achieved

3. Employees are delighted about Methodist Hospital when:
   a. Patients receive high-quality services that are skilled, caring, and effective
   b. All departments work together to improve quality
   c. Leaders understand employee issues, communicate regularly, and recognize employee accomplishments
   d. Processes are made efficient enough to allow requirements to be met with budgeted staffing
   e. New coworkers are carefully selected, highly qualified, and integrated into the workforce, and prove to be long-term employees
   f. Educational and advancement opportunities are readily accessible

4. Payers (employers, insurance companies, Medicare, etc.) are delighted about Methodist Hospital when:
   a. Employees and their dependents are delighted about their care
   b. The value of services received exceeds expectations
   c. The hospital continually demonstrates efforts to reduce costs while improving quality
   d. Indicators of high-quality services are measured and made available
   e. The hospital provides a system for meaningful dialogue between hospital and payer

Measurement Tools

Patients
- Monthly patient satisfaction survey

Physicians
- Semiannual physician satisfaction survey

Employees
- Annual employee satisfaction survey
- Employee evaluation
- Various other internal measurement tools

Payers

- Quality outcome indicators
- Patient satisfaction survey
- Semiannual employer focus groups
- Annual quality perception indicators

Training Objectives

1. Awareness training
   - Ongoing two-day training for all employees (approximately 1,000 have already attended).
   - Remaining employees to complete training by March 3, 1993.
   - After March 1993, monthly awareness training will begin for all new employees.

2. Tools training
   - An eight-hour basic process improvement and problem-solving course will be taught to management council, plus an additional two employees per department—completed by end of 1992.

3. Team leader training
   - A three-day course taught by Dr. Weaver and others. To include team meeting and leading skills and training in FOCUS PDCA problem-solving methodology.
   - Leaders selected for major process improvement teams to be trained by October 1992.
   - Twenty management council members will be trained in each quarter beginning in January 1993.

4. Facilitator training
   - Twenty-four facilitators to be trained in the first quarter of fiscal year 1993.
   - This three-day training to include:
     - Communication skills
     - Total quality management processes
     - Techniques for intervention
     - Practice in process facilitation
     - Additional training in the tools and techniques needed to assist project teams in problem solving

5. Medical staff training
   - Plan still being formed.
   - During interim:
     - Hospital-based physicians (radiologists, pathologists, neonatologists, and emergency physicians) to be involved in monthly staff awareness training and Deming seminars.
   - Spring 1993: Four-day Deming seminar made available to medical staff through satellite downlink.
   - Training to date: Two staff physicians have attended four-day Deming seminar. Five physicians have attended a health care forum on quality.

Activities Objectives

1. Individual efforts
   - Activities carried out by individual employees that evidence their commitment to and participation in TQM. For example:
     - Ways of improving how their jobs are done that are identified, put into practice, and evaluated.
     - Identification of ways in which the jobs of others may be improved, communication of those ideas, and assistance with implementation and evaluation.
     - Suggestions of processes within the department whose examination results in improvement.
     - Active involvement in task teams and department improvement teams.

2. Task teams (TTs)
   - Small groups (three or fewer) addressing processes within given work areas:
     - Processes are predominantly intradepartmental.
     - Customer input is usually required.
     - Limited data collection is usually required.

3. Department improvement teams (DITs)
   - Groups of four or more within the department addressing major intradepartmental processes:
     - Processes are intradepartmental.
     - Customer input is required.
     - Substantial data collection is required.

4. Process improvement teams (PITs)
   - Large groups of eight or more subject-matter experts from two or more departments addressing hospitalwide (macro) processes
     - Processes are interdepartmental.
     - Customer input is required.
     - Gathering of information from subject-matter experts not on the team is required.
     - Data collection is vital and extensive.

5. Activity and time line
   - To assess commitment to and participation in TQM; present employee evaluation tool will be revised by November 1, 1992.
   - During November, input from staff will be sought.
   - The final tool will be circulated in December.
   - Implementation to begin in January 1993.
   - Employee objectives:
     - Employees being evaluated will be expected to demonstrate greater involvement in TQM, evidenced by understanding of the strategic plan; training received; participation in PITs, DITs, and TTs; readings; and examples of individual effort.

Expense Control Objectives

1. Ensure an aggregate growth in hospitalwide operating expenses per patient day of no greater than 2 percent over fiscal year 1992 results.
   - Reductions must come from improvements (efficiency).
   - Quality cannot be compromised.

2. Increases in revenue that are subject to Medicare, Medicaid, CHAMPUS, or managed care discounts may not be used to offset some increases in expenses per patient day.
   - Increases in revenue may come from increased patient admissions or outpatient visits, or
   - They may come from sources unrelated to patient care services, such as paid parking.

3. No quotas are to be established or used.
   - Every department will target improvements that result in overall expense reduction in the processes under study.
     - Expenses can be increased in one part of the process (department) while larger expense reductions result in other parts of the process.

Schedule of Reporting

1. Hospitalwide indicators
   - Monthly reports from patient satisfaction surveys to be disseminated beginning in October.
   - Physician and employee surveys to be initiated by January.

- Payer surveys will be a "Year Two" objective.
- Responsibility for all survey development and reporting: Planning/Marketing Department (Geoff Crabtree).

2. Reports on five core process measures, which cross several departments, are to be reported beginning in the fourth month following the process improvement team's starting. The five process improvement teams for fiscal year 1993:
   - Drug distribution
   - Billing turnaround
   - Admission, discharge, transfer activity
   - Admission process
   - Drug formulary

3. Summary of "Catchball" responses from management council to be reviewed by quality council and returned to departments by October 2, 1992.
   - Follow-up reports on DITs are due from departments by January 15, 1993.

Exhibit D

Customer Demands Matrix

Patient Demands	Strategies 1	2	3	4	5
High-quality care	⊙	○	⊙	○	
Ease of access			⊙	⊙	
Affordable care	⊙	⊙	⊙	⊙	⊙
State-of-the-art facility and service		⊙	⊙	⊙	
Communication in process	⊙		⊙		
Quick service	○	○	○	○	○
Consolidated billing	⊙		⊙		
"Warm fuzzies"					

Physician Demands	Strategies 1	2	3	4	5
Convenient facilities			⊙	⊙	
Quality support staff	⊙		⊙		
State-of-the-art technology		○	⊙		
Hospital–MD support		⊙	⊙		
Efficient systems	⊙		⊙		
Control of documenting			⊙		
Patient compliance	○				

References and Notes

1. Geoffrey W. Crabtree, director of strategic planning and market research, Southwest Texas Methodist Hospital. Interviews by Lisa Boisvert, January 18 and 24, 1994. (Also subsequent quotes.)
2. Hornbeak credits the Peter Block book *The Empowered Manager* (Jossey-Bass) with the original idea for this inverse organizational chart.
3. John E. Hornbeak, FACHE, CEO, Southwest Texas Methodist Hospital. Interview by Lisa Boisvert, February 21, 1994. (Also subsequent quotes.)
4. Brassard, M. *The Memory Jogger Plus.* Methuen, MA: GOAL/QPC, 1989.
5. An affinity diagram is a structured brainstorm, where each idea is recorded on a self-stick note and all notes are sorted to create columns of related items.
6. The interrelationship digraph is a graphic tool that visually represents the cause-and-effect relationships among a group of items.
7. Crabtree, Geoffrey W., and Hornbeak, John E. Paper presented at GOAL/QPC Tenth Annual Conference, Nov. 1993.
8. James Scoggins, Jr., administrator, Southwest Texas Methodist Hospital. Interview by Lisa Boisvert, February 23, 1994.
9. Deming, W. E. *Out or the Crisis.* Cambridge, MA: Massachusetts Institute of Technology, Center for Advanced Engineers Study, 1986, p. 88.
10. Ron Kolar, manager, pharmacy department, Southwest Texas Methodist Hospital. Interview by Lisa Boisvert, Feb. 17, 1994.

CHAPTER FOURTEEN

AT&T Transmission Systems

Louis E. Monteforte, Sr., and Mara Melum

The AT&T Transmission Systems Business Unit (TSBU) is one of six strategic business units within the AT&T Network Systems Group, which is the largest of AT&T's manufacturing groups and a leading worldwide supplier of network telecommunications equipment for public and private telephone networks. The unit's purpose is to deliver the highest-value transmission systems to customers worldwide. The TBSU is the leading supplier of transmission systems within the United States and the second-largest supplier worldwide. If it were a stand-alone company, it would rank roughly 150th among Fortune 500 companies. Headquartered in Morristown, New Jersey, the company employs 7,500 people in the United States and another 2,500 people around the world.

The Transmission Systems Business Unit designs, manufactures, sells, and supports equipment and systems used to deliver telephone calls, data, and video from customer locations to the central office (access systems) or between central offices (transport systems). A 1992 winner of the Malcolm Baldrige National Quality Award, the TSBU aspires to be an overachiever in the eyes of its customers. At least once a year, many of TSBU's major customers issue detailed, individualized "report cards" grading the equipment supplier on the product and service characteristics they deem most important. Driven from this customer-specific information – from measures of product quality to responsiveness of customer-support services – TSBU's integrated strategic planning process ensures that performance improvement goals contribute directly to increases in customer satisfaction and gains in the market.

For telecommunications companies, reliability is the top priority for transmission equipment. The reliability of TSBU products exceeds customer expectations in all of the company's markets. On the basis of that record and continuing improvement in product quality, TSBU has the longest warranty in the industry and warranty expense has decreased even as warranty length has been extended. Further, since 1989, TSBU has cut new-product development time in half and realized cost savings totaling over $400 million.

Reasons for Choosing Hoshin Planning

In April 1989, AT&T announced that it was restructuring the company into 20 business units, one of which was the TSBU. As a developer and manufacturer of systems for transporting voice and image data, TSBU serves a global market and competes head-on with some of the best-known electronics manufacturers in the world. Emerging from a predivestiture monopolistic environment, the new TSBU leadership team, headed by the president of the unit, realized that, to retain and strengthen its position as an industry leader, the company had to revamp its management system.

Although quality-related activities, such as teams, had been in place for some time in TSBU's factories, these efforts were deemed insufficient to provide the results that were required in an increasingly competitive global market. The unit needed to develop a vision of its future and a management system to achieve it. Management wanted to build on the AT&T tradition of quality and its existing team activities. At a decision point at which many companies discard their quality programs, the TSBU examined its management system's gaps to determine causes and formulate actions to improve.

During 1989, TSBU leadership formulated a vision of what they wanted the organization to become. This vision, however, was not just to be engraved on another plaque on the wall. It was going to become a dominant theme that would unite all associates toward a common goal. The TSBU's vision calls for:

- Being the best at everything it does, exceeding customer expectations
- Expanding its business to increase in value to customers, associates, shareowners, and communities in which the TSBU works
- Remaining integral with Network Systems in the achievement of AT&T's mission and values

Because many visions come and go, a process had to be found to enable the TSBU to achieve its vision. During 1990, TSBU management learned of a process that worked for some companies, including Florida Power & Light, 1989 winner of the Japanese Deming Prize. Called strategic policy management, or policy deployment, the process was a lot like management by objectives (MBO) as practiced in many large corporations, but with a few key differences. Basically, policy deployment (or hoshin planning) differs from MBO in its emphasis on process improvement to achieve results, in the level of executive participation, and in its focus on customer satisfaction. It is not about finding out who did not succeed (MBO). Policy deployment is about everyone working together to guarantee success.

Eventually, AT&T decided to adopt policy deployment (the term used throughout this case study for AT&T's hoshin planning activities), which it defines as "an organizationwide and customer-focused management approach aimed at planning and executing breakthrough improvements in business performance":

- An organizationwide activity that requires participation from many members of the organization
- A customer-focused activity driven by an emphasis on meeting current and future customer needs
- A management approach that aligns all associates with the strategic direction of the business and keeps associates informed of their contributions to the results
- An approach aimed at dramatic breakthrough improvements in business performance, which require intense and focused improvement efforts

Hoshin Implementation

In May 1990, the TSBU leadership team had its first policy deployment workshop. Armed with little more than its vision and plenty of skepticism, the group struggled for three days but came to some harsh realizations regarding:

- *Customers:* Who are our customers, anyway, and what do they want?
- *Teams:* We have lots of quality teams already, but they're not able to give us the bottom-line impact we need.
- *Rabbits:* We already have too many priorities to chase, and now we have to do this quality stuff.

Overview

The executive team began to address these critical issues one by one. This was done in the context of the total quality management (TQM) system.

1991: Making Progress toward Winning the Baldrige Award

By the fall of 1990, the TSBU had developed its purpose, vision, and shared values and was on the way toward incorporating them into that TQM model. By February 1991, some progress was being made in a few areas, but TQM system integration was not complete. There was engagement of only a limited set of leaders. Middle management and working-level associates needed to be engaged in policy deployment. To this point, only the specific team working on the policy deployment projects had been trained to work on improving their specific activities. Everyone who had been trained in policy deployment – the executives and the specific teams – believed this was the way to help the organization achieve its vision.

Now it was time to engage the rest of the organization. Management felt that committing the organization to a time line would spur it to rally behind the cause. To jump-start the process, the policy deployment training was rolled out to more than 700 middle managers. Also, the 66 team leaders were trained to create the "Golden Threads." A Golden Thread is the link from the customer through management to all the people on teams working to satisfy customers. In addition, to accelerate the process, TSBU executive management announced that it would submit an application for the 1991 Malcolm Baldrige National Quality Award.

Progress was evident in two ways: the self-assessment scores against the Baldrige Award criteria increased significantly in six months, and continued improvements to the business were made. The TSBU did receive a Baldrige site visit but did not receive an award. Still, the challenge was considered a success because it raised the level of awareness, excitement, and performance – and self-expectation – throughout the organization.

During the winter of 1991, the TSBU continued to make progress in improving product and service quality. Return rates on one key product decreased by more than 50 percent in less than nine months, and on-time delivery performance improved significantly. But some parts of the organization were still not fully engaged. Without them, system integration and maximum gains could not be achieved.

1992: Winning the Baldrige Award

Providing customers with maximum utility for hardware requires high-quality software. The TSBU has an extensive hardware and software development organization of some 850 people. In February 1992, the leaders of the business determined that all senior-level managers and engineers in the organization would be trained in a customized version of the four-day team leader course. Departmental priorities linked to TSBU policies were immediately selected, and the rest of the organization was trained in a customized version of the quality improvement story and quality control tools. The quality improvement story is a seven-step problem-solving tool which is used to analyze and solve a problem. When TSBU adopted the quality improvement story, hardware and software quality began to improve.

At the same time, hardware designers and engineers began linking their goals to factory initiatives, and product quality continued to improve as designs became more robust. Not only were Golden Threads becoming more visible, but more and more associates began to understand their roles in supporting them. Golden Threads were now extending from the customers to the associates on the shop floor, from the marketing specialists to the designers, from the factories to the parts suppliers.

By April 1992, there was a renewed enthusiasm throughout the TSBU. Operational indicators were improving significantly, and associate climate/attitude surveys had shown dramatic improvement in key areas. The momentum was building, and management once again announced that the TSBU would apply for the Malcolm Baldrige National Quality Award. On October 15, 1992, AT&T Transmission Systems was named as one of five winners. It was evident to the examiners that the TSBU management system was the process that led to the many dramatic operational performance improvements and the resulting increase in overall customer satisfaction. Only two and one-half years had passed between the first policy deployment workshop and the award announcement.

Choosing Priority Goals

Priority goals are chosen at AT&T Transmission Systems based on customer, associate, and shareowner needs. As shown in figure 14-1, customers rank "quality/reliability" as their most important need (4.78). Next, the TSBU develops indicators to determine existing TSBU performance levels for each customer need. To help prioritize efforts, it used the approach depicted in figure 14-2. This approach determines priorities by considering the customer's rank of importance and the company's need to improve performance.

Figure 14-1. Customer Priorities

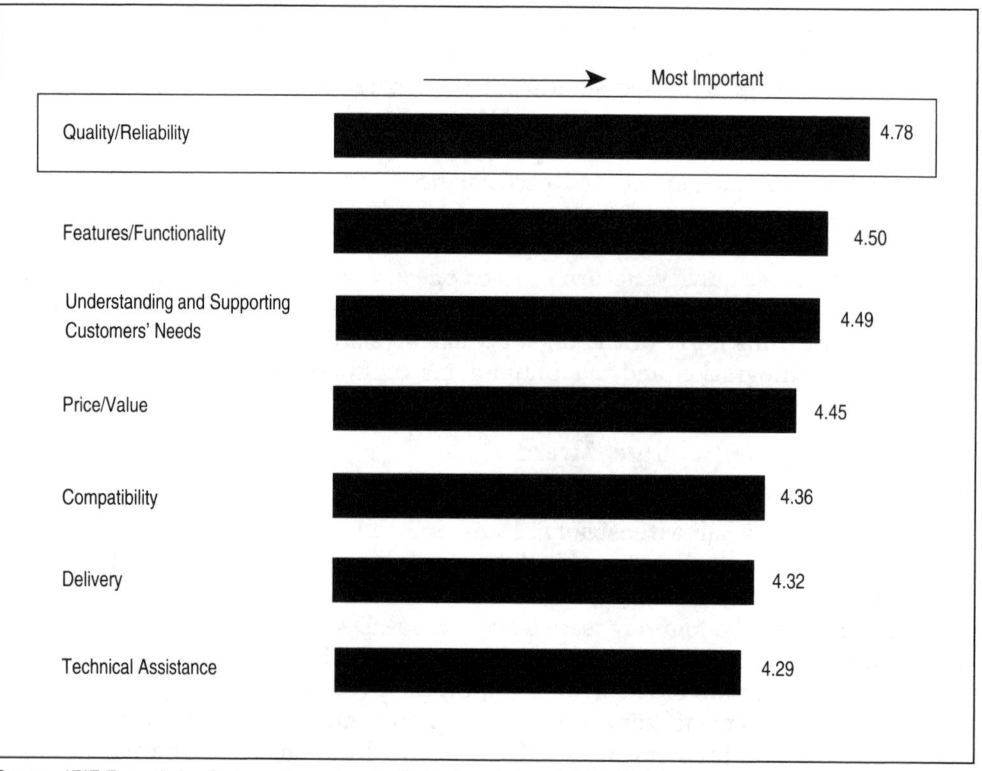

Source: AT&T Transmission Systems. Reproduced with the permission of AT&T.

Figure 14-2. Determining Performance Levels

Customer Need	Importance Weight	× Need to Improve Performance	= Overall Score	
Reliability	4.8	5.0	24.0	→ Priority
Features	4.5	3.2	14.4	
Price	4.4			
Others				

Legend: 1 = low 5 = high
Note: Highest scores are priorities.

Source: *National Productivity Review*, Spring 1993, p. 154. Reprinted by permission of John Wiley & Sons, Inc.

Following are five examples of AT&T Transmission Systems breakthrough goals developed through policy deployment:

1. Achieve 100 percent on-time delivery for all products in three years.
2. Achieve no more than 1 in 10,000 circuit pack returns by 1997 (25 in 10,000 by 1993).
3. Achieve a customer grade of 4.25 (on a scale of 5) on all report cards by 1993.
4. Meet or exceed customer expectations on 80 percent of report card items by end of 1992.
5. Increase responsiveness to customer complaints by 25 percent over a two-year period.

Renewing the Process Annually

Policy deployment begins anew each year. How the process works at AT&T Transmission Systems is described step by step in the following sections.

Choosing the Organization's Focus

As the policy deployment model in figure 14-3 shows, AT&T starts the annual planning process by developing a clear purpose (why we are here) and a shared vision of the business (what we want to be). The purpose and vision—coupled with the knowledge of customer expectations (voice of the customer) and the business environment inside and outside the organization (voice of the business)—guide senior management in establishing a strategic direction for the business. The strategic direction points out the desired future for the business and acts as the compass for the annual policy deployment activities.

Aligning the Organization with the Focus

After this strategic direction is established, the following activities are carried out throughout the year:

1. *Draft annual objectives.* The three- to five-year strategic plan is used to draft annual objectives. Although senior management is responsible for establishing strategic objectives, commitment to and effective implementation of the objectives are enhanced by obtaining input and buy-in from people in the organization during this early stage.

Figure 14-3. Policy Deployment Model

Building on the PDCA cycle shown below, the policy deployment model emphasizes continuous evaluation and improvement of the results and of the process that led to the results. A second PDCA cycle is also carried out during the steps of plan implementation and regular reviews.

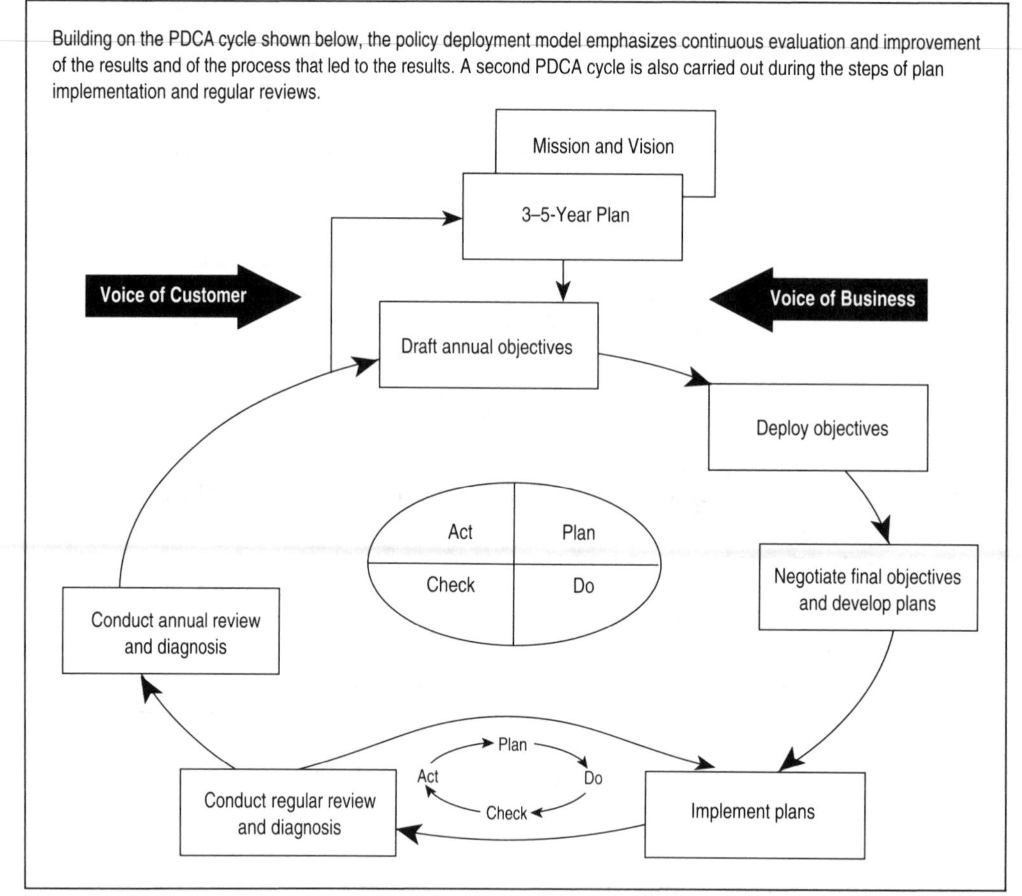

Source: *Policy Deployment Handbook: Setting the Direction for Change,* p. 7. Reproduced with the permission of AT&T

2. *Deploy objectives.* Deployment of objectives occurs through the following channels:
   - Objectives that address individual work or behaviors are deployed down through the business hierarchy to functional organizations or individual associates through the performance management process and cascading of objectives.
   - Most objectives require a collaborative effort by a cross-functional team. This team can be an existing process management team (PMT) or a newly established policy deployment task team (PDTT). This cross-functional team may then form specific PMTs or quality improvement teams (QITs). The PMTs may also lead to the formation of smaller QITs or reengineering teams, depending on the improvement objectives. The team, organization, or individual to whom the annual objective is deployed assesses the impact of the objectives, estimates how much they need to upgrade the current process capabilities to contribute to the objectives, and recommends how and to what extent the objectives can be achieved.
3. *Negotiate final objectives and develop plans.* The "catchball" process is used to communicate the assessment and recommendations upward and then back down through the organization. Analogous to tossing a ball back and forth, catchball is a participative decision-making process based on upward and downward communication and negotiation to determine what the organization should

accomplish, in what time frame, and with what resources. Catchball continues until the "players" resolve major issues, obtain a mutual understanding, and finalize an action plan. The action plan includes specific objectives, measures, assigned resources, clear ownership and accountability, and a schedule.

Implementing the Plan and Monitoring Progress

Each team that develops an action plan has the accountability and authority for its implementation. The team collects data on the implementation process, as well as on the results. Although the data collection methods may vary (for example, interviews, surveys, existing records), a standard format is used for planning, analysis, and reporting – the quality improvement story. This standard format reduces variability and misinterpretation.

Review and Improvement

The team conducts periodic reviews (usually monthly or quarterly) on the progress of the action plan and reports the results to higher-level management. Regularly scheduled reviews are important because they give the team an opportunity to correct problems or adjust action in a timely fashion. These reviews provide the teams an opportunity to make requests of the leadership to remove roadblocks, allocate resources, and receive coaching.

The highest management level is responsible for initiating annual reviews, which start at the operational level of the organization and then progress through the organization. Annual reviews provide an opportunity to evaluate results, synthesize lessons learned during the year, plan for the next year, and examine the deployment process. When examining the deployment process, senior management may ask the following types of questions:

- How effective was the deployment approach?
- How well was catchball carried out?
- Were the improvement targets too ambitious or not ambitious enough?
- Did the action planning process encourage innovative thinking?
- How was the coordination among various improvement teams?
- How effective were the regular reviews and follow-ups?
- What are the organizational barriers to effective policy deployment?

The cycle then begins again for a new year. Each new year of planning begins with a review of the past year's results, the latest three- to five-year strategic plan, and an assessment of the latest customer satisfiers and expectations, and competitor capabilities and strategies.

In the annual cycle, some activities – such as drafting annual objectives, deploying objectives, and conducting annual reviews – occur only once a year. Other activities – such as implementing plans and conducting regular reviews and diagnosis – require monthly or quarterly measurements and adjustments relative to the milestones of the action plans. The annual policy deployment cycle – from drafting objectives to the process review and diagnosis – should coincide with the business planning cycle. The timetable shown in figure 14-4 is based on the AT&T business planning schedule.

Policies are selected during the three- to five-year strategic planning process. These policies are reviewed every year during spring planning, when annual objectives are drafted. In the fall, after rounds of catchball, the participating teams agree to the final action plans. When these action plans are implemented during the next year, the teams also begin to think about year 2 objectives. The year 2 objectives are modified as the regular reviews yield more information about the progress of the year 1 objectives.

Figure 14-4. Policy Deployment Timetable

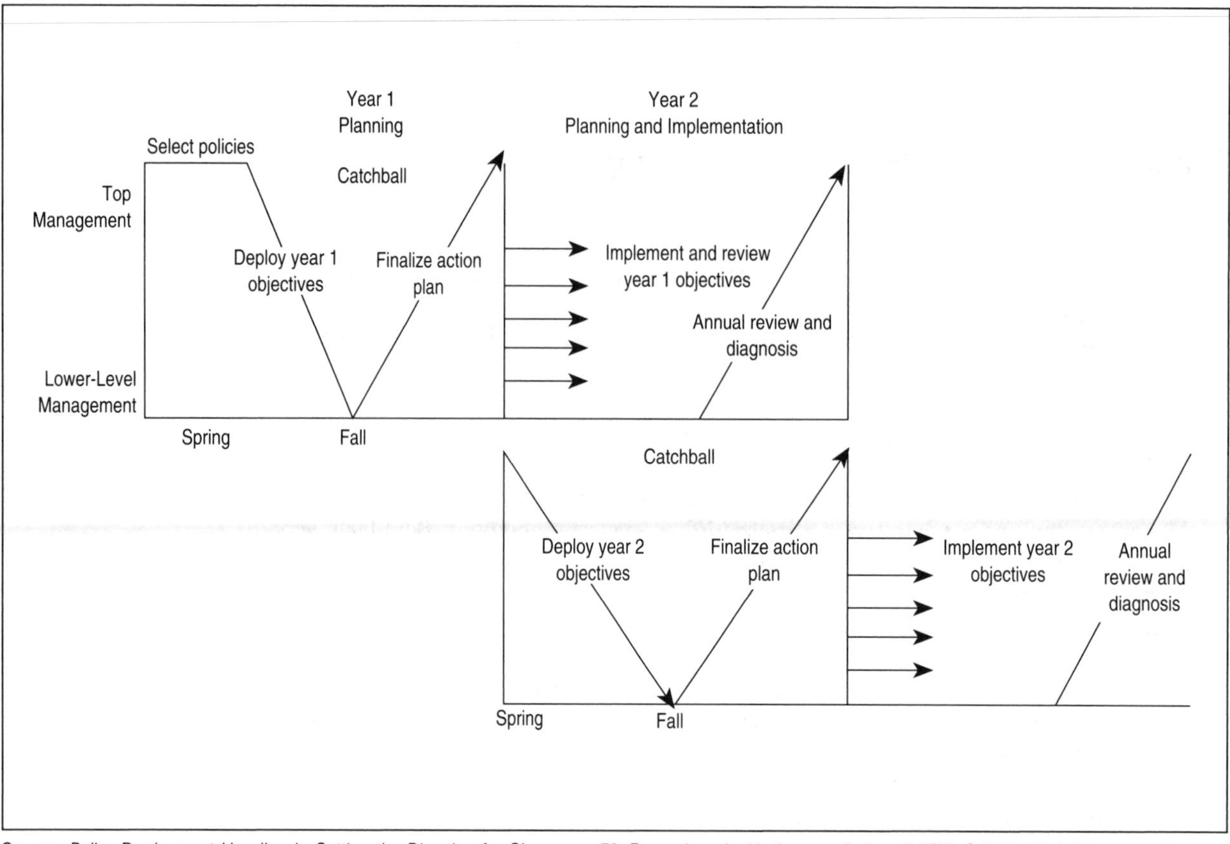

Source: *Policy Deployment Handbook: Setting the Direction for Change*, p. 72. Reproduced with the permission of AT&T ©1992. All rights reserved.

How a TSBU Golden Thread Leads to Improvement

Golden Threads are created when the TQM business structures and principles are in harmony with the company's purpose, vision, and shared values. Effective application of the TSBU's quality improvement story process helps integrate these components to produce dramatic improvement. The fictional example in figures 14-5 and 14-6 detail the improvements created when a Golden Thread linked the TSBU vision, customer, and associate with data. Following is an explanation of these figures:

- In *section 1 of figure 14-5*, the stakeholders' needs and the TSBU's strategic intent are evaluated with respect to purpose, vision, and shared values. Policy is formulated and fundamental objectives are developed. Fundamental objectives are measurable components of the vision.
- In *section 2, Reason for Improvement*, the fundamental objectives are documented along with the corporate-level detailed objectives and individual projects on the quality planning matrix. Also included are the means by which the project will be measured and the goal. Task teams, along with subject-matter experts, analyze the gap to determine where deployment, or the Golden Threads, should go to have the greatest impact. The circuit pack return rate is 145 per 10,000. The benchmark goal for 1993 is 25 per 10,000, with a target of 1 per 10,000 by 1997.
- In *section 3, Current Situation*, the gap is stratified and more teams are formed to address the various bars in the Pareto charts – for example, components and transformers.

Figure 14-5. Example of a Quality Improvement Story

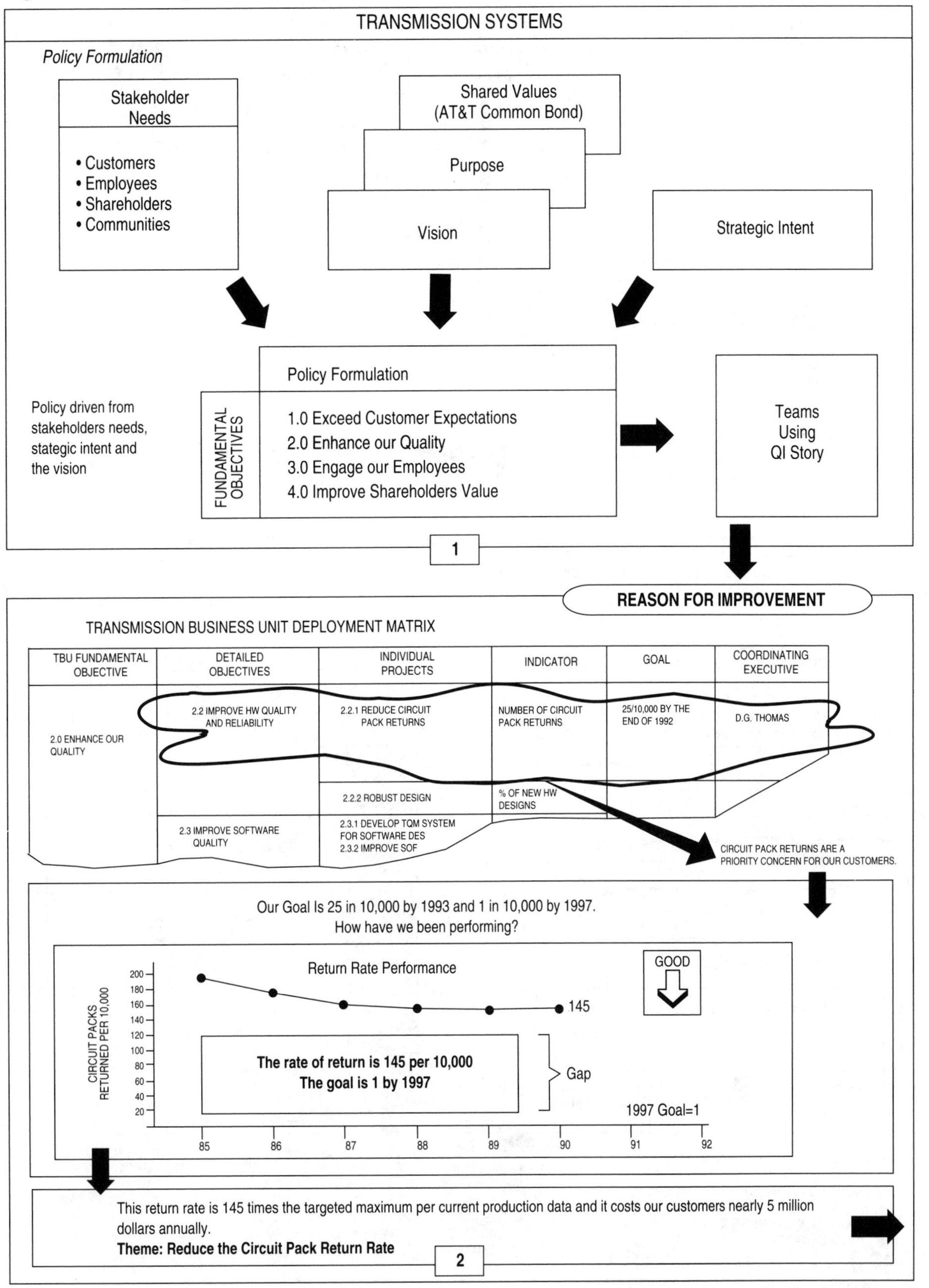

(Continued on next page)

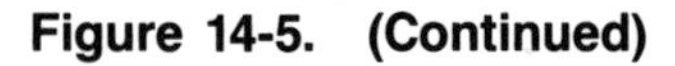

Figure 14-5. (Continued)

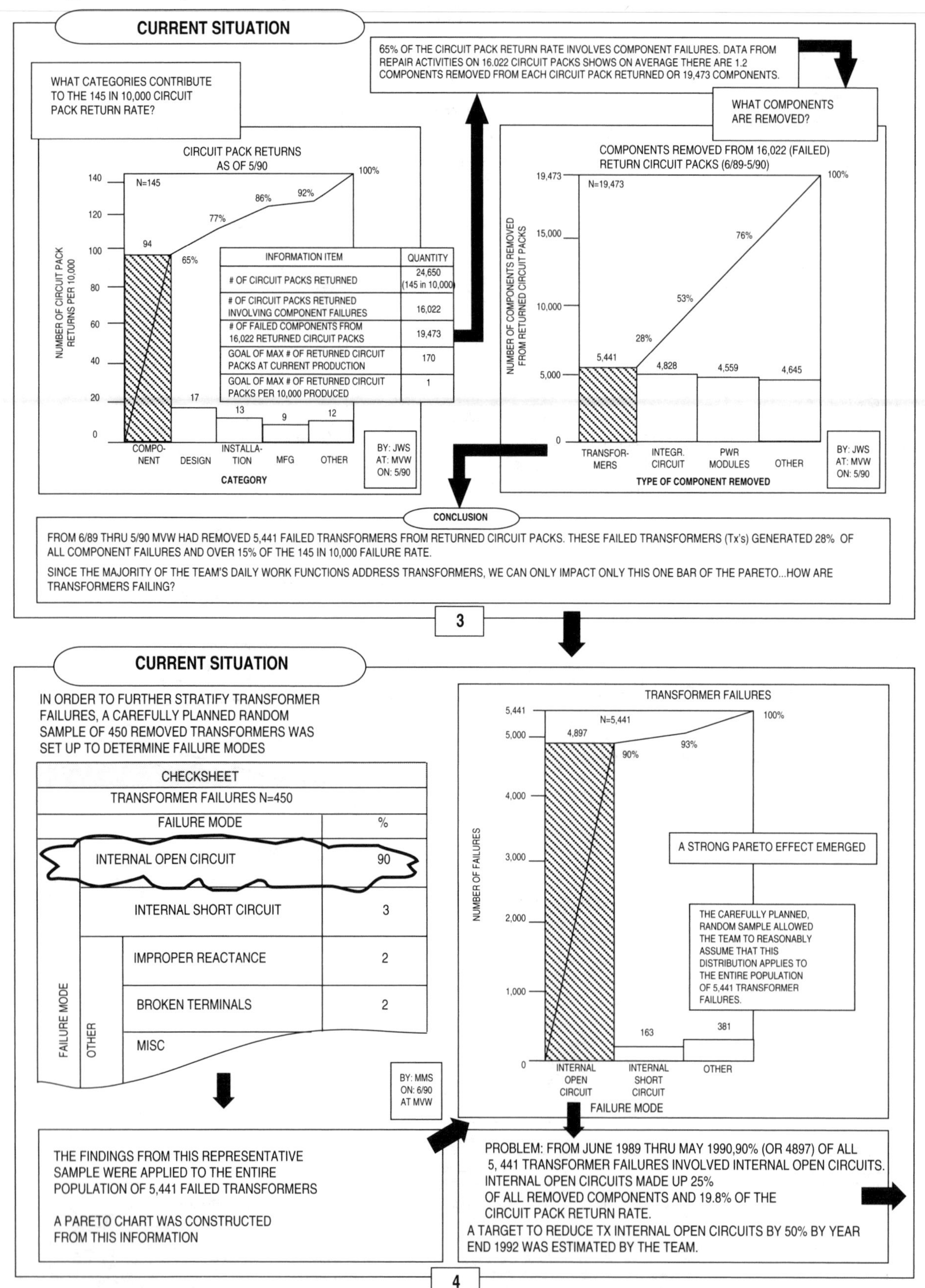

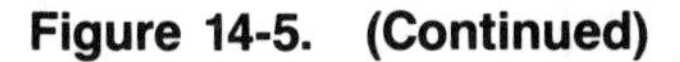

Figure 14-5. (Continued)

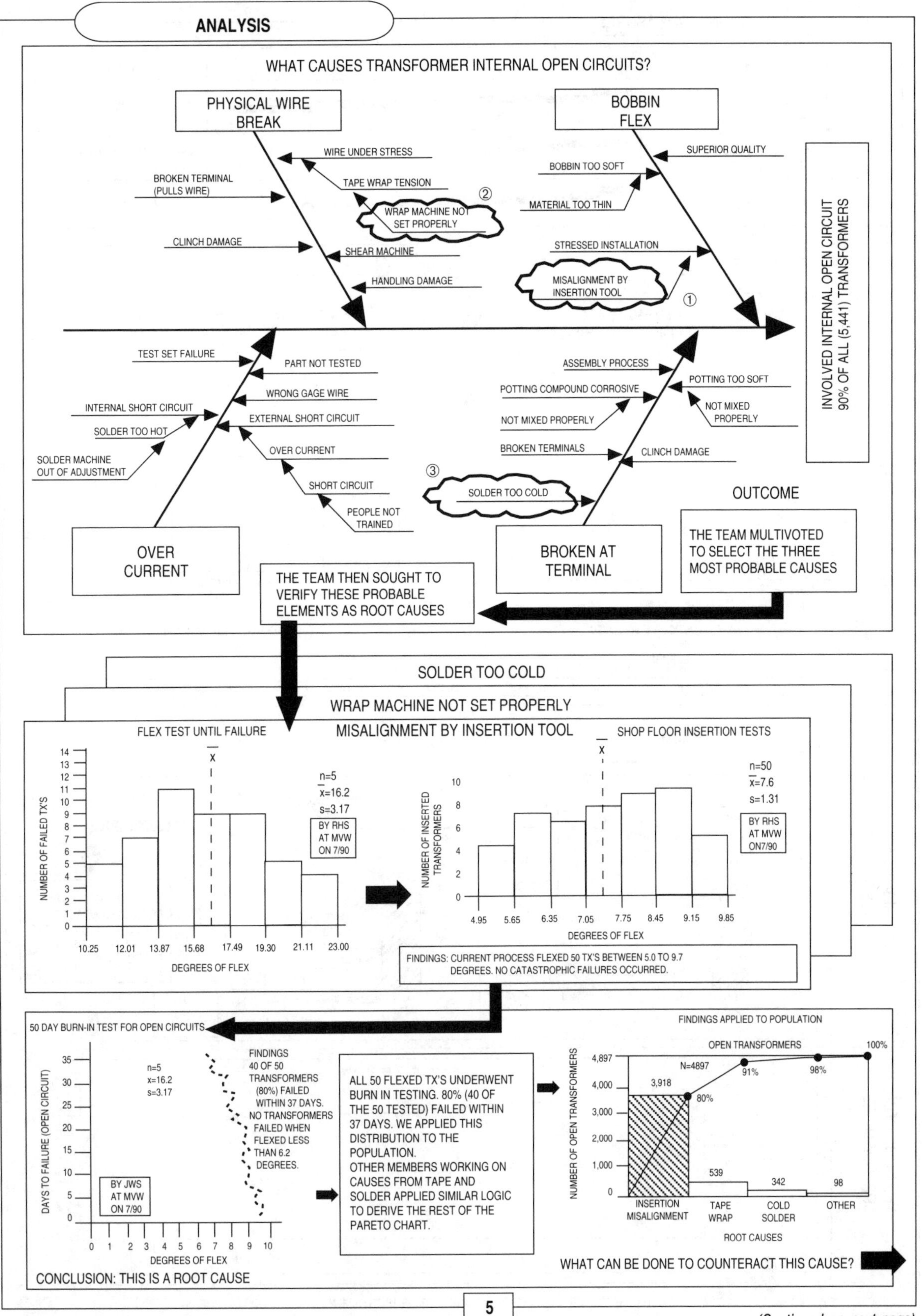

(Continued on next page)

Figure 14-5. (Continued)

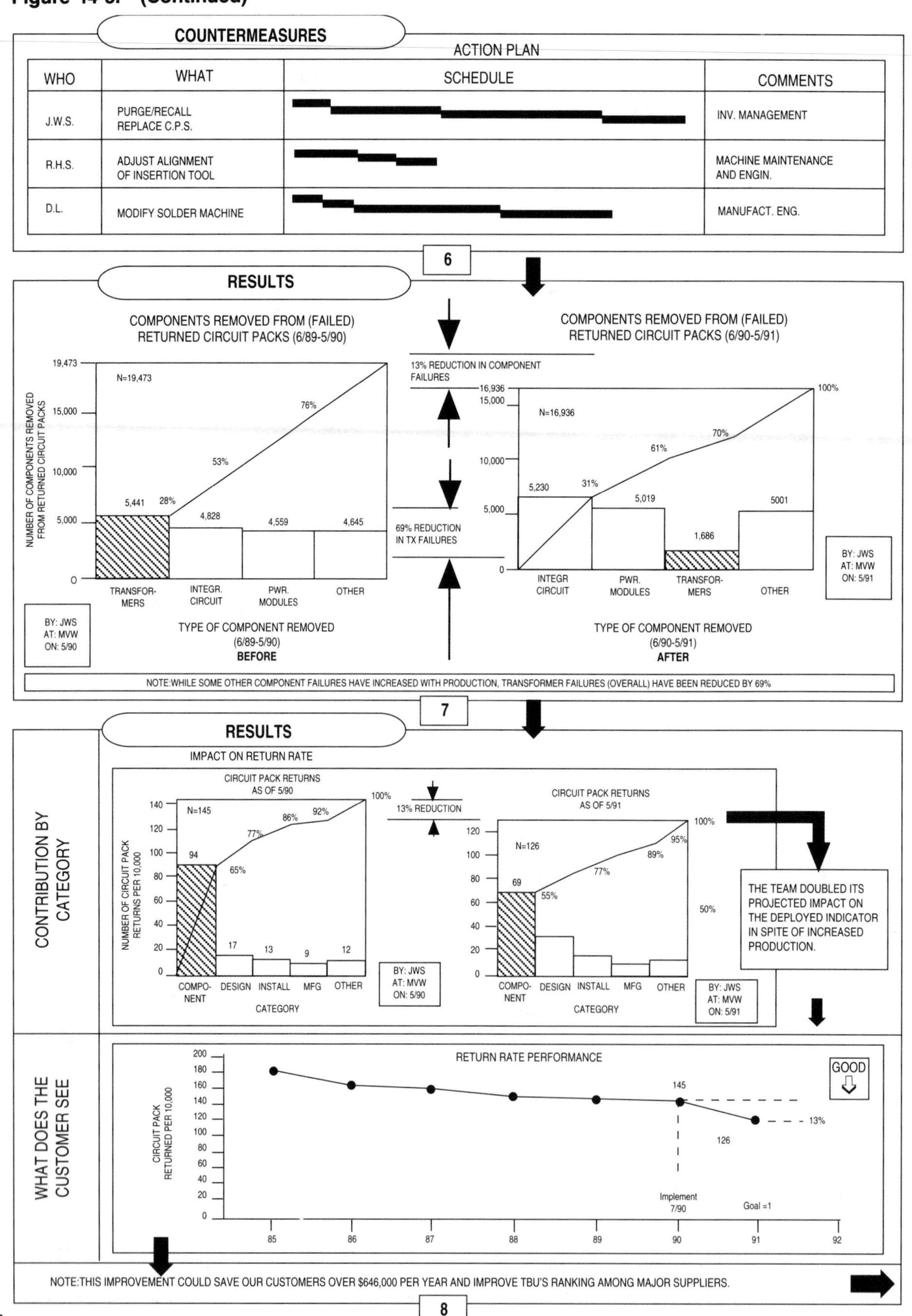

Figure 14-5. (Continued)

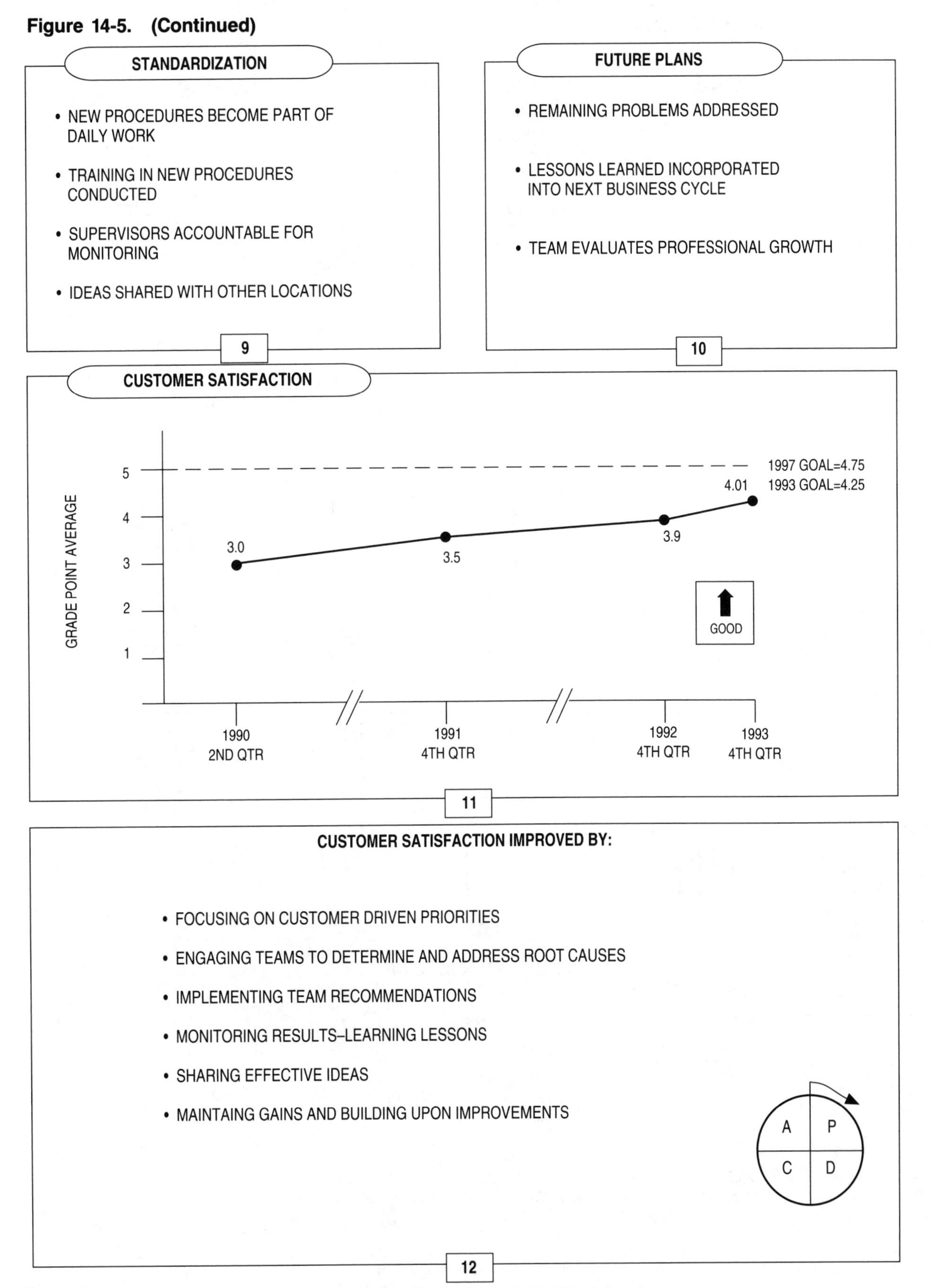

STANDARDIZATION
• NEW PROCEDURES BECOME PART OF DAILY WORK
• TRAINING IN NEW PROCEDURES CONDUCTED
• SUPERVISORS ACCOUNTABLE FOR MONITORING
• IDEAS SHARED WITH OTHER LOCATIONS
9
FUTURE PLANS
• REMAINING PROBLEMS ADDRESSED
• LESSONS LEARNED INCORPORATED INTO NEXT BUSINESS CYCLE
• TEAM EVALUATES PROFESSIONAL GROWTH
10
CUSTOMER SATISFACTION
GRADE POINT AVERAGE
1
2
3
4
5
1997 GOAL=4.75
1993 GOAL=4.25
3.0
3.5
3.9
4.01
GOOD
1990 2ND QTR
1991 4TH QTR
1992 4TH QTR
1993 4TH QTR
11
CUSTOMER SATISFACTION IMPROVED BY:
• FOCUSING ON CUSTOMER DRIVEN PRIORITIES
• ENGAGING TEAMS TO DETERMINE AND ADDRESS ROOT CAUSES
• IMPLEMENTING TEAM RECOMMENDATIONS
• MONITORING RESULTS–LEARNING LESSONS
• SHARING EFFECTIVE IDEAS
• MAINTAING GAINS AND BUILDING UPON IMPROVEMENTS
A
P
C
D
12

National Productivity Review, Spring 1993, pp. 160–64. Reprinted by permission of John Wiley & Sons, Inc.

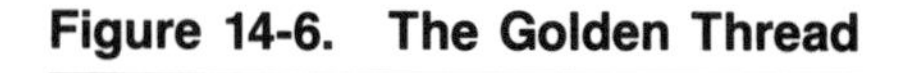

Figure 14-6. The Golden Thread

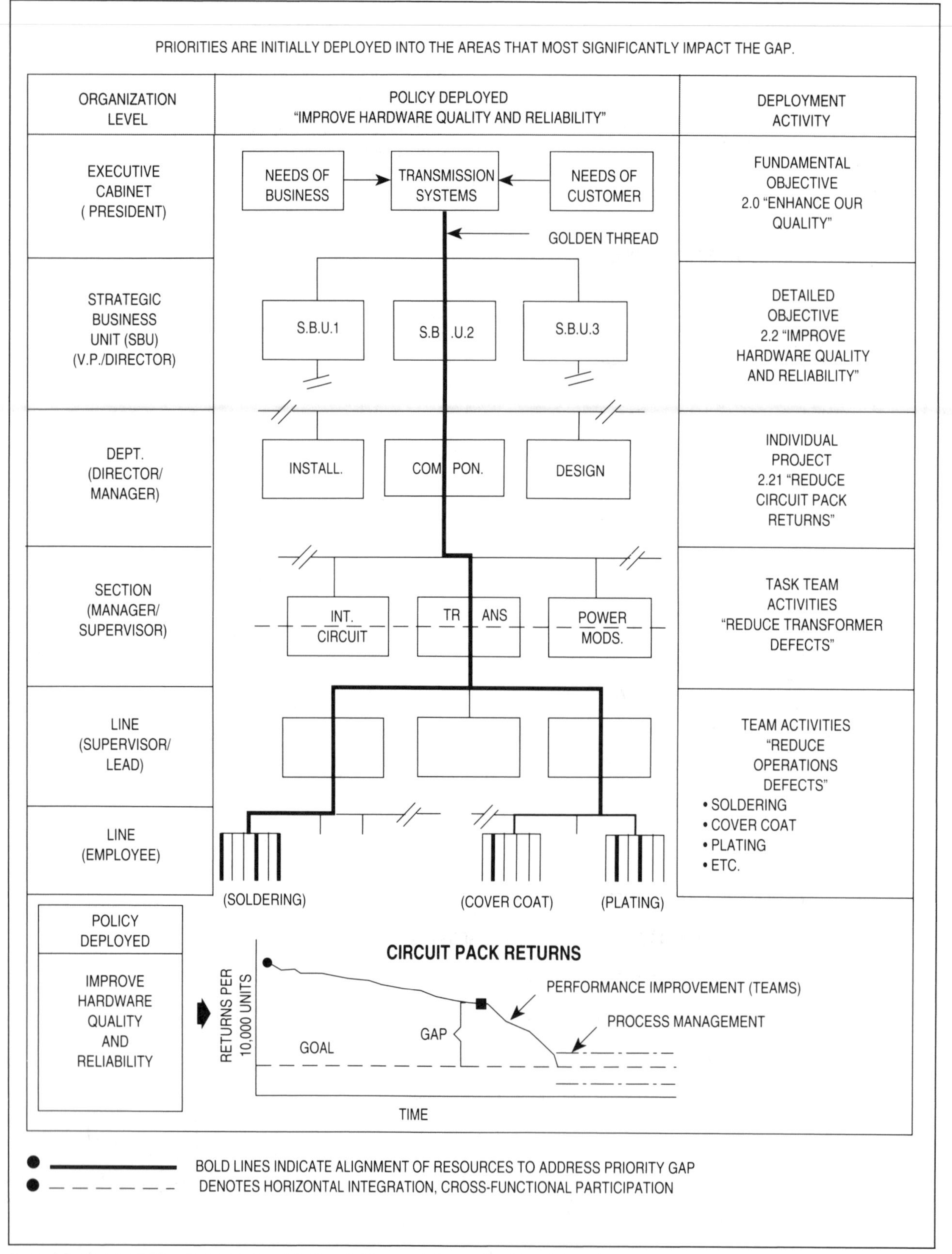

National Productivity Review, Spring 1993, p. 165. Reprinted by permission of John Wiley & Sons, Inc.

- *Section 4, Current Situation,* shows how a team will evaluate the situation to identify a problem that is significant – for example, internal open circuits – and try to determine its root causes.
- In *section 5, Analysis,* the team uses creative and subjective tools, such as brainstorming, consensus voting, and the fishbone diagram, to determine potential root causes. Other quality control tools, such as histograms, scatter diagrams, and Pareto charts, help verify the root causes and assess the impact of each root cause on the internal open circuit problem.
- In *section 6, Countermeasures,* cost-effective countermeasures with an action plan are developed to attack the verified root causes. Accountability, schedule, and contingencies are also established to ensure success.
- *Section 7, Results,* measures results in the same key terms in which the root causes and problems are quantified in the current situation and analysis steps (sections 3, 4, and 5).
- In *section 8, Results,* the impact on the policy deployment indicator is finally determined. In this example, just one team was able to reduce the circuit pack return rate from 145 per 10,000 to 126 per 10,000, a 13 percent reduction.
- In *section 9, Standardization,* improvements are standardized to prevent problem recurrence and are then shared with other locations to prevent duplication of efforts.
- In *section 10, Future Plans,* remaining problems are addressed, and lessons learned are incorporated into future plans.
- *Sections 11 and 12, Customer Satisfaction,* show that when many teams improve operational performance in policy-focused areas, it can have significant impact on customer satisfaction.
- Finally, *figure 14-6* shows the route of one Golden Thread from the customer to associates on teams.

Overall Benefits and Results

The leaders of AT&T's TSBU believe that policy deployment has been key to the success of the business. Among the benefits that they have observed are the following:

- Aligned, engaged, and empowered associates
- A stronger focus on satisfying the customer
- An excellent management system that allowed Transmission Systems to communicate key customer priorities to all associates and to track progress on customer-focused projects
- Continued financial success in a highly competitive environment, with TSBU products considered best in class in their markets

Benefits

Policy deployment enables an organization to implement a results-oriented approach to planning and management. The benefits include:

- A focus on strategic and operational priorities
- Resource alignment independent of organizational boundaries
- Enhanced management involvement – because management's priorities receive attention in policy deployment, and it provides an explicit way to involve executives in the work of the teams
- Translation of key components of the organization's vision into priorities and actions that are deployed into the business

- Successful performance of the activities throughout the organization, enabling the vision to be achieved
- A way to establish the most effective linkage between a strategic quality plan and a strategic business plan
- A system to drive customer priorities and organizational objectives throughout the business
- A constant reference point to keep the company's goals and resources focused on key customer satisfiers

By identifying and directing attention to the right things, strategic policy management and deployment provides a systematic process to achieve the company's vision. Through it, the organization's focus is directed toward stakeholder-oriented operational improvements and strategic growth opportunities.

Results

The results of policy deployment at AT&T since 1990 are dramatic. For example, in the first year, return rate performance improved 33 percent, from 90 to 60. This improvement is estimated to save customers millions of dollars per year. By mid-1992 the circuit pack return rate was further reduced to 35 per 10,000. This is well on the way to reach the previously unbelievable goal of 1 per 10,000 by 1997.

Most important, TSBU customers consider the reliability of the company's products as critical to their success. Some customers compare vendor circuit pack return performance to determine which vendor should be selected. In figure 14-7, one TSBU customer compares vendors' products to determine the benchmark for return rates. The best vendor's performance was used (figure 14-8) to determine how any other vendor performs and how much extra another vendor's products would cost because of higher return rates. In this example, a vendor having 70 returns per 10,000 would have an additional cost of more than $340,000 associated with that rate. The customer's analysis is performed during the purchasing decision on the product. It is obvious from this example why customers can rate the quality and reliability of TSBU products so highly. By reducing circuit pack return rates, the company is potentially saving its customers millions of dollars. There was also a 30 percent improvement in on-time delivery performance over a one-year period, from 1991 to 1992.

The TSBU receives feedback from customers in the form of a report card, each of which is developed jointly with each customer for that customer's needs. The TSBU then combines all the data for each attribute to determine overall satisfaction. The overall score, called "grade point average," is plotted on a five-point scale. The TSBU's report cards measured additional exciting results: customer satisfaction, measured by aggregating all customer report card input on a five-point scale, improved from a rating of 3 in 1990 to 4.01 in 1993, a 25 percent improvement.

Key Success Factors

Six key factors have contributed to the success of policy deployment at AT&T Transmission Systems:

1. Strong leadership from top executives
2. Standardization of processes
3. Golden Thread connecting process to customers
4. Customer-driven objectives
5. Management by fact
6. Involvement of everyone

Strong Leadership

In the TSBU, the executives lead by example. This means they lead teams and own the key customer satisfiers. They form a council and review progress against the policy deployment matrix. Executives communicate these key customer satisfiers and projects to all staff. They also state how important it is to them and to the business for everyone to work on these items.

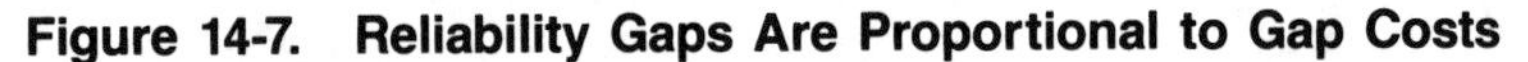

Figure 14-7. Reliability Gaps Are Proportional to Gap Costs

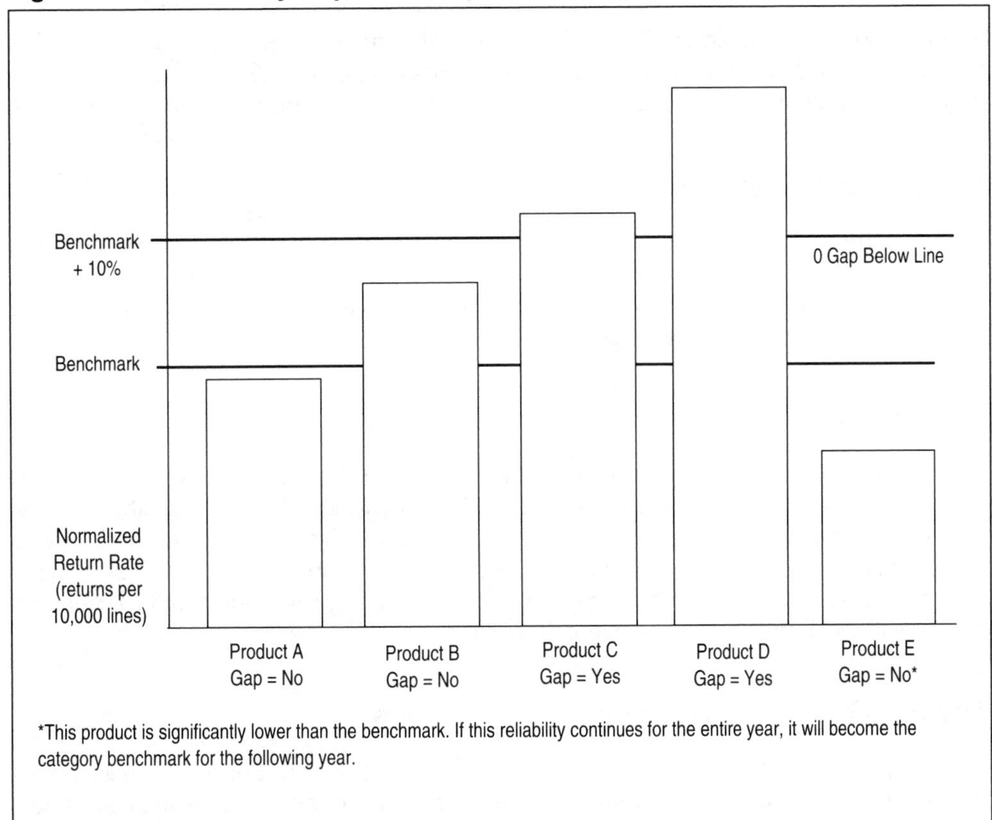

*This product is significantly lower than the benchmark. If this reliability continues for the entire year, it will become the category benchmark for the following year.

Figure 14-8. Simplified Gap Cost Analysis

PRP Benchmark	18.2
PRP Benchmark Window	20.0
Actual Returns	70.0
PRP Gap (excess returns)	50.0
Total Lines per System	150
Average Total Cost per Return	$400.00
Gap Cost per Line/Year	$2.00
Lines Installed	171,450.0
Gap Cost All Installed Lines per Year	$342,900.00

Standardization of Processes

The quality improvement story has become a problem-solving tool and the way company associates communicate with one another. The TSBU identified high-level projects to work on across the business and formed cross-functional teams to address a particular problem for the entire business unit. This was a major improvement over separate functional units' developing separate solutions.

Golden Thread Connection

The concept of the Golden Thread is to "tie a thread" from each customer satisfier to company leaders, to managers, to all associates. Thereby, all company people are linked to key customer satisfiers. Linking people to customers is like finding *gold.*

Customer-Driven Objectives

Using customer input to identify key policy deployment projects, the TSBU develops indicators, objectives, and goals that will help satisfy its customers. In the past, some objectives were internally focused on the priorities of those who ran the business, rather than on the priorities of customers.

Management by Fact

It is important to get away from making decisions emotionally in the heat of the moment. By identifying the company's objectives and goals, the TSBU is able to track its progress and manage the projects by fact. In addition, by using the quality improvement story, the company began to solve problems by having teams analyze current data and then develop corrective measures. This is an improvement from just having managers decide what is wrong and how to fix it.

Involvement of Everyone

It is very important to have everyone involved in the process. The TSBU uses policy deployment as a way to communicate to everyone what the key customer satisfiers are and how the company is solving related problems. It is used as a way to excite people and to change the organization to be more customer-focused. That got people involved; they now know how to satisfy a customer. They know satisfied customers vote with their dollars and, if happy, will buy TSBU products again. They know this means jobs and security.

However, not everyone is on a team linked to a policy deployment project. About 10 percent of the company's associates work directly on a team tied to the policy deployment projects. However, many other self-managed teams are formed to solve problems, and they now know what is important to the customer, because the company has communicated to everyone what its customers say is important to them. Therefore, everyone is helping satisfy the company's customers by solving day-to-day problems.

Problems and Challenges

Problems and challenges were encountered by the TSBU in four basic areas: customer needs, policy deployment priorities, team effectiveness, and associate commitment. The following sections describe how these hurdles were addressed.

Determining Customer Needs

When the TSBU began using policy deployment in 1990, customer needs were known in the general sense, but not specifically in many cases. In addition, the customers' weighting of specific needs was not known, and the TSBU's performance in meeting the needs was not well understood or quantified. Many performance measures were internally focused and did not take into account the customer's viewpoint. This helped explain some of the discrepancy between performance indicators and customer feedback report cards.

To overcome this information shortcoming, the management team tentatively spoke for the customer by developing an initial list of specific needs and ranking their performance. Next, they developed indicators to determine existing TSBU performance levels for each one. To help prioritize their efforts, they considered the customers' rank of importance and the company's need to improve performance for each need.

At first glance, this approach appears to be in direct conflict with the TQM principle of management by fact. However, developing this information through formal market research would have taken many months. Moreover, marketing and management already had a strong sense of the customers' needs and felt that they knew enough or could collect sufficient data to get started. Finally, there was a good chance that the right ones would be selected anyway; just the order of importance might be different. It was either start now or wait until next year. Management developed a list of deployment candidates by collecting sufficient marketing and performance data to validate preliminary conclusions. They also included business improvement priorities derived from Baldrige assessment feedback from qualified examiners. The customer- and assessment-driven priorities formed TSBU's first quality planning matrix.

Selecting Policy Deployment Priorities

Enthusiasm to move forward was so great that priorities multiplied like rabbits. The management team knew that not all ideas could receive priority treatment. A coordinating executive was assigned to each "rabbit." The coordinators' mission was to use data to identify the fat rabbits. The management team used the resulting information to prioritize activities for incorporation into the business plan. The fat rabbits were selected for policy deployment, and accountability was initiated to ensure that Golden Threads were created. Benchmarking was used to establish world-class performance targets.

By early July 1990, the management team had achieved some critical milestones established during the policy deployment workshop. For example, it finalized policy deployment priorities with which to engage the organization. The management team also developed an education and training plan to enable the appropriate parts of the organization to competently address the priorities. The education and training plan required the following:

- All coordinating executives of policy deployment initiatives and their respective teams would receive policy management, quality improvement story, and quality control tools training.
- More than 700 middle-management associates would receive policy management overview, quality improvement story, and quality control tools training.
- More than 2,000 associates at all levels from the top floor to the shop floor would receive customized quality improvement story and quality control tools training.
- Sixty-six team leaders with a vested interest in the policy deployment priorities would initially be trained in an intense four-day team leader skills workshop. They would be expected to coach their team members in the application of the quality improvement story process on Golden Thread issues. Reviews were scheduled for every four to six weeks to enable management to coach and advise the teams, thus facilitating progress.

As part of the training, an explanation of how initial TSBU policy – the common bond of shared values, vision, and purpose – was developed and was provided to the associates to help them understand the origins of the TSBU Golden Threads and why they are so critical.

Utilizing Teams More Effectively

How can teams be better utilized to get results focused on customers? Up to this point, associates had received training in team-building skills, but little training in structured problem solving and root-cause analysis. Teams had used fishbone (cause-and-effect) diagrams before, but fishbones did not help verify root causes. Teams that did develop seemingly good recommendations often had difficulty communicating their ideas through multiple layers of management. A method was needed to think logically and analytically about issues and then communicate ideas in a common language. The answer to this problem was the quality improvement story.

During the initial policy deployment workshop, one TSBU executive said that performance breakthroughs on corporate issues could be achieved if there was a way to:

- Prioritize vision-driven policy issues
- Engage teams to work on these issues using data to determine root causes
- Provide recommendations that will have impact

Management came up with the term *Golden Thread* to identify and make visible the link between the customer-focused priority on the top floor and the associates working on data-driven issues on the shop floor to improve the quality of the product or service to that customer. The management team members were now on a mission to create Golden Threads from their vision-driven stakeholder policies. They had a reason to be excited, for people working on teams would be addressing issues critical to the success of the company. In a sense, associates could influence their own future by knowing how to satisfy customers.

Engaging Associates

One of AT&T's toughest challenges has been to truly engage associates so they become personally committed to policy deployment. Many of the associates in AT&T's TSBU are engineers, so policy deployment represents a dramatic cultural change and shift in approach to work. Design engineers tended to work independently and were not linked in general to what customers needed. In addition, engineers worked on improvements focused on their individual work area and would innovate new solutions and procedures for a portion of the TSBU. With policy deployment, we began to look at problems across the business unit that were aligned with customers' needs. The implementation of policy deployment and the use of the quality improvement story helped to change the culture among AT&T's engineers.

AT&T has worked hard to build up the level of engagement, but it is a long process. Its approach is:

- To develop a shared vision that these are the right organizational priorities and, therefore, that associates need to be on teams to have an impact on the priorities.
- To nurture, reward, and recognize the initially small core of associates who are actively engaged. This is done through public acknowledgments, performance appraisals, informal expressions of appreciation from the president, team rallies, and similar actions.
- To persistently keep going back, year after year, to engage more people – to try to get more people involved.

It is estimated that in the first year of policy deployment, about one-third of the associates were strongly committed. In the second year, this increased to about two-thirds. After about four years of hard work, perhaps 80 to 90 percent of all associates are really engaged in this effort.

Roles and Responsibilities

AT&T's TSBU executives must take on roles and responsibilities to ensure the success of policy deployment. Those directly involved include the TSBU president, steering committee, cross-organizational teams, and the director of transmission quality planning.

The President

The role of AT&T Transmission Systems' president in policy deployment is to clearly communicate the quality planning matrix to all associates either directly or through his direct reports. He leads the quality council, consisting of the company's top management executives, which reviews key projects. He also supports the teams along with providing input on the development of the yearly changes to the matrix. The president leads by example, always talking about policy deployment and its importance to business. He holds performance review conversations individually with his direct reports on how they helped and supported the key projects and what their plans are to continue the effort in the future.

Management within Units

To achieve the TSBU purpose, vision, and values within the policy deployment framework, coordinating executives lead a steering committee. The steering committee consists of approximately seven other senior executives, who support task teams responsible for individual policy deployment projects. Each steering committee also includes a unit adviser who is an expert trained in quality techniques and policy deployment.

Each management layer has cascaded goals to the next layer, and each manager has defined objectives that contribute to these goals. The TSBU has defined the following management roles and responsibilities:

- *Directors and second- and third-level managers* establish specific teams and plan, identify, direct, and track quality improvement projects.
- *First-level supervisors, engineers, and occupational associates* participate on teams to control and improve processes, suggest quality improvement projects, and operate processes according to description.

Cross-Organizational Teams

To promote cooperation among different units, managers participate in *cross-organizational teams.* For example, the steering committees and task teams include managers and associates from many different organizations. They promote cooperation by focusing each person on the achievement of a common goal. Figure 14-9 describes in more detail the policy deployment accountabilities of coordinating executives, the steering committee, the quality team leader, and the unit adviser.

Director of Transmission Quality Planning

The director of transmission quality planning has the following policy deployment responsibilities:

- Identifies training needs and implements quality training activities
- Administers and manages projects and tracks results
- Coaches and advises the quality council and the president of AT&T Transmission Systems
- Supports unit advisers and coordinating executives
- Is accountable to the president for successful projects
- Owns the yearly process to revise the matrix
- Brings policy deployment issues to the quality council for review and closure
- Leads the yearly review of the business against the Baldrige criteria to improve the business

Lessons Learned

The TSBU learned three crucial lessons in its experience with policy deployment:

- Get going on policy deployment.
- Develop a common language and good communication vehicles.
- Work with individuals to provide lots of hands-on, personalized training and support.

Get Going on Policy Deployment

It is important to resist the temptation to analyze policy deployment to death and worry about having a perfect system in place. Start by doing some benchmarking. Then get executives engaged so that this will work for you. After that, learn as you go.

Develop a Common Language

The QI story has proved to be a very helpful common language. It was a critical component to the TSBU's success. It is the way the company communicates.

Figure 14-9. TSBU Accountabilities in Policy Deployment

Coordinating Executives
- Get accountabilities defined and installed within their detailed objective area
- Creating the structure of fulfillment
  —What are the parts and how do they relate?
  —What is the structure for communication?
  —Making it clear to all people on how they can participate
- Reaching the overall results/targets
- Recruiting steering committee members
- Coaching steering committee members
- Ensuring that accountable people receive training
- Doing QI story reviews

Steering Committee
- Replicating what works in their reporting organization
- Coaching designated quality teams
- Designing the structure, recruiting quality team leaders
- Getting trained in the QI story
- Doing QI story reviews

Quality Team Leader
- Getting trained in QI story, policy deployment, and leadership
- Managing their project to close the gap
- Reporting the results
- Requesting coaching

Unit Advisers
- Coaching all positions in the detailed objective structure in use of:
  —Common language
  —Quality tools
  —PAL
- Replicating what works within the project structure
- Supporting the coordinating executives and steering committee members
  —Results reporting
  —Communication
  —QI story training and reviews
- Supporting other unit advisers
  —Replicate what works
  —Resolve overlap

Source: AT&T Transmission Systems. Reproduced with the permission of AT&T.

Provide Plenty of Training and Support

At AT&T TSBU, every associate receives 20 to 40 hours of quality-related training each year. Policy deployment training was one type of training given to executives first. Excerpts from the participant workbook used in the early AT&T policy deployment training sessions for executives are shown in figure 14-10.

Figure 14-10. Quality Planning Participant Workbook (Excerpts)

Outline

Unit 1: Introduction to Quality Planning
Unit 2: Project Planning Exercise
Unit 3: Building the Mission and Vision
Unit 4: Developing Quality Fundamental Objectives (Midterm Plan)
Unit 5: Identifying Problem Areas and Prioritization
Unit 6: Developing Detailed Objectives (Short-Term Plan)
Unit 7: Starting the Deployment Process

Foreword

A. About This Workbook

1. This workbook follows the outline of the course roadmap and the preliminary reading. It summarizes the preliminary reading and provides space to take notes as the instructors discuss aspects of quality planning.
2. The preliminary reading is a prerequisite that will enable you to get the most from this course.
3. The next few days will be your "first lap around the track" with respect to quality planning. Further refinement, consistent with PDCA, is necessary.

B. Course Goals

1. Understand the quality planning model and its components.
2. Understand the concept of synergy through teamwork and the generic steps necessary for planning and implementing improvement projects.
3. Develop a mission and a vision for the organization; and, from these, a set of fundamental objectives.
4. Develop a set of short-term (detailed) objectives based on identification of major problems that have an impact on the fundamental objectives.
5. Understand the concepts involved in initiating team activities.

C. Teaching Method

1. Define the concept.
2. Discuss the team exercise.
3. Test for understanding.
4. Do the team exercise.
5. Consolidate the team results.

D. Course Roadmap

Day 1	**Day 2**	**Day 3**
Introduction	Review	Review
The Quality Planning Model	Fundamental Objectives	Detailed Objectives
Project Planning Exercise	Problems/Issues	Starting the Deployment Process
Mission	Evaluation	What Happens Next?
Vision		Course Summary
Evaluation		Evaluation

E. Expectations

1. Individually, list the expectations you have for this course.

____

____

____

2. In teams, combine your expectations and prioritize the top three or four.(List all expectations for your group on a flipchart.)

Source: AT&T Transmission Systems. Reproduced with the permission of AT&T.

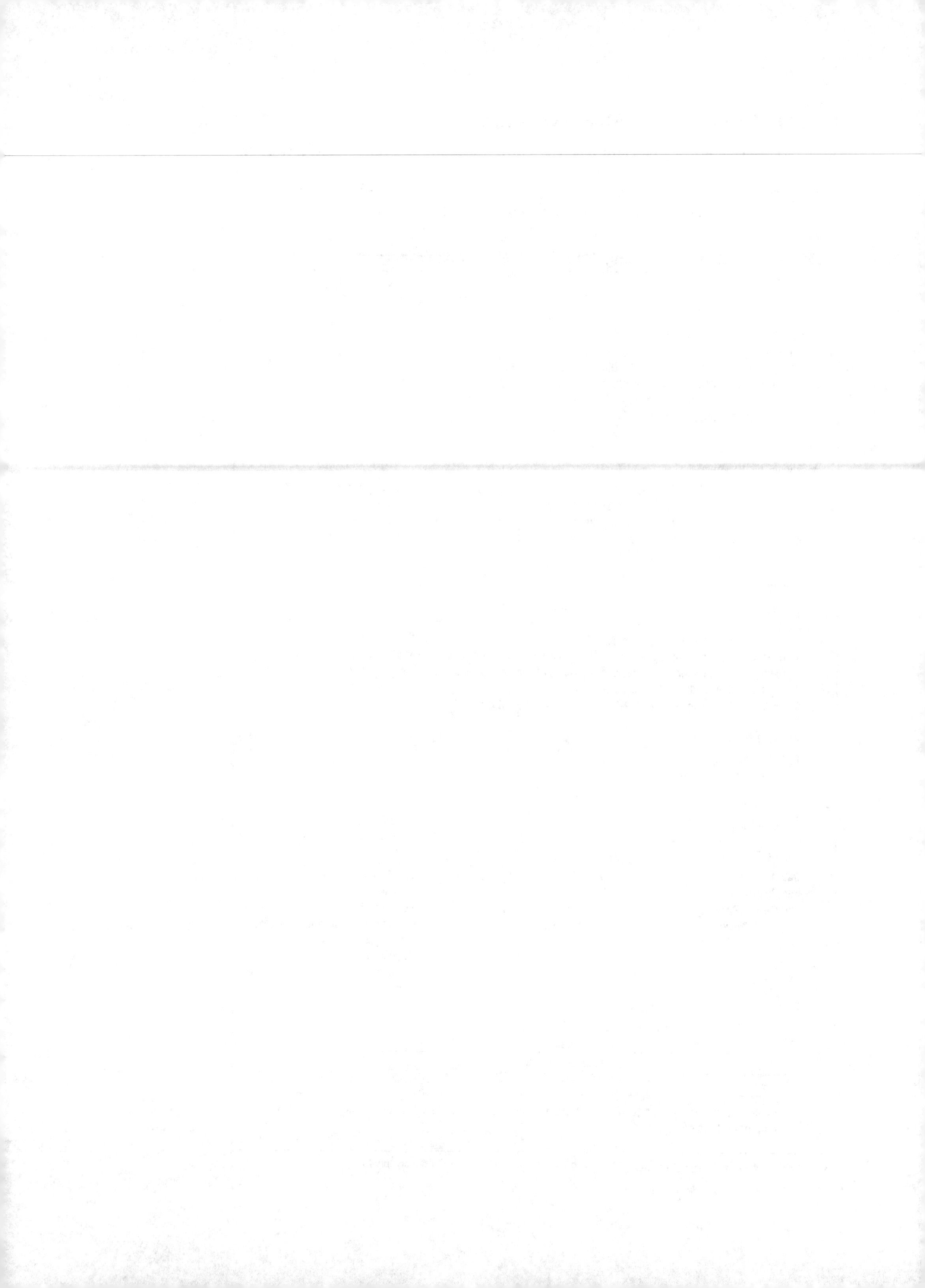

CHAPTER FIFTEEN

Hewlett-Packard Company Medical Products Group

Brad Harrington, Lois Gold, and Casey Collett

A pioneer of hoshin planning in the United States, the Hewlett-Packard Medical Products Group (MPG) ranks as one of the world's largest manufacturers of non-X-ray electromedical devices and systems. Its 1993 revenue of $1.2 billion accounted for 6 percent of the total revenue of the Hewlett-Packard Company. With the 1961 acquisition of the Sanborn Company, Hewlett-Packard inherited a 40-year legacy of excellence, health care experience, and innovation that formed the foundation of the Medical Products Group. The 5,200 employees are organized into field sales and six applications business units, including intensive care, coronary care, clinical information systems, diagnostic cardiology, neonatal care, and obstetrics. The MPG markets more than 900 medical products and supplies internationally. The group is number 1 worldwide in patient-monitoring systems, cardiac ultrasound imaging, Rappaport-Sprague stethoscopes, and clinical information systems for the intensive care unit.

Medical Products Group leadership developed a mission statement that includes the following key points:

- To ensure customer satisfaction as the top priority
- To provide leadership for quality within the group
- To push for continuous improvement of processes, products, and services

This mission is consistent with the Hewlett-Packard reputation as an innovative manufacturer that values quality and excellent service. The mission also set the stage for hoshin planning to flourish.

Reasons for Choosing Hoshin Planning

For the Hewlett-Packard Company, hoshin planning began in the early 1970s within the Yokagawa Hewlett-Packard (YHP) division in Japan. Experiencing difficulties with product quality, sales, and profits, YHP was in danger of being driven out of business by its competitors. In response to this threat to the division's survival, the leadership of the YHP division decided to begin a systematic, divisionwide implementation of total quality improvement. The YHP division used the hoshin planning framework to coordinate the comprehensive total quality implementation. The approach worked.

Yokagawa Hewlett-Packard went from being one of the least successful divisions in the company to winning the coveted Deming Prize in 1982. The YHP hoshin methodology was used as a model for other Hewlett-Packard divisions interested in implementing hoshin planning.[1]

In the mid-1980s the MPG was experiencing severe competitive pressures from firms more attuned to changing customer needs. Top management within the group needed a systematic methodology to address key breakthrough issues, such as significantly reducing new-product introduction time. Hoshin planning was that methodology.

Medical Products Group perceives hoshin planning as "a means to get the organization to focus on a few breakthrough issues which are of strategic importance in accomplishing our long-term plans." This definition is consistent with the Hewlett-Packard Company definition, which is "a process for annual planning and implementation which focuses on areas needing significant levels of improvement."

Hoshin Implementation

Hoshin implementation at Medical Products Group occurred in three phases:

- *Phase 1:* The first phase began when Hewlett-Packard began its official companywide rollout of hoshin. In 1985 the company translated hoshin materials from YHP for use in U.S. divisions. At the annual meeting of quality managers in 1986, Medical Products Group quality managers were among those who received the training in hoshin. They began implementing hoshin in their home divisions in 1986–87. Some developed the use of hoshin extensively, but many others perceived hoshin as a variation on the Hewlett-Packard tradition of management by objectives (MBO). Eventually, everybody "had a hoshin plan," but the rigor with which those plans were developed, deployed, and reviewed varied widely among organizations. Hoshin was viewed as simple and straightforward – a management exercise without a lot of power.
- *Phase 2:* In the late 1980s hoshin entered a transition phase when MPG developed a breakthrough objective aimed at improving the product generation process. This hoshin objective generated a fair amount of activity, but because it was developed and owned more by staff people (for example, planning or quality departments) than by line people (for example, manufacturing or marketing departments), it was not seen as a powerful tool to drive organizational change.
- *Phase 3:* The third phase of hoshin implementation began in 1991 when MPG empowered a management task force to investigate ways to improve total quality management (TQM) within MPG. Data from surveys and interviews pointed to the need for a more structured, "top-down" TQM strategy. As the leaders of YHP had done in the early 1970s, MPG leaders decided that hoshin planning was the best methodology to deploy such a comprehensive quality improvement strategy. A critical feature of this phase of hoshin implementation was that the line people owned both the creation and adoption of the hoshin objective.

Overview

Within Hewlett-Packard, the term for the current year's breakthrough focus is "the hoshin objective," or "the hoshin" for short. Hoshin objectives are derived from a long-term (three- to five-year) planning process, known within Hewlett-Packard as the 10-step planning process or the business strategy review (BSR). One month after the completion of the BSR each year, MPG holds a management meeting to select two breakthrough issues considered most critical to achieving the longer-term plan. Although a true breakthrough may be a multiyear task, hoshin objectives are framed in one-year increments, with midyear milestones and reviews.

Breakthrough Goal

In response to the recommendation of the 1991 management task force, MPG selected the following hoshin objective for FY 1992: "Establish total quality management as the management methodology within Medical Products Group." (See the hoshin planning table in figure 15-1.) In so doing, Medical Products Group leaders were saying that they wanted to make TQM the pervasive way to manage the organization. This goal was consistent with the mission element "to push for continuous improvement of Medical Products Group processes, products, and services."

Measures of Success

Medical Products Group decided that the best way to measure the success of the hoshin would be to utilize the Hewlett-Packard quality maturity system (QMS), a companywide mechanism for assessing progress in applying TQM principles in each operating unit. Similar in nature to the Malcolm Baldrige National Quality Award, the QMS bases its scores on the unit's performance in the following areas of TQM application:

- *Customer focus:* Data from customer needs and satisfaction driving quality improvements

Figure 15-1. Annual Hoshin Planning Table

Prepared by: MPG Exec Comm	Date: 8/24/91	Fiscal year: FY 1992	Division: MPG	Location: Group Headquarters

Situation: MPG competes in a global marketplace with serious competitors who have committed time, people, money, and resources to the pursuit of total quality. QMS reviews have shown that MPG is still lagging the corporation in its execution of TQM.To improve our operating results, we believe that institutionalizing TQM is the key strategy that needs to be employed.

Objective	No.	Strategy (Owner)	Performance Measure
1.0 Establish TQM as the management methodology within MPG.	1.1	Develop an MPG quality strategy that is integrated with MPG's mission, vision, and BSR objectives. Owner: Holmes	1.1 — Document ratified by (Q1) — Communicated to all employees in all-hands meetings/a document (Q1)
	1.2	Implement a customer feedback system worldwide. Owner: McDonald	1.2 — Concept defined (Q1) — Start implementation (Q3)
Target/Goal	1.3	Improve the effectiveness of MPG's annual planning process. Owner: Langan	1.3 — Calendar and process published (Q1) — Quarterly reviews conducted
QMS score > 2.5 by end of FY 1992.	1.4	Create an effective infrastructure to support TQM at all levels. Owner: B. Harrington	1.4 — Quality charter established (Q1) — Quality function resources in place (Q2) — Quality training curriculum developed (Q1)
	1.5	Establish a recognition and reward system that supports TQM. Owner: J. Halloran	1.5 — Scope defined (Q1) — Proposals (Q2) — Quarterly reviews
	1.6	Develop an improvement process strategy. Owner: Kyle	1.6 — Proposal (Q1)
	1.7	Develop an approach for improving MPG's horizontal processes. Owner: Rankin	1.7 — % Execution versus Plan

- *Planning:* Strategic, hoshin, and business fundamentals (operational management) systems integrated and driven, in part, by customer data
- *Improvement cycle:* Systematic detection of and response to needed improvements
- *Process management:* Key processes identified, measured, controlled, and improved
- *Total participation:* Teams and individuals involved in systematic, ongoing improvement activities

There is also a composite (or average) score for the five areas that gives an overall rating quality performance for the unit. (See the radar chart in figure 15-2.) At the time the hoshin was initiated, the average composite score of the MPG operating units was 1.8 on a 5.0 scale. Medical Products Group leaders decided that they wanted to achieve a half-point (0.5) improvement within the first year (moving their average score from 1.8 to 2.3), with a goal of exceeding 3.0 for the product group by 1994. (See figure 15-3.) When Medical Products Group set its improvement target of 0.5 point in one year, the Hewlett-Packard Company's average improvement was about 0.45 in two years. With this breakthrough goal, MPG was aiming at an improvement rate that was more than twice the speed of the rest of the company.

Choosing the Organization's Focus

Medical Products Group begins its strategic planning process cycle in January of a given year. By mid-May, the strategic (10-step) plan is completed and presented to the Hewlett-Packard CEO and staff. Within a month (by mid-June), Medical Products Group holds a meeting of the top 80 to 100 managers. At this meeting, the MPG leadership presents the long-term strategic view for the group.

After the management team has listened to and read through the strategic view, it breaks up into 10 smaller groups, each of which is facilitated by a member of the Medical Products Group executive committee. The subgroups use a modified affinity diagram approach, with voting and prioritization, to identify what the 100 managers think are the most significant issues MPG has to address in a given year. (See appendix B, "Hoshin Toolbox," for instructions on completing the affinity diagram.) Each subgroup identifies its top two issues to report to the larger management team. Acting as representatives of their groups, the executive committee members collect all 20 top issues, categorize them, and label the themes. These themes become background and justification for potential hoshin items. The executive committee then prioritizes these "situation statements" and chooses the top two as the hoshin items for the year. It is apparent that there is consistency between the issues identified by the 10 small groups and the hoshin items chosen by the executive committee.

Aligning the Organization with the Focus

Once the executive committee develops the annual planning table (figure 15-1, p. 243) and assigns one of its members to "own" each strategy, the hoshin plan is deployed using the implementation planning table shown in figure 15-4 (p. 246).

Once the hoshin objectives are determined, a cause-and-effect analysis is conducted to determine how the objectives will be accomplished. Three to five strategies (methods or means) for archiving the objectives are selected. Strategies, in turn, get deployed in implementation plans.

The implementation plan (figure 15-4) is synonymous with an action plan. It provides the specific details or tactics for accomplishing the hoshin strategy and assigns specific ownership and a time line for the tasks.

Figure 15-2. Quality Maturity System Review Radar Chart

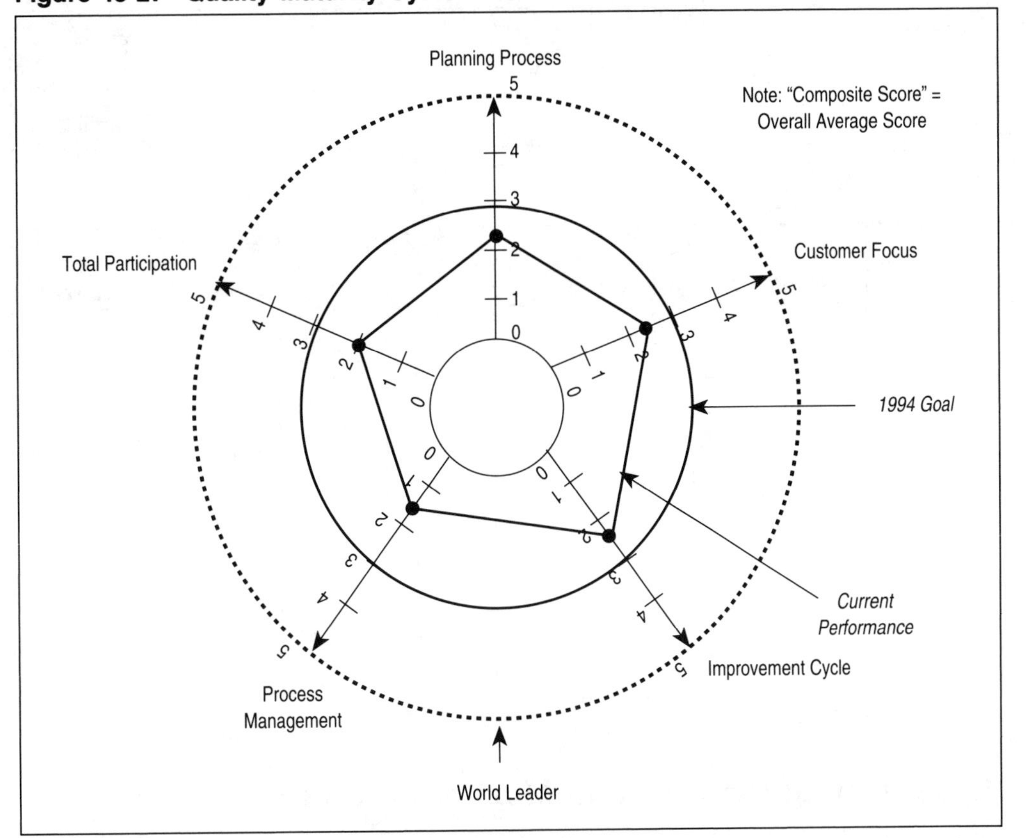

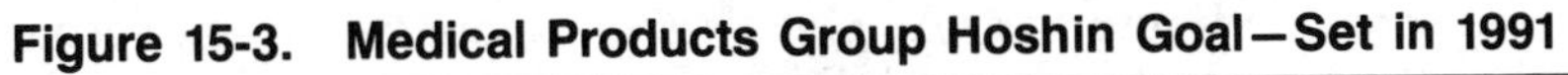

Figure 15-3. Medical Products Group Hoshin Goal—Set in 1991

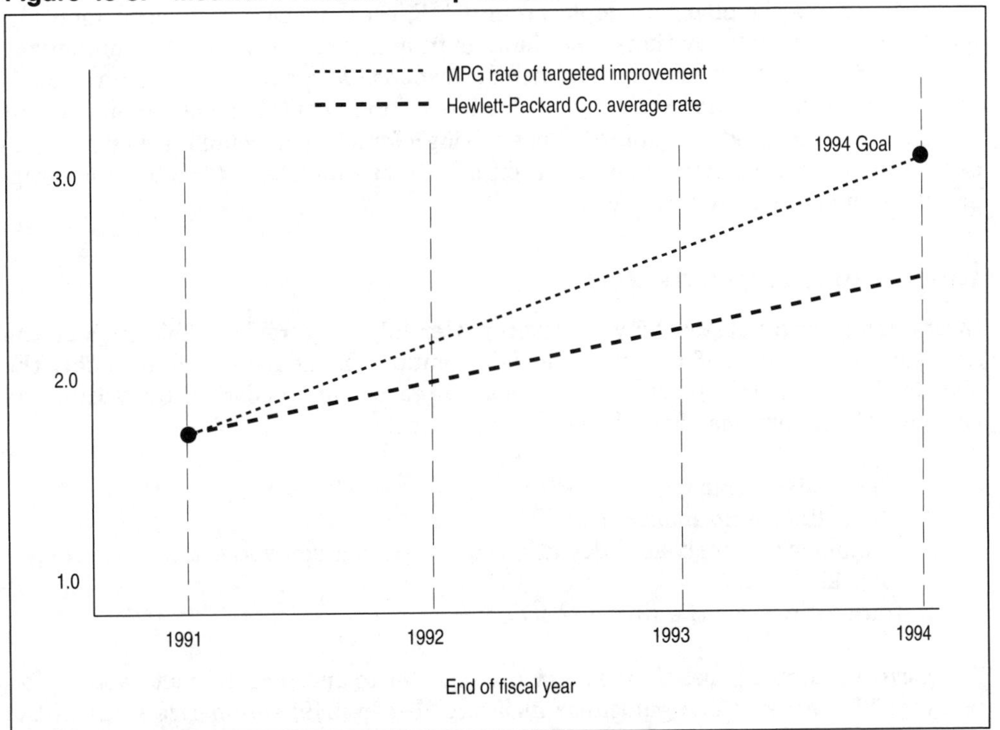

Figure 15-4. Implementation Plan

Implementation Plan	Department: Manager:	FY 1993 04/13/93
Reference Number and Strategy:		

Ref. No.	Tactics	Resp. Person	Q1			Q2			Q3			Q4			Date Completed	Remarks
			N	D	J	F	M	A	M	J	J	A	S	O		

Implementing the Plan and Monitoring Progress

Participants in the hoshin and business fundamentals (daily management) planning processes receive a handbook that describes key terms, roles, and procedures, such as the review process shown in figure 15-5. As plans are implemented, reviews occur regularly. Where the plans are deployed in detail, these reviews may occur monthly, following regular staff meetings. The findings from monthly reviews are summarized in entitywide quarterly reviews. The person responsible for reporting at a review is the owner of the hoshin strategy or business fundamental. (Daily management processes are discussed in chapter 5, Robert King's foreword, appendix A, and the glossary.) Where multiple owners are listed on a plan, one member of the team is designated to report at quarterly reviews.

Review and Improvement

In preparing for a quarterly review, the reporter fills out a review table such as the ones shown in figure 15-6 (p. 248). The wide columns on the review tables reflect the plan-do-check-act (PDCA) cycle for continuous improvement popularized by W. Edwards Deming. These columns allow the reporter to record:

1. The strategy (Plan)
2. The actual performance (Do)
3. A summary of analysis of deviations between strategy and actual performance (Check)
4. Implications for the future (Act)

The narrow columns (labeled "M") allow the reporter to encode comments about plan progress. The review table guidelines in figure 15-7 (p. 249) summarize some of the comments commonly used.

Reporters at the reviews bring updated plans, the appropriate review tables, and all relevant data. The hoshin handbook lists the following uses for data:

- To accurately state actual performance
- To delineate solutions
- To sort out possible solutions
- To sort out possible causes
- To identify and assess potential actions
- To identify and justify permanent solutions

Figure 15-5. Hoshin/Business Fundamentals Review Process

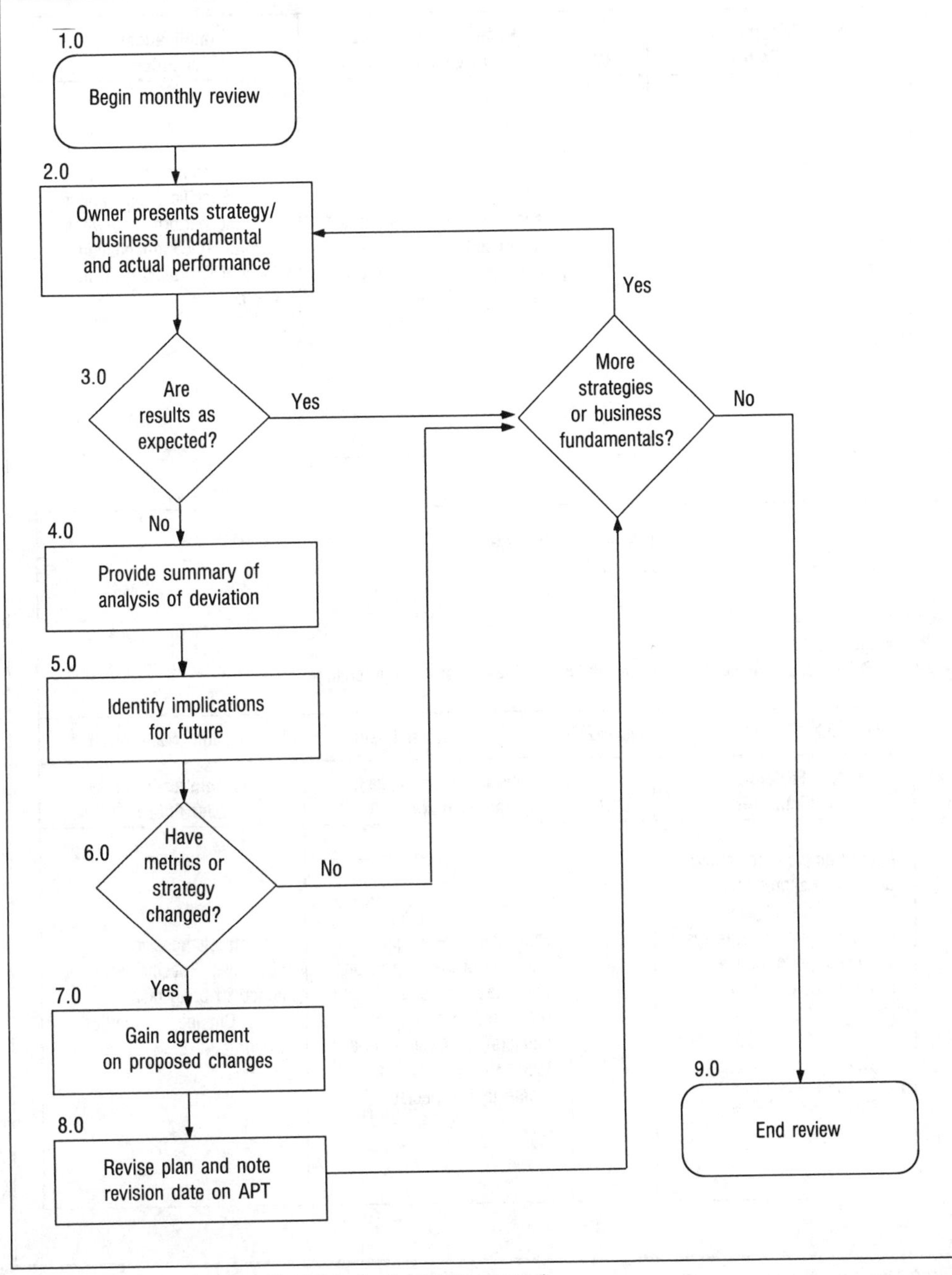

Figure 15-6. Review Tables

Business Fundamentals Each business owner/reporter will review business fundamentals out of limit by presenting the information on a completed *business fundamental review table.* (shown below)

MONTHLY HOSHIN REVIEW TABLE
MONTH 199X

Legend
Trend (T): ↓↑ Change since last review
Concern (C): **H** High **M** Moderate **L** Low
Status (S): ○ On target ○ Behind plan ● Far below expectations ⊜ Metrics or strategy change

Prepared by: J. Shea | Date: July 15, 199X | Year: FY9X | Div: Waltham | Location: Manufacturing

Objective/Strategy (P)	Actual Performance & Limits (D)	* S/C/T	Summary of Analysis of Deviations (C)	Implications for Future
CATEGORY: 1. Business Fundamental (Numbered)	List goal and limit vs. actual performance. Goal: 10 / Limit: 13 / Actual: 14.2	○ M ↓	Summarize the major cause(s) of the deviation and attach the analysis and data used to determine cause(s). A deviation is a result significantly better or worse than expected.	Indicate changes to goal or limit. Specific tactics added to bring performance within control. Recommendation for a TQC Project or Task Force.

MONTHLY HOSHIN REVIEW TABLE
MONTH 199X

Legend
Trend (T): ↓↑ Change since last review
Concern (C): **H** High **M** Moderate **L** Low
Status (S): ○ On target ○ Behind plan ● Far below expectations ⊜ Metrics or strategy change

Prepared by: J. Shea | Date: July 15, 199X | Year: FY9X | Div: Waltham | Location: Manufacturing

Objective/Strategy (P)	Actual Performance & Limits (D)	* S/C/T	Summary of Analysis of Deviations (C)	Implications for Future
1.0 List Hoshin Objective 1.1 Links strategy to appropriate objective.	Review progress to Target/ Goal when appropriate List performance measures vs. actual performance using words or graphs. PM	○ M ↑	Summarize the major cause(s) of each deviation and attach the analysis and data used to determine cause(s). A deviation is a result significantly better or worse than expected.	Indicate changes to strategies. Specific tactics added to bring plan on track. Changes to metrics or strategy.

Figure 15-7. Review Table Guidelines

Element:	Explanation:
Objective/Strategy	Same as under Annual Plan.
Status	○ ON TARGET means proceed according to plan. Target = Actual, executing Implementation Plan as scheduled. ○ BEHIND PLAN indicates minor adjustment to objectives, strategies, performance measures, or targets/goals may be required. Potential for getting into serious trouble exists. Results sliding—negative trend. Exceeded action limits; behind schedule in Implementation Plan or not executing. ● FAR BELOW EXPECTATIONS means progress is unacceptable. Data indicated objective/strategy in danger of not being met. Revision of objective/goal/strategy required. Data/changing circumstances determine what action is required. ⊜ METRICS OR STRATEGY CHANGE means wrong or incomplete metric in place. Analysis indicates a strategy needs to be changed or one added. ↑ Data show improvement in performance since last review. ↓ Data show decline in performance since last review.
Concerns	LOW CONCERN (**L**)—Slightly behind in implementation schedule but tactics put into place will bring it back on track. Operating within natural variation of process; within action limits. MODERATE CONCERN (**M**)—Exceeded action limits. Significant slippage in implementation plan. Ongoing tactics not being executed. HIGH CONCERN (**H**)—Significant deviation from target; implementation plan not being executed.
Actual Performance & Limits	For each objective list the performance measure, target/goal and actual performance. Deviations can be expressed as a percentage or illustrated in an appropriate table, graph, or chart, highlighting the deviation. For Business Fundamentals list GOAL/LIMIT/ACTUAL.
Summary of Analysis of Deviations	Summarize the major cause(s) of each deviation and attach the analysis and data used to determine cause(s). A deviation is a result significantly better or worse than expected. Ask "why" 5 times.
Implications for Future	List any changes in objective, strategies, performance measures, targets/goals, or tactics. Specify the actions proposed to eliminate or minimize the impact of problems on next period's performance.

Reprinted, with permission, from Hewlett-Packard.

The handbook maintains that reviews typically identify one of three major problems:

1. Inappropriate plans, performance measures, and/or goals
2. Plans that are appropriate but poorly executed
3. Plans that are appropriate and executed satisfactorily, but processes that are interfered with by "extra" unanticipated variables

The reviews test for these problems and approve the plan as appropriate, even up to the top-level annual planning table.

Reviews typically result in one of the following actions for problem resolution:

- *Emergency countermeasures:* Actions taken to alleviate the immediate problem—putting a finger in the dike

- *Short-term fixes:* Actions taken that are slightly more permanent and prevent the problem from recurring in the short run – patching the dike
- *Permanent elimination of root causes:* Actions taken that eradicate root causes of problems and prevent their recurrence permanently – studying or locating the stresses on the dike and removing them

Quarterly reviews are focused on elimination of root causes and prevention of further problems, but there are times when short-term fixes are necessary. Once root causes are identified and solutions proposed, the solutions are standardized and documented as part of the quarterly review process. Standardization and documentation allow the participants in a hoshin planning system to learn from past experiences – both positive and negative. Learnings from the quarterly reviews are summarized in the annual review and used to feed the front end of the next year's hoshin planning cycle.

Overall Benefits and Results

Hoshin planning in Medical Products Group has provided numerous benefits and tangible (statistical) results. The following sections detail these positive outcomes.

Benefits

Among the benefits to Medical Products Group that stem from hoshin planning, two stand out. These are increased alignment and greater customer focus.

Increased Alignment

As a complex, global organization, Medical Products Group uses the hoshin process to involve the top 100 managers in selection of its key business issues. This structured method of gathering input during the selection of the hoshin issues also functions to improve the level of understanding and commitment to the issue.

According to the quality manager for the Americas Geographic Business Unit (AGBU), "The critical benefit is alignment – providing a mechanism that all managers use to look at cross-functional issues in a way they had never done before." She cites the fact that three major manufacturing organizations within MPG achieved International Standards Organization (ISO 9000) certification in one year. "They could not have accomplished that without hoshin. It was a priority that people took seriously and reviewed regularly. Hoshin provided alignment."

Over the past few years, Medical Products Group has made a major shift in its focus from being a clinical products company to one that specializes in both computers and clinical solutions. Again, hoshin was instrumental in providing the alignment necessary to accomplish that transition in a complex, global organization. The (10-step) business strategy review process is credited with contributing to the change – and the BSR is operationalized through hoshin.

Greater Customer Focus

Medical Products Group has always been very sensitive to its customers. However, in the 1990s, the competitive environment has heated up. The competition is also listening to the customer. Whoever can be most agile in responding to customer needs and the competitive environment will succeed. What hoshin planning provides is a methodology for systematically translating the voice of the customer into plans. It also provides the means for effectively communicating the plans to all parts of the organization that need to be involved. The review process provides a rigorous mechanism for assessing the impact of the plans and for revising them in response to changing conditions.

The MPG leaders acknowledge that in any given year many challenges confront an organization which, if it does not use customer data to help set priorities, may become inwardly focused. It may be so consumed with efficiencies of internal processes that it loses perspective. The key focus should be on enabling the organization's core processes to meet its external customer needs. The test of a good objective is whether it reflects the essence of the problem as perceived through the customer's eyes. Customer data are driving MPG's hoshin objective on order fulfillment, data that led the group to select ISO certification as a strategy in the 1993 hoshin plan.

Other Benefits

Hoshin made a clear statement about strategic focus – not just for the executives, but for everybody within the group. Stating what the focus would be also provided clarity about what the focus would *not* be. Another benefit, then, is that hoshin created disciplined review and follow-up sensitization.

Results

Medical Products Group achieved dramatic results. Within one year, the average quality maturity system scores went from 1.8 to just under 2.5, an improvement of more than 0.6 (better than the aggressive 0.5-improvement target, as illustrated in figure 15-8). Fueled by the already significant improvement, MPG decided to carry TQM implementation through into a second-year hoshin objective, with the goal of improving average scores from 2.5 to 2.8, another 0.3-point improvement. At the end of 1993, with all but one of the product-generation businesses having received their annual QMS reviews, the average score stood at 3.0, yet another 0.5-point gain.

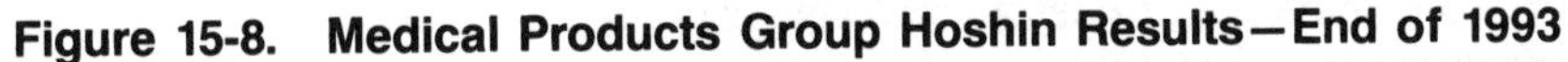

Figure 15-8. Medical Products Group Hoshin Results – End of 1993

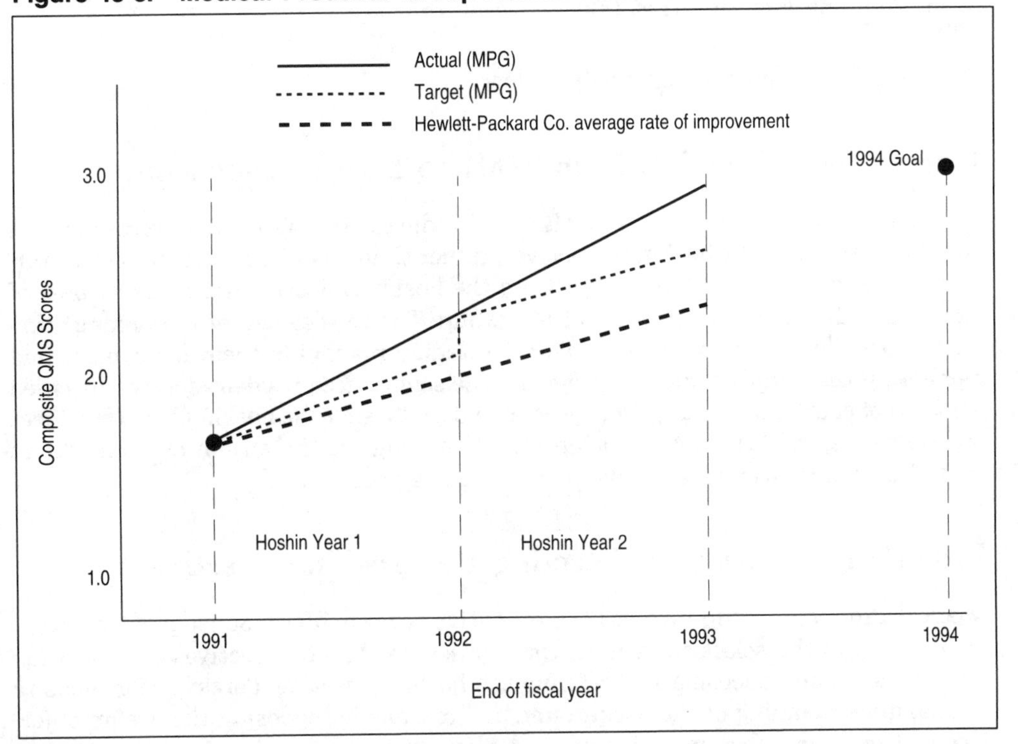

Medical Products Group received additional validation of the success of its hoshin effort from an unexpected source. In 1993 operations within the group earned two of seven Hewlett-Packard President's Quality Awards. Designed to recognize the top organizations within Hewlett-Packard on all-around quality performance, this award requires minimum QMS scores of 3.0 to determine eligibility. In addition, entities must achieve established levels of customer satisfaction, meet financial objectives, and earn above-average scores on the *HP Way* employee survey.

Of the 150 Hewlett-Packard entities that were QMS reviewable, 12 exceeded the 3.0 score required for award eligibility. At the time of the award selection, Medical Products Group had 3 of the 12 eligible entities and 2 of the 7 that won. This means that MPG, which represented 5 percent of the reviewable entities, collected 30 percent of the president's awards.

Since the awards were granted, six of the seven Medical Products Group entities have achieved a QMS score of 3.0. In response to another hoshin strategy, those same six entities have become certified by the ISO 9001 to position the product group for doing business in 21st-century Europe.

Key Success Factors

With eight years of experience to draw upon, the Medical Products Group has identified five factors as key to the successful implementation of hoshin planning:

1. Transferring ownership from staff to line management
2. Developing broad participation in the selection of the hoshin objective
3. Changing the timing and emphasis of executive committee meetings to coincide with the rhythm of the hoshin process reviews
4. Choosing appropriate, meaningful, and challenging measures that related to quality performance and customer satisfaction
5. Building a culture that takes reviews seriously

These KSFs are summarized briefly below.

Transfer of Ownership from Staff to Line Management

A primary factor in the success of Medical Products Group's hoshin process is that line managers write the hoshin themselves, rather than delegating that task to a staff function. The top leadership team selects the hoshin objective with a great deal of input from the management staff of the group. The top leaders of the organization take responsibility for the major hoshin strategies, managing their deployment and monitoring their implementation progress. The senior vice-president devotes specified amounts of each staff meeting to reviewing and discussing the hoshin plan. This direct involvement gives MPG leaders a working knowledge of the hoshin plan and direct control over improvements in the hoshin planning process.

Broad Participation in Selecting the Hoshin Objective

Medical Products Group involves the executive team and two subsequent management layers in the selection of breakthrough issues. The perspectives of more than 100 people go into choosing and refining the hoshin objective. Participation leads to a fuller understanding of the background and reasons for choosing the hoshin objective and to a smoother, more informed deployment process.

Timing and Emphasis of Executive Committee Meetings

Executive committee meetings within the Medical Products Group are scheduled to coincide with the key events (selection, deployment, and review) in the hoshin planning cycle. The general manager of MPG dedicates 25 percent of the ongoing meetings of top leaders to reviewing the hoshin and business fundamentals (daily management) processes. This action has both symbolic and practical value. Time symbolizes importance, and the leadership team is modeling how important these two critical management systems really are. On a practical note, it takes a great deal of leadership time to operate these systems effectively – to plan, review, and improve the systems by which the group achieves breakthrough and incremental improvements.

Measures Related to Quality Performance and Customer Satisfaction

The quality maturity system of scoring quality performance was a well-tested companywide measure. Like the Malcolm Baldrige system, the QMS review procedure is rigorous and thorough. Quality maturity system scores are based on five factors:

1. Planning process
2. Customer focus
3. Improvement cycle
4. Process management
5. Total participation

Together, they give a business unit an overall rating of its quality performance. Individually, they assess the critical elements of a total quality management system, such as the customer feedback loop.

Medical Products Group leaders knew that they were setting a hoshin improvement goal that more than doubled the rate at which the rest of the Hewlett-Packard divisions were improving their overall quality performance. The group used its prior experience with hoshin planning and continuous improvement efforts to exceed the stretch goal.

A Culture That Takes Reviews Seriously

Perhaps most critical to hoshin success are the structured periodic reviews. Review schedules are set well in advance and are adhered to faithfully. Unlike the traditional results-focused MBO reviews, the hoshin reviews cause Medical Products Group to focus on in-process activity as well as on plans outcomes.

Problems and Challenges

Medical Products Group experienced problems with the timing of the hoshin process – synchronizing planning, deployment, review, and planning for next year's cycle across a large and complex organization. Another major problem was the apparent simplicity of the hoshin planning process.

Timing and Logic in Deployment

Reflecting on the evolution of the hoshin process, the Medical Products Group quality manager notes that timing and logic in deploying the objectives is much "trickier" than one might think. Having picked a certain objective and strategies, it is not easy to know what the next two tiers down will need to do. "Everybody is trying to understand how to let the high-level plan align their activities. It becomes a staging problem." The quality manager gave the following example: If the Medical Products Group hoshin is to implement a customer feedback system worldwide, the people in the next tier of the organization have two options: to repeat this objective verbatim and begin immediately developing supporting strategies or to wait until someone else comes up with a strategy that affects them. If they duplicate the objective, they may run the risk of redundancy or wasted effort. If they fail to repeat the objective, they may risk misalignment. Therefore, "one of the biggest problems is how to get deployment to work in a logical, nonredundant fashion, such that timing of everything works most efficiently."

Medical Products Group has developed a simple coding system to address the problem of redundancy, as illustrated in figure 15-9. As the executive team develops strategies, it labels each one with an *I* for "implement" or a *D* for "deploy." An *I* indicates that the strategy can go directly to an implementation plan at the operational level and not be deployed further by the executive team. A *D* means that the executive team wants the strategy to be deployed (repeated verbatim) down to the next level, which means all the operating units work on the same thing. This system helps people understand whether they should be working on the same strategies as others in the organization.

Medical Products Group is still dealing with the timing problems inherent in deployment. Difficulties arise in staggering the start times of strategies so that the people who designed the strategies really understand what needs to be done before the people in the next tiers begin to do the work.

Timing and Logic of Planning and Review Processes, Year to Year

Another hurdle is the effort it takes to synchronize the timing and execution of the planning and review processes. Medical Products Group leaders had to ask themselves,

Figure 15-9. Coding System

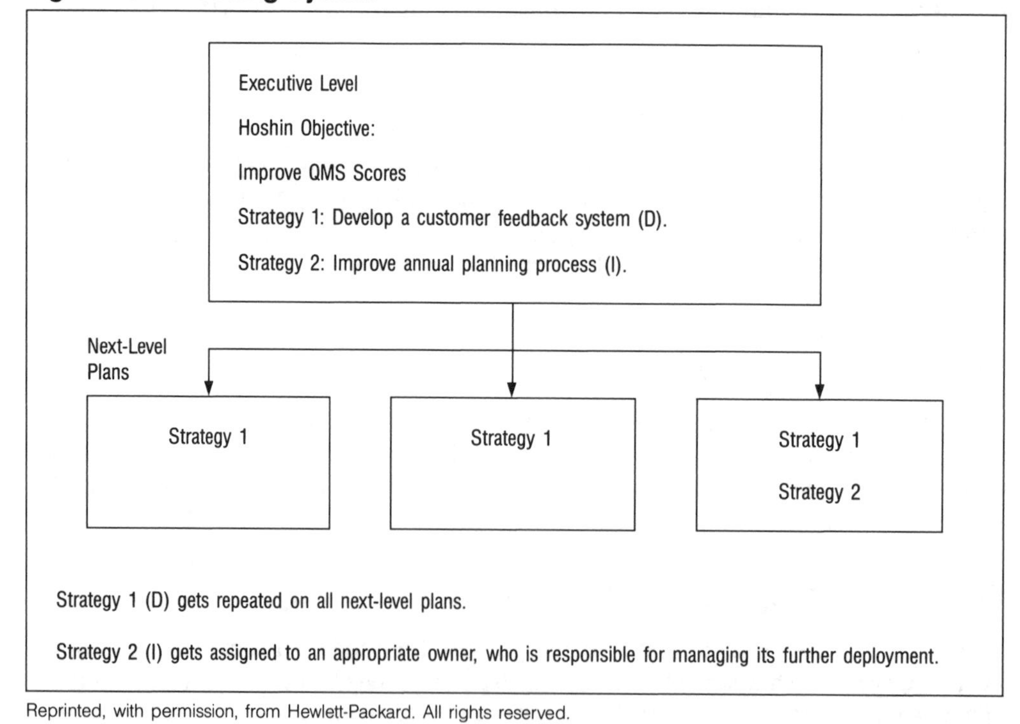

Executive Level
Hoshin Objective:
Improve QMS Scores
Strategy 1: Develop a customer feedback system (D).
Strategy 2: Improve annual planning process (I).
Next-Level Plans
Strategy 1
Strategy 1
Strategy 1
Strategy 2
Strategy 1 (D) gets repeated on all next-level plans.
Strategy 2 (I) gets assigned to an appropriate owner, who is responsible for managing its further deployment.

"When do we want to draft the objectives? When do we want to have a final version of the strategies? When do we want the plan deployed to the next levels? When should quarterly reviews start, and at which level, in order to have a roll-up that works?" (A *roll-up* is a coordinated collection of data in preparation for a review, beginning with the most detailed level of the plan and summarizing level by level upward.) To further complicate matters, the rolling nature of a hoshin system allows for some plans to be developed as others are still being executed and reviewed.

To address this issue of synchronicity, MPG developed a detailed planning process (figure 15-10) with a calendar of dates and times for completion of each major step. Within the first year, Medical Products Group adjusted its management meetings to coincide with the hoshin reviews. For example, the ideal time for the top-level hoshin review was the sixth week after the end of each quarter. The traditional timing of the quarterly executive meeting had to change to make sure the right people were present for the hoshin reviews.

Deceptive Simplicity of Hoshin

The last difficulty hoshin posed was that "it looked too simple." Deceived by the apparent simplicity of the planning tables, people questioned the need for two days of training – or even a half day – if all hoshin amounted to was filling out some tables. Even when they understood the mechanics of the planning and deployment processes, people grossly underestimated the time it would take to execute them. In hindsight, MPG's quality manager believes that the Medical Products Group could have used a week's worth of training, but they did not know it at the time.

The assumption may have been made that the difficulty in the hoshin process lay in filling out the tables. Instead, the real difficulties were twofold:

- Choosing the right strategies and measures
- Reviewing the plan as a process rather than as a collection of results

The quality manager asserts that "if you really believe in the hoshin method and you use it, you are going to drive massive amounts of organizational activity. The activity is not in filling out the forms. Instead, the activity is what the forms stimulate, and you have to think very carefully about how you structure that action for its maximum effect. As you stimulate all the action, you need to be clear about what action you want and how you will measure it. Picking the wrong measure, for example, could cause a lot of people to do the wrong thing."

Roles and Responsibilities

Three roles that are vitally linked to the success of hoshin planning within Medical Products Group are the general manager, the quality manager, and the owner/leader of the strategy deployment effort.

Top Executive

With hoshin, the Medical Products Group general manager (who is also a Hewlett-Packard vice-president) has become increasingly more comfortable with using a structured process to solicit input and then to roll up issues that need to be addressed by the group. He believes that involvement of the management team yields a better outcome than if he and his staff had selected the breakthrough issues themselves. He now relies on the broad participation of the management team in the hoshin selection process to test whether Medical Products Group is focusing on the right issues. Exhibiting strong

Figure 15-10. MPG Hoshin Planning Process

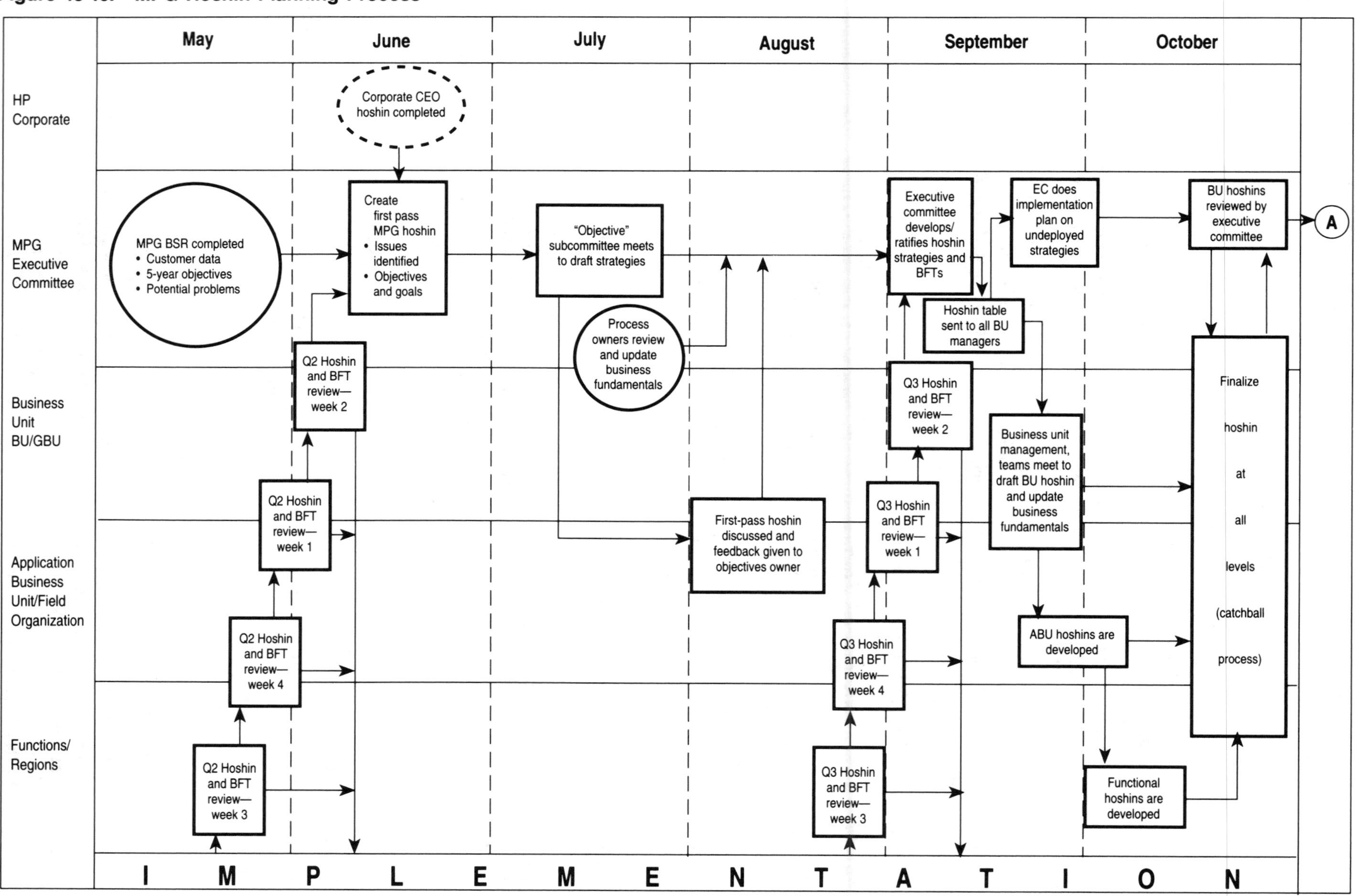

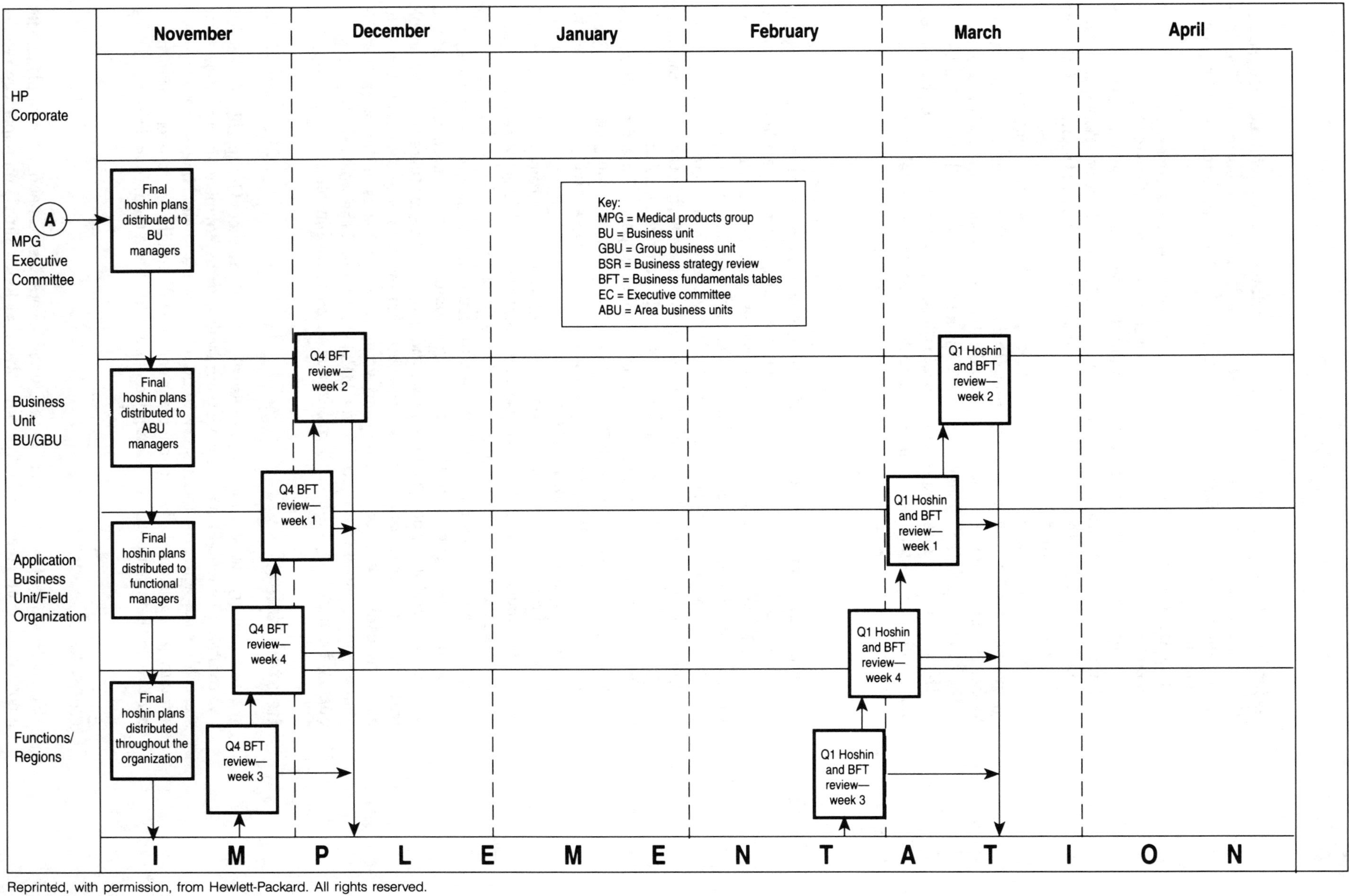
November
December
January
February
March
April
HP Corporate
A
MPG Executive Committee
Business Unit BU/GBU
Application Business Unit/Field Organization
Functions/ Regions
Final hoshin plans distributed to BU managers
Final hoshin plans distributed to ABU managers
Final hoshin plans distributed to functional managers
Final hoshin plans distributed throughout the organization
Q4 BFT review—week 2
Q4 BFT review—week 1
Q4 BFT review—week 4
Q4 BFT review—week 3
Key:
MPG = Medical products group
BU = Business unit
GBU = Group business unit
BSR = Business strategy review
BFT = Business fundamentals tables
EC = Executive committee
ABU = Area business units
Q1 Hoshin and BFT review—week 2
Q1 Hoshin and BFT review—week 1
Q1 Hoshin and BFT review—week 4
Q1 Hoshin and BFT review—week 3
I M P L E M E N T A T I O N

leadership of the hoshin process, the MPG general manager has required that the first 25 percent of each of his management meetings focus on the hoshin and "business fundamentals." (*Business fundamentals* is the Hewlett-Packard terminology for process of daily management.)

The MPG general manager and his staff meet five or six times annually for 16 to 20 hours at a time. The first four hours of those meetings are divided equally between hoshin and business fundamentals. Each quarter the general manager discusses his hoshin and business fundamentals items with the CEO of Hewlett-Packard. In addition, he uses hoshin as a communication vehicle at various gatherings of Medical Products Group staff during the year.

From her observations across many Hewlett-Packard business entities, the quality manager for the Americas Geographic Business Unit finds that "the time required for hoshin planning to take hold and sustain itself varies as a function of leadership. If the top leader doesn't believe that hoshin is a critical methodology for implementing the two or three most important priorities, hoshin won't work. Further, that leader must build in a formal review process and hold people accountable to it."

Hoshin Process Owner

In every hoshin implementation, there is a need to make someone responsible for the overall hoshin planning cycle. That person ensures that important milestones (such as planning and review meetings) occur on schedule, that new people are trained in the process, and that problems within the process are addressed on an ongoing basis. In the Medical Products Group, that person is the quality manager.

The quality manager coordinates hoshin activities with the group controller, who is responsible for the integration of all planning processes within the group, including 10-step strategic planning, hoshin, business fundamentals, and financial targets. In a given year, the general manager assigns ownership for specific hoshin objectives and strategies to members of the executive committee (including the general manager). From year to year, the group quality manager assumes responsibility for the integrity and improvement of the hoshin process.

Medical Products Group leaders view hoshin as a change process. As hoshin process owner, the quality manager sees himself as a manager of change. When MPG picks a hoshin item, it is a breakthrough – something the group has never done before. The quality manager encourages MPG leaders to think about their goals for change as well as about the organizational infrastructure, training, and communication patterns needed. As curator of the hoshin process, the quality manager talks to many people within Medical Products Group to make sure that everybody understands what the executive committee is trying to do and what everyone's role is in the big picture. He answers questions of interpretation for MPG staff around the world. In so doing, the quality manager plays a critical role in aligning the hoshin plan.

Related Roles

Where a strategy owner/leader (in the case of Medical Products Group, this is an executive committee member) is assigned a team facilitator, deployment seems to flow more smoothly than when the leaders try to do all the work alone. Now, when a top-level strategy gets assigned, the leaders are given the OK to hire or transfer a staff member to help them structure the strategy and put together a team to address the issues.

Lessons Learned

Medical Products Group leaders have learned several lessons about the ripple effects a hoshin plan can create. A hoshin objective that looks simple on paper can require a tremendous amount of activity and significant realignment of resources. Hoshin also tests the organization's ability to make and sustain incremental improvement in its important processes.

Hoshin Objectives Stimulate Action

It took Medical Products Group leaders years to learn how powerful the hoshin process really was. Early in the implementation process, hoshin was viewed as a simple documentation exercise. Once MPG leaders realized that they were stimulating "tons of action" with the hoshin process, they began to think very carefully about how they structured their strategies and measures.

Hoshin Plans Require Resource Realignment

The emergence of a role such as strategy facilitator exemplifies one of the lessons Medical Products Group has learned – that working to achieve breakthrough will involve a shift in resources. Breakthroughs require an organization to develop a new and sometimes fundamentally different set of skills or competencies from its current ones. These skills come with a price. Because people are so involved in their day-to-day responsibilities, the organization cannot assign them additional responsibility for hoshin and just ask them to work harder. Doing so usually means that some things go undone. Rather, the assignment of a hoshin responsibility needs to be accompanied by appropriate resources – either newly developed or realigned.

Familiarity with Continuous Improvement Methodologies Facilitates Hoshin Planning

Another lesson Medical Products Group has learned is that, because hoshin is not as simple as it may first appear to be, it helps if an organization understands fairly intimately the construct of the plan-do-check-act cycle. Hoshin requires the capability to critique *both* the planning/implementation process *and* the results the plan yields – a capability many U.S. managers need to develop. An illustration of this point involves a Japanese company and a U.S. company both doing hoshin planning. If the Japanese company were to exceed its hoshin goal using insufficient strategies, that company would be very troubled by its inability to draw cause-and-effect relationships between the strategies and the outcome. On the other hand, this same case of blind luck would thrill an American company. One of the weaknesses of U.S. managers using hoshin is that they are good at measuring results and not so good at measuring the process. They are not rigorously testing cause and effect – asking themselves, "Did the execution of our strategies account for the outcome, or was it sheer luck?" Unless managers understand plan-do-check-act and the importance of measuring process as well as outcome, hoshin will become simply a documentation template by which to measure the results of a plan.

What Made Hoshin Work

During the past eight years within the Medical Products Group, hoshin evolved from the latest version of management by objectives, imported from the corporate offices, to a powerful, locally owned planning infrastructure. This infrastructure took a great deal of time and commitment to build and to maintain. The hoshin process within Medical Products Group became rigorous and more robust when the general manager "became very serious about hoshin."

Taking hoshin seriously from the onset coupled with more extensive training may have accelerated Medical Products Group's learning of the process. The group quality manager maintains that an organization "just has to do hoshin to understand the idiosyncrasies of the approach. That learning takes time – probably three or four years to achieve mastery." As the AGBU quality manager put it, "The first year or two may not be very pretty. You may not achieve all you had hoped. But you are learning all along, and the system is better than it would have been without a hoshin plan."

For Hewlett-Packard's Medical Products Group, taking the time to learn the essence of hoshin as well as the mechanics paid double dividends. The group has an established framework for hoshin planning and total quality management, both powerful forces in the design and realization of a favorable future.

Reference

1. Chang, Y. S. *Case Study: Hoshin Planning at Hewlett-Packard.* Boston, MA: Boston University Asian Management Center, 1990, p. 2.

CHAPTER SIXTEEN

The Wright Brothers: A Hoshin Metaphor

On the blowing sands of the North Carolina Outer Banks stands a monument to American ingenuity and determination. At that site, on a windy December day in 1903, two bicycle mechanics from Dayton, Ohio, completed the first powered test flights in a heavier-than-air machine. With singular vision, Orville and Wilbur Wright developed a breakthrough in the direction of human transportation technology, on a total four-year budget of just over $1,000!

The story of the Wrights is an apt metaphor for hoshin planning. Responding to a need for improved understanding and control of heavier-than-air flying machines, the Wrights *chose a focus* and stuck with it. The focus guided their studies, through which they amassed an impressive number of previously unknown facts. The focus encouraged them through the hundreds of preliminary test flights.

They *aligned their organization,* albeit small, with the focus. This took the form of commandeering their sister's sewing machine to sew the muslin wing coverings, obtaining resources and space to build full-size models and engines, and enlisting the help of a man who had never seen a camera to snap a picture of their historic first flight.

In *implementing the plan,* the Wrights used every opportunity to monitor and learn from their progress. So meticulous were their notes that when the Kitty Hawk memorial was dedicated in 1928, Orville could mark the exact takeoff and landing points of the four test flights that had occurred 25 years earlier.

The Wrights also knew how to *review and improve* their own performance. Taking turns piloting the plane in their business suits and starched collars, the brothers learned to adjust their methods so that the fourth test flight, of 852 feet, was already four times longer than the first.

This breakthrough – this apparent quantum leap – was preceded by three years of study and painstaking experimentation. Even if the historic test flights near Kitty Hawk had failed, the list of the brothers' accomplishments would have been daunting. While pursuing their dream, the Wrights had built their own wind tunnel, designed the first propeller, and developed a control system that operated on the same principles as that of a modern 747.[1] While pursuing their focus, many hoshin practitioners also realize unexpected benefits – some tangible and some intangible – that add to the positive effect of the hoshin planning experience.

The story of the Wrights illustrates timeless qualities of leadership – simplicity, creativity, tenacity, openness, reflection, learning, and good humor. The story even more dramatically illustrates the power of clear vision. Like the Wrights, today's leaders need to begin with a vision that is informed but not fettered by current knowledge. That vision provides the power and the lift necessary for the creation of the hoshin plan. And once the plan is launched, it is the vision that helps leaders to maintain a panoramic view, to stay the course, and to adapt successfully to a rapidly changing environment.

Reference

1. Zinsser, W. *American Places.* New York City: HarperCollins Publishers, 1992, pp. 117–27.

PART FOUR

Appendixes, Resources, Glossary, and Index

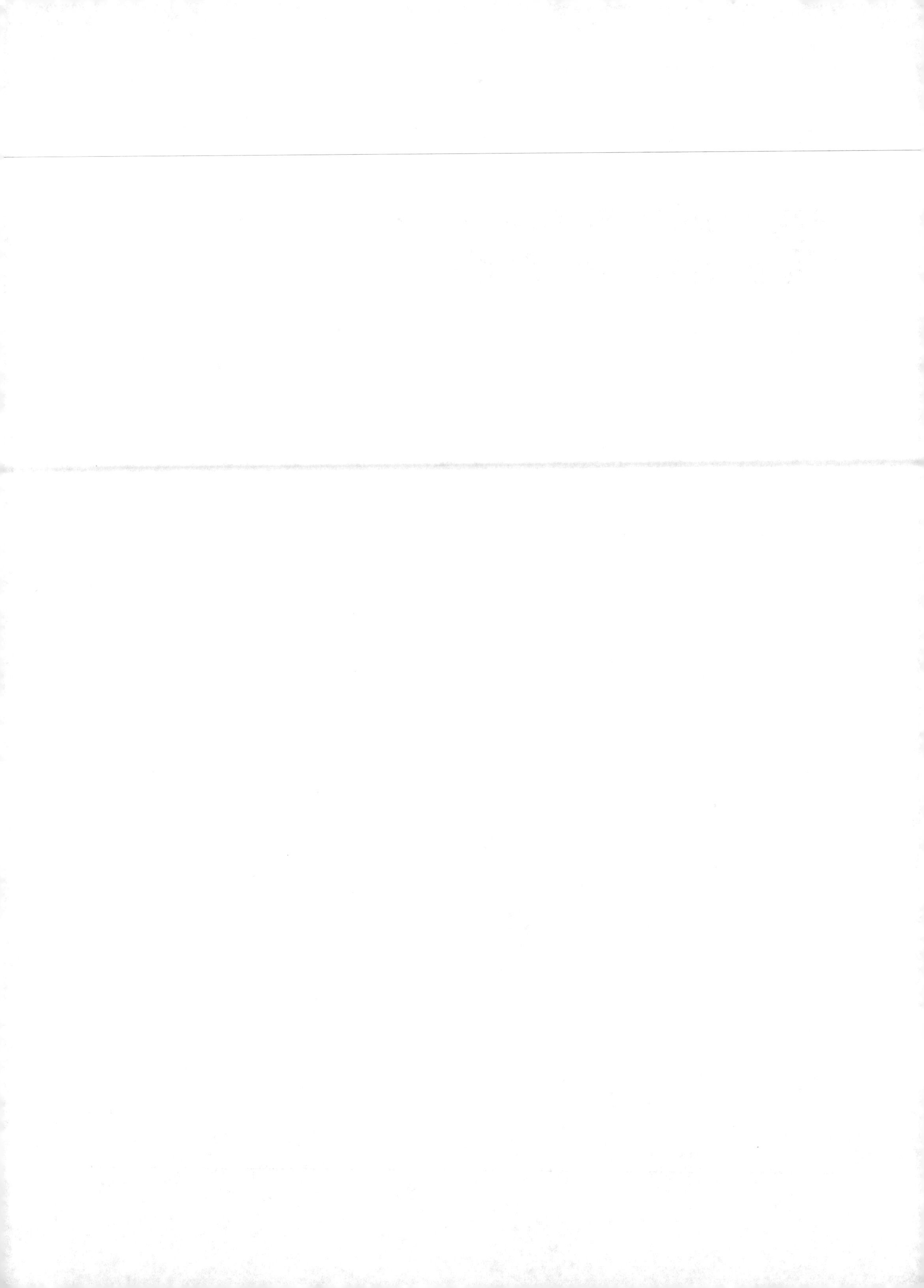

APPENDIX A

Establishing Mission, Values, and Vision

Chapter 6, "Step 1: Choose the Focus," provided a discussion of how to get hoshin planning started in an organization. The initial two substeps (1.1 and 1.2—also referred to in the chapter as task 1 and task 2) so closely resemble traditional strategic planning that they were summarized only briefly in the chapter. For the reader who wants more detail, this appendix expands on the concept of establishing mission, values, and vision statements.

Step 1.1: Make the Current State of the Organization Visible

The first step in choosing the organization's focus is to make the current state of the organization visible through statements that define its mission and values. (See the micro flowchart in figure A-1.) Carrying out this step requires three actions:

1. Revisit why the organization exists: its mission and values.
2. Identify trends regarding the major customers, suppliers, and competitors.
3. Analyze the current state of the business.

Revisit Why the Organization Exists: Its Mission and Values

Each hoshin planning process needs to begin with a review of the mission to remind the top leadership team of the reason the organization exists. Mission statements are stable over time, but they must be reviewed and refined periodically to be kept alive. They carve out a broad arena in which the hoshin plan will operate. The hoshin plan must be congruent with the mission.

Mission Statement

A mission statement describes in clear, brief terms the purpose of an organization and the customers it serves. Here are two examples of mission statements:

- To provide high-quality, affordable health care to the residents of greater Gotham City

- To develop and distribute vegetable seeds for home gardeners in the northwest maritime climate

To construct a first-draft mission statement, follow these steps:

1. Ask the members of the leadership team and any stakeholders (customers, suppliers, or other interested parties you may have asked to join you) to describe in one sentence or a few phrases what they think is the purpose of the group (or organization, activity, or effort). As a beginning point for this discussion, the group may benefit from asking, "Who are our customers? What are their needs?"
2. Chart each member's response for all to see.
3. Identify the "common ground" or themes in the responses.

Figure A-1. Micro Flowchart of Step 1

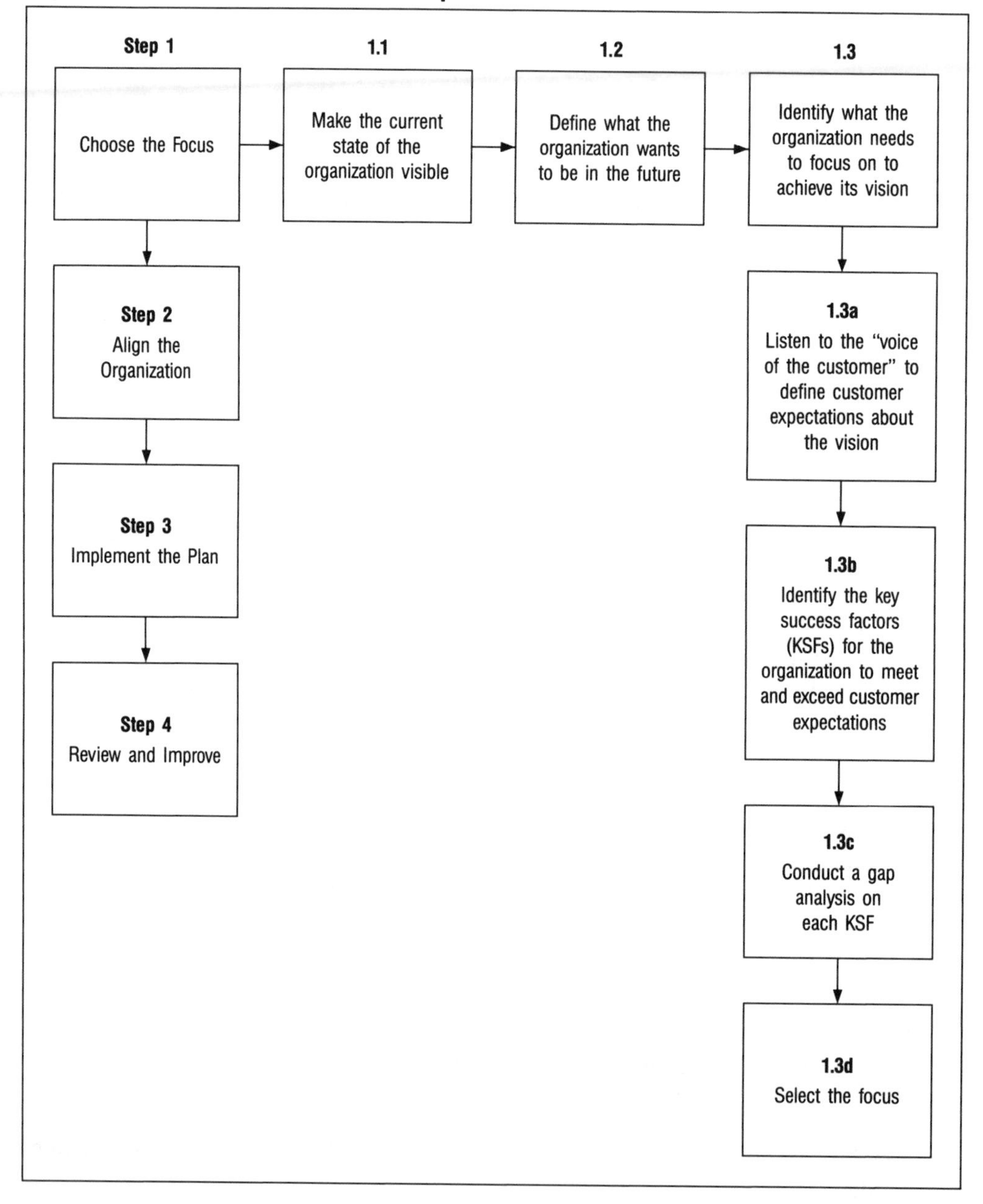

4. Ask participants to identify those words or phrases from the chart that best capture the purpose, those that embody the "heart" of the enterprise.
5. With the group, begin to weave those words or phrases into a single statement, keeping these suggestions in mind:
   - Eliminate redundant words or phrases so that each word chosen is rich in meaning.
   - Sometimes this feels like a struggle. That's OK! It is not unusual for the group to search for the right words for some time and then to have them fall into place quite suddenly.
   - If the group is large, consider having a subgroup "wordsmith" the statement and bring it back to the larger group for approval.[1]
6. (Optional) Use a worksheet like the one in figure A-2 to build a new mission or to revise an existing one. The sheet can be given out ahead of time to allow people to write down their thoughts.

Statement of Values

Values (such as compassion or treating the patients like family) are statements of belief that guide decision making across an organization. Like the mission statement, a statement of values is an enduring document. The review of organizational values at the beginning of a hoshin planning process reminds the top leadership team of the kind of organization it wants to build. The hoshin plan must produce actions that are consistent with organizational values.

To develop a first-draft set of shared values, follow this process:

1. Prepare for the values development session by gathering the appropriate leaders. Determine the key customer and stakeholder groups (such as patients, physicians, employees, board members, or payers).
2. If necessary, survey the groups to determine their opinions on the values.
3. Share survey data with the values development team.

Figure A-2. Mission Statement Worksheet

The mission of the

____

(*Who:* Name of your group or team)

is to produce or provide

____

____

____

(*What:* Your product/service)

to or for

____

____

____

(*Whom:* your customers and, if appropriate,
where: The customers' geographic scope or location)

(Optional) so that they can

____

____

____

(*Why:* The reason or purpose for your work)

4. Give each team member three large self-stick notes (minimum size 3″×5″). Ask the members to think of the three top-priority values for the organization and to record each one in large, bold print on a sticky note. Values may be single words (such as *compassion* or *integrity*) or short phrases (such as *Put the patient first*).
5. On a separate sheet of paper, ask the individuals to write the answers to these questions to clarify the meaning of their values:
   - How does this value look in action? (Here, you are looking for behavioral definitions or examples of the value.)
   - What happens when this value is not present? (This question may help clarify a value that is hard to define behaviorally.)
6. Ask for a volunteer to post his or her values on a flipchart in the front of the room, leaving some space between the sticky notes. Ask for a one-sentence definition of each value as it is posted.
7. Continue posting values, but ask people to begin clustering their values with similar ones of the other team members. This clustering will indicate congruence of opinions. Each cluster (or stand-alone sticky note) represents a value.
8. When the posting activity is done, ask team members to review the list of values (clusters and stand-alone ideas) and ask for clarification if they need it. Give each cluster a single title (word or short phrase).
9. Narrow the list, if you choose, by:
   - Consensus discussion, or
   - Giving each team member three to five votes to cast for the key values. Have the members cast their votes using colored markers or colored adhesive dots.
10. When the list is complete, assign a subgroup to write a draft statement of organizational values. The statement should include three things:
    - The value,
    - A brief definition
    - Behaviors that exemplify the value

Review of Mission and Values

Together, the mission and values statements define the organization and its character. They establish the background and constancy of purpose for the hoshin plan. In reviewing the mission and values, the top leadership team may ask itself the following questions:

- How clear are the statements of mission and values to the people who must use them?
- Has every employee received a copy of these documents along with a chance to discuss what they mean?
- How well do these documents describe the principles that determine how we treat our customers and how we treat one another?
- Could we go anywhere within the organization, ask any employee to describe the mission and values, and get consistent answers?
- Considering some recent organizational behaviors, such as the action items in last year's plan or an organizational response to a recent crisis, how consistent were those actions with the mission and values?

Identify Trends Regarding Major Customers, Suppliers, and Competitors

This task requires the top leadership team to collect and review important anecdotal and trend data in preparation for the selection of the organization's focus. The data collected are historical and are extracted from existing sources. If systems do not exist for collecting customer, competitor, and supplier data, this step suggests the types of questions the organization needs to ask.

Customer Trend Data

The hoshin planning process relies strongly on solid customer data. In establishing a customer data-gathering system, the leadership team will need to:

- Identify the customers, both current and future (potential).
- Group the customers into meaningful segments. Customers may be grouped by characteristics (such as gender or age) or by need (such as use of a product or service produced by the organization).
- Prioritize customers. If there are too many customers for the organization to serve effectively, or if some customers' needs outweigh others, priorities need to be stated clearly.

Once the leadership team knows who the customers are, it can gather customer data in three domains: customer needs/wants, customer satisfaction, and customer follow-up. Years of work in building customer data systems helped Fox Valley Technical College to develop a concise way of selecting the best method of gathering data, based on the data domain. Figure A-3 is a summary of "what works when."[2]

All forms of data – formal or informal, qualitative or quantitative – are aimed at answering these kinds of questions on an ongoing basis:

- What are our customers' needs? Expectations?
- How well are we doing at meeting their needs? Expectations?
- What are their priorities?
- What are the problems they are trying to solve for themselves? For their customers?
- What are their dreams and visions?
- How can we go beyond what they expect so as to delight them? To anticipate their future needs?

In analyzing customer needs, it may be helpful to think of what customers want on three levels:

1. What they *assume* and don't even think of mentioning, such as "Please use sterile procedures."

Figure A-3. Gathering Customer Input: What Works When

	What Do Customers Need/Want?	How Satisfied Are Customers?	What Is Happening to Our Customers?
One-on-One Interview	Excellent		
Focus Group	Excellent		
Survey (Phone, Mail, Classroom)	Excellent	Excellent	Excellent
Point-of-Service Evaluation		Excellent	
Suggestion System	Excellent		
Observation of Customers			Excellent
Records/Database Analysis			Excellent

Source: The Academy for Quality in Education.

2. What they *want* and can think of mentioning, such as "Serve me promptly."
3. What they *would love* but can't even imagine yet, such as "Call me at home periodically to see if I need anything."

Traditional customer survey techniques zero in on level 2. They miss the assumed needs, which can be big dissatisfiers if unmet. They also miss the things the customer would love but cannot articulate. If the organization can identify and satisfy level 3 needs before the competition does, it is poised for breakthrough.

The use of a customer data table, such as the one in figure A-4, may help the organization to learn about customer needs on all three levels. The table can be used when a team is trying to project what customers will say their needs are. It can also be used in face-to-face interviews with customers to validate the needs projected by the team.

Verbatim comments (or things the team believes the customers would say their needs are) go into column 1. The demands these needs place on the organization's products and services go into column 2. The next four columns are designed to identify assumed needs (level 1) and things the customer would love (level 3). By asking about the use of the current product or service offering in a variety of ways (Who? How? When? and Where?), the interviewer may elicit needs the customer did not think about mentioning. Finally, column 7 provides a place to record ideas for how to measure success of the product or service from the customers' point of view.

As the top leadership team members analyze customer needs information and trend data, they should summarize important observations and patterns. A data collection worksheet like the one in figure A-5 provides a vehicle for recording important findings about customers.

Supplier Trend Data

In addition to customer data, supplier trend data can help planners identify potential opportunities and barriers that may affect the selection of the organization's focus. Some of the same questions the top leadership team asked about customers apply to suppliers as well:

- Who are our key suppliers?
- What do they need to be in a successful partnership with our organization?

Figure A-4. Customer Data Table

Column 1	Column 2	Column 3	Column 4	Column 5	Column 6	Column 7
Customers' Words: What they say they need/want in a product/service (P/S)	Customers' Words: Translated into organizational language	Who will use the P/S?	How will they use the P/S?	When will they use?	Where will they use?	Potential Measures or Indicators
We need the ability to offer new and different services	Spectrum of services	All physicians in clinic without walls	To gain networking opportunities	—	—	Number of formal networking opportunities
Instructions: Interview customer. Record verbatim responses in column 1. Translate customer words into organization language in column 2. Continue to probe customer need with questions in columns 3 through 6. Record possible measure in column 7.						

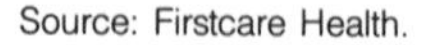
Source: Firstcare Health.

Figure A-5. Worksheet: Data Collection and Analysis for Selection of Focus

Column 1	Column 2	Column 3	Column 4
Observations about the current state of the organization Include themes, observations, or issues about: • Current strategy • Customer needs • Supplier data • Competitor data • External environment • Internal environment	Observations about the future Record "short list" of future customer needs Record future demands/issues related to: • Competitors • Suppliers • External environment • Internal environment	Key Success Factors (KSFs) 5–6 or fewer The few important things the organization must do well to meet customer needs and to achieve the vision	Ideas for potential breakthrough (focus) Record ideas for possible hoshin focus items
Examples: Strategy: Tertiary care Customer base aging (*B) Two new competitors (*A)	Anticipate increased local competition for recruiting geriatric care specialists	Retraining, reallocating workforce Understanding and meeting needs of the specialists	New levels of specialist recruitment/retention

***Note:** You can use an "A, B, C" system to indicate the impact of each observation you write in columns 1 and 2:
A = High impact item B = Medium impact C = Minimal impact

- How well are we working in partnership now?
- How can we improve?
- What are the strengths of our suppliers? Their weaknesses?
- What can we do together in the future to improve the products and services that we give our customers?

The top leadership team can record their observations about suppliers on the data collection worksheet (figure A-5).

Competitor Trend Data

The top leadership team needs to understand both the strategies and positioning (product/service and financial) of competitors. In addition, the leaders must know how the competitors are perceived by the customers and how they fit into the customers' strategies.[3] In its research report on integrated planning, GOAL/QPC recommends the following questions for competitor analysis:

- Who are our major competitors?
- What products/services do they offer?
- What are their market shares/market presence?
- What is each competitor's intent?
- How does our performance rate against that of the competitors?[4]

Conclusions drawn from the competitor data can be recorded on the data collection worksheet (figure A-5).

Analyze the Current State of the Business

To stay current with the rapidly changing environment in which the organization exists, the leadership team will need to perform both external and internal analyses of the state of the business. Information from these analyses will shape both the selection of the organization's focus and the extent of "stretch" in setting the goal.

External Environment

The GOAL/QPC integrated planning research report suggests the following questions for examining the external environment:

- What technological issues affect the industry?
- What economic issues?
- What political, governmental, or legal issues?
- What social, cultural, demographic, or geographic issues?
- What market trends will affect the industry?
- What is the current industry structure?
- What factors drive inherent profitability?
  - Stakeholder bargaining power
  - Stability of competitors and products/services
- What trends are likely to change the industry structure?
- How will the industry evolve in response to the trends?[5]

Internal Environment

Just as the top leaders looked for trends in customer, supplier, and competitor data, they need to look for trends in data generated by the internal processes of their organization. These data help the leaders to identify common weaknesses across businesses and specific weaknesses within a given unit, product line, or process. Even more important, the leadership team needs to understand why weaknesses exist or targets were missed. The "whys" may point to a serious deficit in the organization's systems that can be turned into a golden opportunity for breakthrough improvement.

The organization's leaders can simplify their search for internal trend data by creating a *daily management* system. If hoshin is like converting a barn to a house, daily management is like keeping the current house in order during the building process. In addition to "feeding" the hoshin planning process, daily management provides "effective management of routine processes, discovering abnormalities, and preventing their recurrence."[6]

Daily management is focused primarily on the work-unit level, with some amount of cross-unit coordination. To set up a daily management system, a work-unit manager would have to:

- Define the mission and customers of the unit
- Define customer needs and current products and services
- Define the most important work processes in the unit – those critical to meeting the mission and customer needs
- Select measures or indicators to track the critical work processes over time
- Identify and prioritize improvement opportunities
- Improve the processes and monitor progress

The last three steps above are often associated with continuous quality improvement (CQI) activities.

A healthy by-product of the daily management system is the accumulation of vital process data. Ongoing reviews of daily management data from within the various work units and across the organization are summarized on quarterly and annual bases and are used as inputs to the hoshin planning process. Observations from the analyses of the external and internal environments can be recorded on the data collection worksheet (figure A-5).

Step 1.2: Define What the Organization Wants to Be in the Future

This step involves developing or refining a vision – the dream of what the organization will become. Visions should create mild discomfort, in a good way. If they do not engage and compel the organization to reach and grow beyond its current capabilities, they are not "visionary" enough. The vision is the "pull factor" or positive tension for change in the hoshin plan. Within the vision is the seed of the organization's priority focus.

Create a Vision Statement

There are various methods for creating a vision statement, from brainstorming and consensus discussion to the use of specific tools or discussion aids. One such structured approach is known as the affinity diagram. (See appendix B, "Hoshin Toolbox," for instructions on the affinity diagram and other processes suggested in the following text.)

Method 1: Affinity Diagram

Known as one of the management and planning (MP) tools, the affinity diagram asks the team to think of as many answers as possible to questions about the future. The team then groups the responses into like categories, or vision elements, and analyzes further.

Hoshin stakeholders in the Vermont Academic Medical Center used an affinity diagram and the following question to generate a vision: "What would the organization look like 10 years from now if it were meeting and exceeding the needs of its customers, responding to the issues in the outside environment, ideally positioned within the marketplace, and capitalizing on its strengths and weaknesses?" The resulting vision is made up of multiple elements, such as "products and services, organizational structures, human and financial resources, or relationships with customers and the community." The exploration of these elements and their relationship to one another leads to the identification of "key vision elements," which form the basis for the organization's hoshin priorities.[7]

Method 2: Graphic Images

Another process for developing a first-draft vision statement involves having small groups create graphic images. Following are suggested guidelines:

1. Work in small groups (three to five persons).
2. Give each group creative tools – colored markers, crayons, scissors, tape, and other materials as desired.
3. Ask each group to create a graphic image of its vision for the group (or organization, project, or other unit).
4. The final product must represent ideas from all team members.
5. Allow 20 to 40 minutes for this activity.
6. Each group shares its visual image with the large group, explaining what it represents.
7. Chart the key elements of the visions described by each group.
8. Look for common themes.
9. This work may be useful in a number of ways; for example:
   - Use the ideas to construct a vision statement. (Follow step 5 from the mission statement section earlier in this appendix.)

- Use the elements as a basis to develop specific strategies and action plans.
- Keep the pictures posted to communicate the vision to others.[8]

Note: This process may be modified by substituting other approaches for steps 2 and 3.

Other Methods for Developing a Vision

Following are some additional approaches for developing a vision:

1. Write an imaginary journal article for your favorite business publication. Set the story from 2 to 10 years into the future. Chronicle your success.
2. Build a discussion around your values or your customers' needs.
3. Use analogies to build a verbal picture of your vision. Complete the following sentence: "If I were to describe my work group as a [fill in with one of the categories suggested below], I would say it is . . ."
   - Vehicle
   - Color
   - Season
   - Food or beverage
   - Song
   - Movie
   - Machine
   - Emotion
   - Geographic location
   - Any other category of your choice

   An example of a completed sentence would be, "Our team is like a sports car–polished, tuned up, and ready to race."[9]

Take the Next Step

With the vision defined or refined, the top leadership team has created positive tension for change. It is now ready to take the next step toward selecting the breakthrough goal or goals that will bring about that change.

References

1. Vicky Willis, assistant to the president, personal communication with Casey Collett, Apr. 1994.
2. Mishler, C. J. Practicing what we teach: five years of implementing a continuous improvement initiative at Fox Valley Technical College. Presentation, Conference on TQM in Colleges and Universities, Michigan State University, Troy, MI., Mar. 30–31, 1992.
3. Soin, S. *Total Quality Control Essentials.* New York City: McGraw-Hill, 1992, p. 52.
4. Hsiang, T., Siira, M., Kotecki, M., and Hotopp, D. *Integrated Planning Model.* GOAL/QPC Research Report No. 92-01R. Methuen, MA: GOAL/QPC, 1992, p. 21.
5. Hsiang and others.
6. Soin, p. 74.
7. Demers, D. Tutorial: Implementing hoshin planning at the Vermont Academic Medical Center. *Quality Management in Health Care* 1(4):64–72, 1993.
8. Willis.
9. Whiteley, R. *The Customer-Driven Company.* Reading, MA: Addison-Wesley, 1991, pp. 227–28.

APPENDIX B

Hoshin Toolbox

The hoshin planning process provides a rich forum for discussion of opinions and facts. Tools such as the ones in this appendix can be invaluable means of aiding the discussions and recording them for later use. No one tool or combination of tools is absolutely necessary to make the hoshin process work, but some of the more widely used tools include the following:

- Affinity diagram
- Cause-and-effect diagram
- Flowchart
- Force field analysis
- Interrelationship digraph
- Matrix diagram
- Prioritization matrix
- Process decision program chart (PDPC)
- Radar chart
- Tree diagram

The material in the Hoshin Toolbox is reprinted from the GOAL/QPC publication *The Memory Jogger II.* It describes the tools listed above, which are 10 of the 26 continuous improvement concepts covered in the publication.

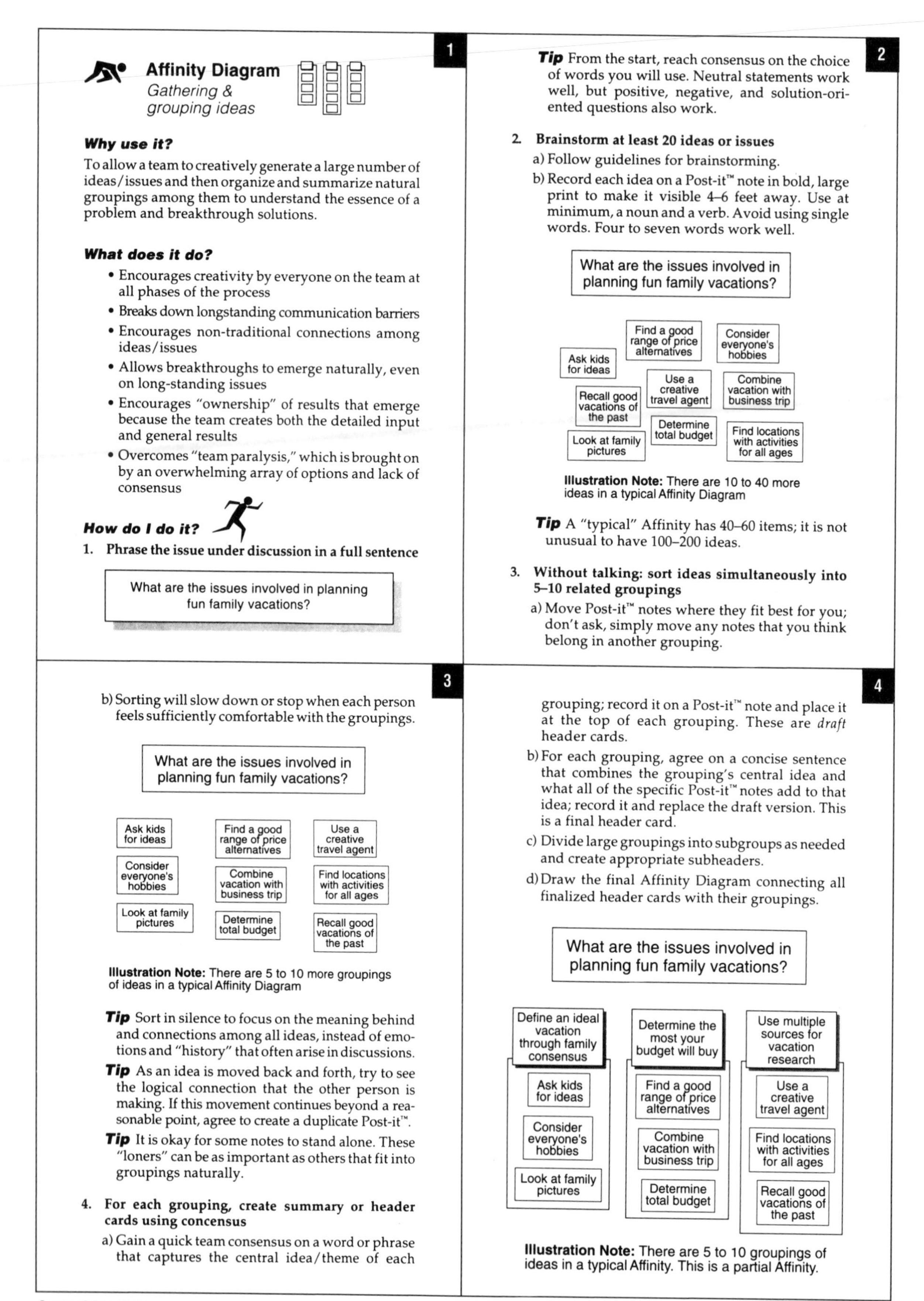

1

Affinity Diagram

Gathering & grouping ideas

Why use it?

To allow a team to creatively generate a large number of ideas/issues and then organize and summarize natural groupings among them to understand the essence of a problem and breakthrough solutions.

What does it do?

- Encourages creativity by everyone on the team at all phases of the process
- Breaks down longstanding communication barriers
- Encourages non-traditional connections among ideas/issues
- Allows breakthroughs to emerge naturally, even on long-standing issues
- Encourages "ownership" of results that emerge because the team creates both the detailed input and general results
- Overcomes "team paralysis," which is brought on by an overwhelming array of options and lack of consensus

How do I do it?

1. **Phrase the issue under discussion in a full sentence**

What are the issues involved in planning fun family vacations?

2

Tip From the start, reach consensus on the choice of words you will use. Neutral statements work well, but positive, negative, and solution-oriented questions also work.

2. **Brainstorm at least 20 ideas or issues**

   a) Follow guidelines for brainstorming.

   b) Record each idea on a Post-it™ note in bold, large print to make it visible 4–6 feet away. Use at minimum, a noun and a verb. Avoid using single words. Four to seven words work well.

Illustration Note: There are 10 to 40 more ideas in a typical Affinity Diagram

Tip A "typical" Affinity has 40–60 items; it is not unusual to have 100–200 ideas.

3. **Without talking: sort ideas simultaneously into 5–10 related groupings**

   a) Move Post-it™ notes where they fit best for you; don't ask, simply move any notes that you think belong in another grouping.

3

   b) Sorting will slow down or stop when each person feels sufficiently comfortable with the groupings.

Illustration Note: There are 5 to 10 more groupings of ideas in a typical Affinity Diagram

Tip Sort in silence to focus on the meaning behind and connections among all ideas, instead of emotions and "history" that often arise in discussions.

Tip As an idea is moved back and forth, try to see the logical connection that the other person is making. If this movement continues beyond a reasonable point, agree to create a duplicate Post-it™.

Tip It is okay for some notes to stand alone. These "loners" can be as important as others that fit into groupings naturally.

4. **For each grouping, create summary or header cards using concensus**

   a) Gain a quick team consensus on a word or phrase that captures the central idea/theme of each

4

grouping; record it on a Post-it™ note and place it at the top of each grouping. These are *draft* header cards.

   b) For each grouping, agree on a concise sentence that combines the grouping's central idea and what all of the specific Post-it™ notes add to that idea; record it and replace the draft version. This is a final header card.

   c) Divide large groupings into subgroups as needed and create appropriate subheaders.

   d) Draw the final Affinity Diagram connecting all finalized header cards with their groupings.

Illustration Note: There are 5 to 10 groupings of ideas in a typical Affinity. This is a partial Affinity.

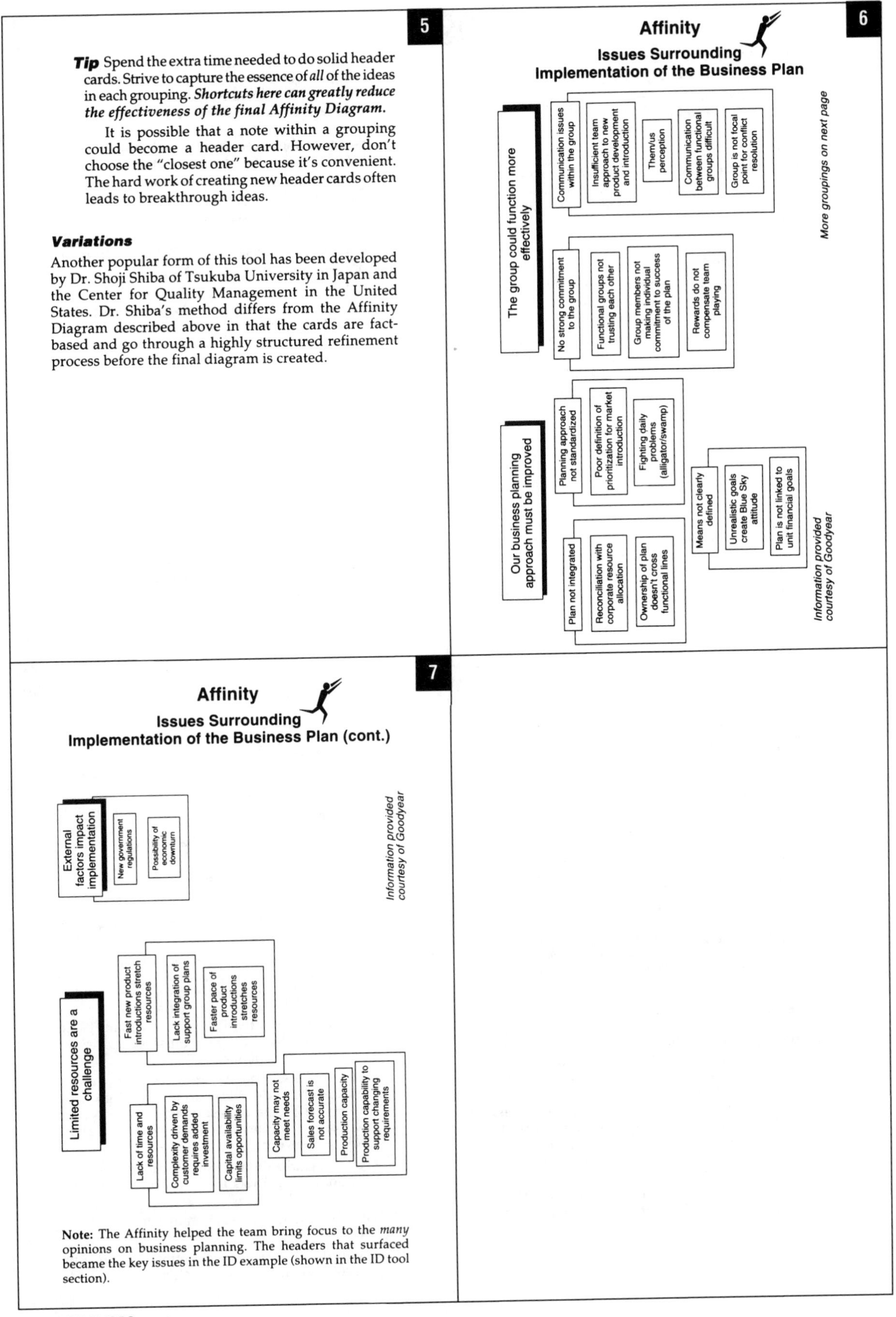

5

Tip Spend the extra time needed to do solid header cards. Strive to capture the essence of *all* of the ideas in each grouping. ***Shortcuts here can greatly reduce the effectiveness of the final Affinity Diagram.***

It is possible that a note within a grouping could become a header card. However, don't choose the "closest one" because it's convenient. The hard work of creating new header cards often leads to breakthrough ideas.

Variations

Another popular form of this tool has been developed by Dr. Shoji Shiba of Tsukuba University in Japan and the Center for Quality Management in the United States. Dr. Shiba's method differs from the Affinity Diagram described above in that the cards are fact-based and go through a highly structured refinement process before the final diagram is created.

Note: The Affinity helped the team bring focus to the *many* opinions on business planning. The headers that surfaced became the key issues in the ID example (shown in the ID tool section).

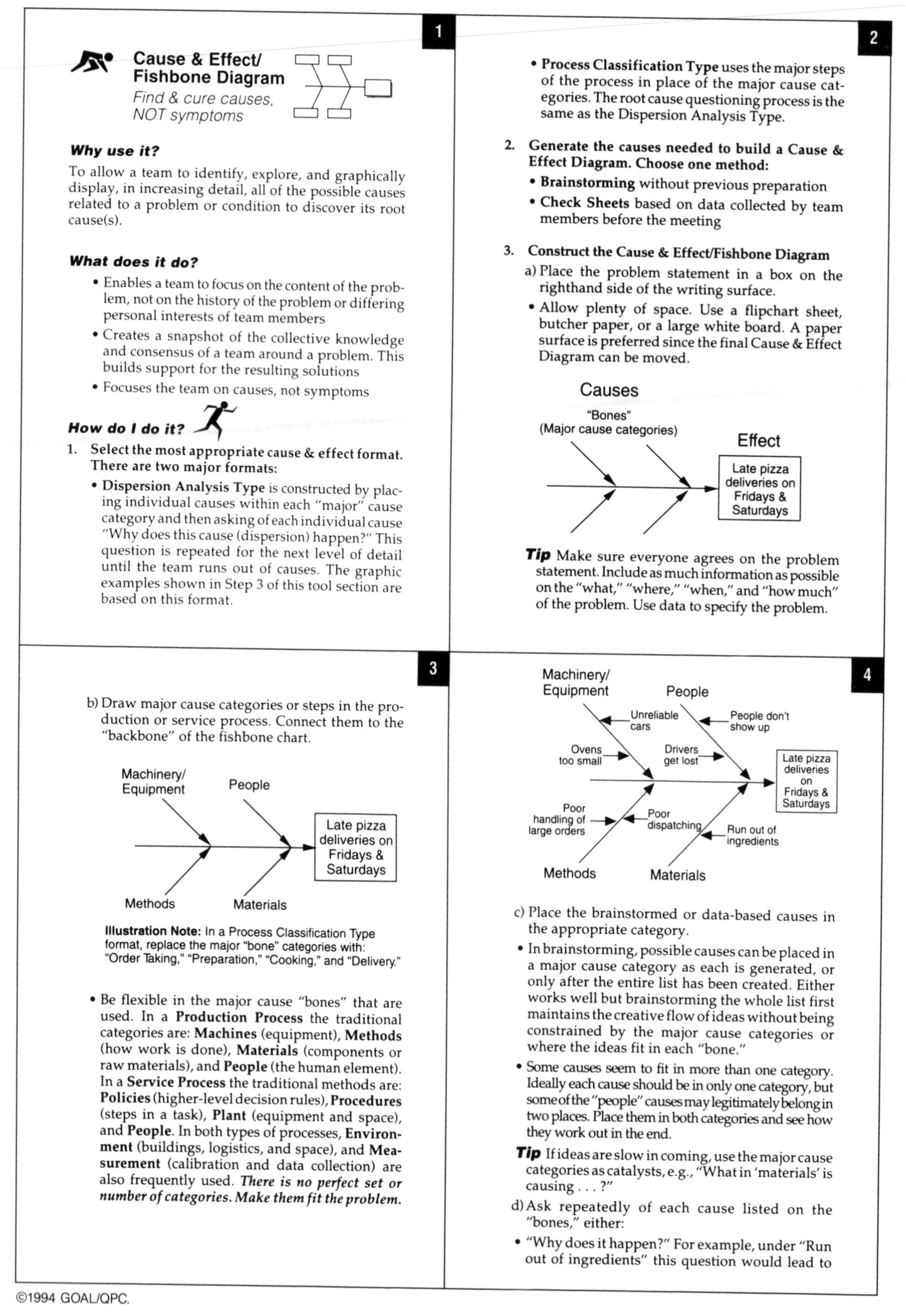

1

Cause & Effect/ Fishbone Diagram

Find & cure causes, NOT symptoms

Why use it?

To allow a team to identify, explore, and graphically display, in increasing detail, all of the possible causes related to a problem or condition to discover its root cause(s).

What does it do?

- Enables a team to focus on the content of the problem, not on the history of the problem or differing personal interests of team members
- Creates a snapshot of the collective knowledge and consensus of a team around a problem. This builds support for the resulting solutions
- Focuses the team on causes, not symptoms

How do I do it?

1. **Select the most appropriate cause & effect format. There are two major formats:**
   - **Dispersion Analysis Type** is constructed by placing individual causes within each "major" cause category and then asking of each individual cause "Why does this cause (dispersion) happen?" This question is repeated for the next level of detail until the team runs out of causes. The graphic examples shown in Step 3 of this tool section are based on this format.

2

   - **Process Classification Type** uses the major steps of the process in place of the major cause categories. The root cause questioning process is the same as the Dispersion Analysis Type.

2. **Generate the causes needed to build a Cause & Effect Diagram. Choose one method:**
   - **Brainstorming** without previous preparation
   - **Check Sheets** based on data collected by team members before the meeting

3. **Construct the Cause & Effect/Fishbone Diagram**

   a) Place the problem statement in a box on the righthand side of the writing surface.
   - Allow plenty of space. Use a flipchart sheet, butcher paper, or a large white board. A paper surface is preferred since the final Cause & Effect Diagram can be moved.

Tip Make sure everyone agrees on the problem statement. Include as much information as possible on the "what," "where," "when," and "how much" of the problem. Use data to specify the problem.

3

b) Draw major cause categories or steps in the production or service process. Connect them to the "backbone" of the fishbone chart.

Illustration Note: In a Process Classification Type format, replace the major "bone" categories with: "Order Taking," "Preparation," "Cooking," and "Delivery."

- Be flexible in the major cause "bones" that are used. In a **Production Process** the traditional categories are: **Machines** (equipment), **Methods** (how work is done), **Materials** (components or raw materials), and **People** (the human element). In a **Service Process** the traditional methods are: **Policies** (higher-level decision rules), **Procedures** (steps in a task), **Plant** (equipment and space), and **People**. In both types of processes, **Environment** (buildings, logistics, and space), and **Measurement** (calibration and data collection) are also frequently used. ***There is no perfect set or number of categories. Make them fit the problem.***

4

c) Place the brainstormed or data-based causes in the appropriate category.
- In brainstorming, possible causes can be placed in a major cause category as each is generated, or only after the entire list has been created. Either works well but brainstorming the whole list first maintains the creative flow of ideas without being constrained by the major cause categories or where the ideas fit in each "bone."
- Some causes seem to fit in more than one category. Ideally each cause should be in only one category, but some of the "people" causes may legitimately belong in two places. Place them in both categories and see how they work out in the end.

Tip If ideas are slow in coming, use the major cause categories as catalysts, e.g., "What in 'materials' is causing . . . ?"

d) Ask repeatedly of each cause listed on the "bones," either:
- "Why does it happen?" For example, under "Run out of ingredients" this question would lead to

5

more basic causes such as "Inaccurate ordering," "Poor use of space," and so on.

6

- "What could happen?" For example, under "Run out of ingredients" this question would lead to a deeper understanding of the problem such as "Boxes," "Prepared dough," "Toppings," and so on.

Tip For each deeper cause, continue to push for deeper understanding, but know when to stop. A rule of thumb is to stop questioning when a cause is controlled by more than one level of management removed from the group. Otherwise, the process could become an exercise in frustration. Use common sense.

e) Interpret or test for root cause(s) by one or more of the following:

- Look for causes that appear repeatedly within or across major cause categories.
- Select through either an unstructured consensus process or one that is structured, such as Nominal Group Technique or Multivoting.
- Gather data through Check Sheets or other formats to determine the relative frequencies of the different causes.

Variations

Traditionally, Cause & Effect Diagrams have been created in a meeting setting. The completed "fishbone" is often reviewed by others and/or confirmed with data collection. A very effective alternative is CEDAC®, in which a large, highly visible, blank fishbone chart is displayed prominently in a work area. Everyone posts both potential causes and solutions on Post-it™ notes in each of the categories. Causes and solutions are reviewed, tested, and posted. This technique opens up the process to the knowledge and creativity of every person in the operation.

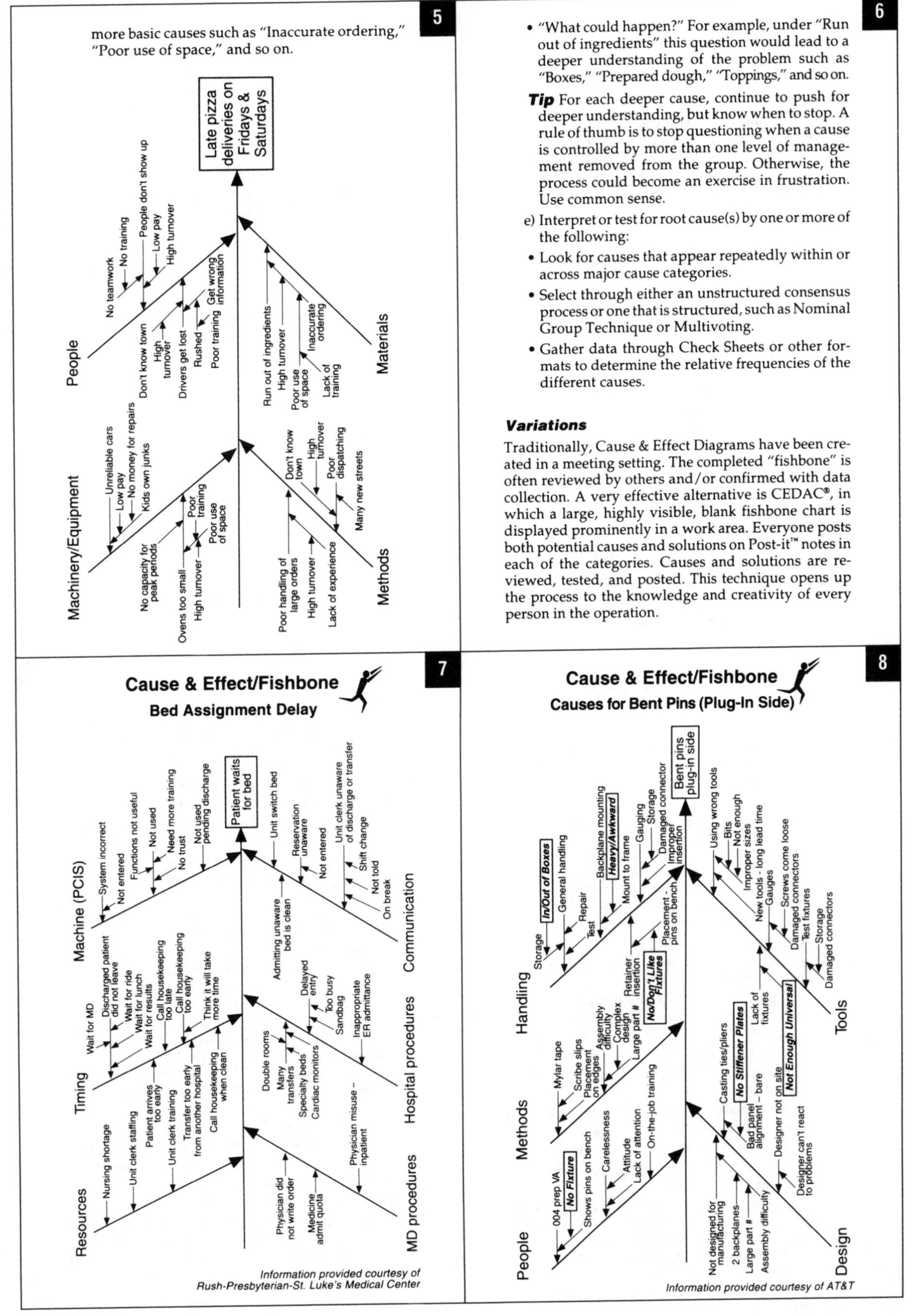

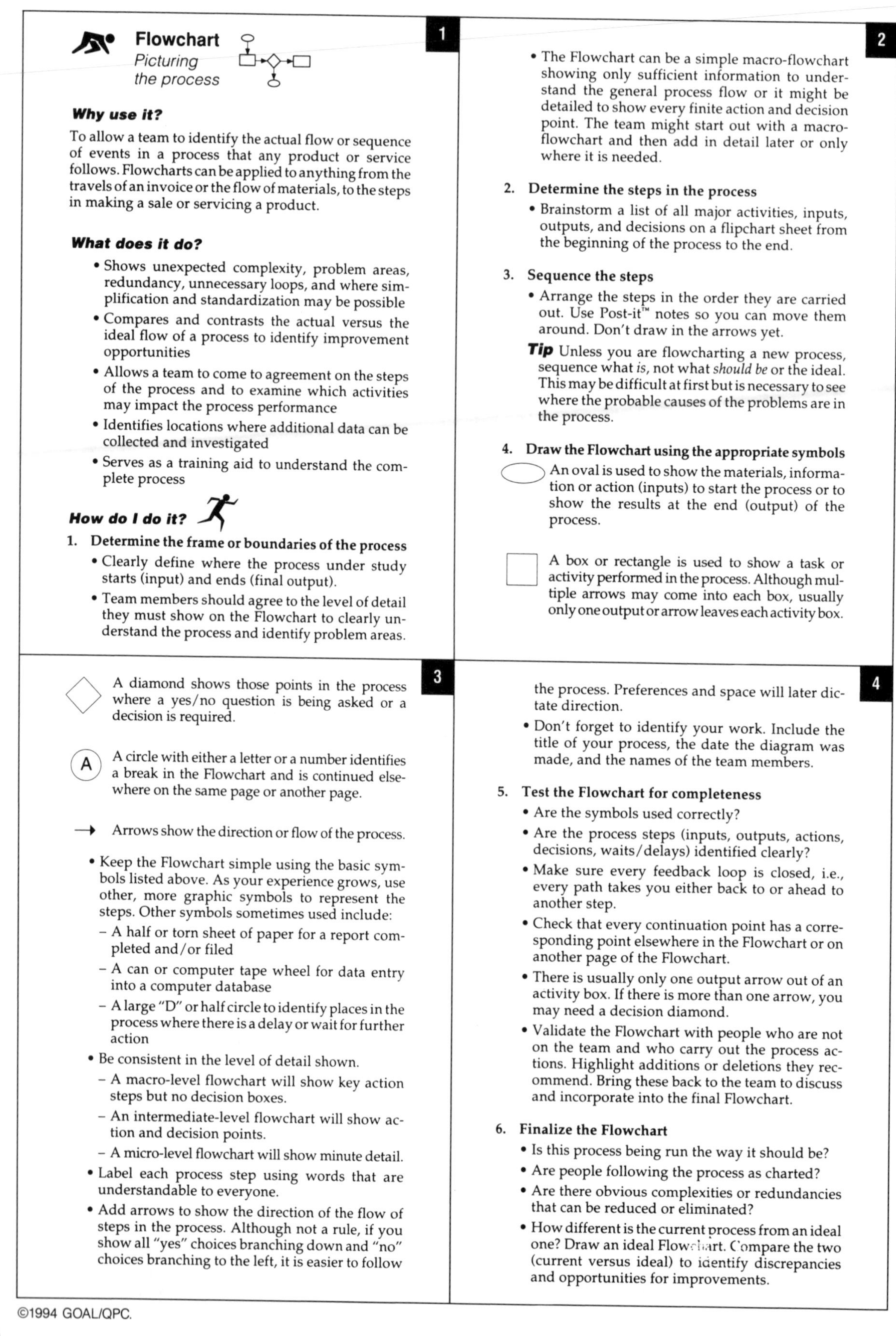

Flowchart

Picturing the process

Why use it?

To allow a team to identify the actual flow or sequence of events in a process that any product or service follows. Flowcharts can be applied to anything from the travels of an invoice or the flow of materials, to the steps in making a sale or servicing a product.

What does it do?

- Shows unexpected complexity, problem areas, redundancy, unnecessary loops, and where simplification and standardization may be possible
- Compares and contrasts the actual versus the ideal flow of a process to identify improvement opportunities
- Allows a team to come to agreement on the steps of the process and to examine which activities may impact the process performance
- Identifies locations where additional data can be collected and investigated
- Serves as a training aid to understand the complete process

How do I do it?

1. **Determine the frame or boundaries of the process**
   - Clearly define where the process under study starts (input) and ends (final output).
   - Team members should agree to the level of detail they must show on the Flowchart to clearly understand the process and identify problem areas.
   - The Flowchart can be a simple macro-flowchart showing only sufficient information to understand the general process flow or it might be detailed to show every finite action and decision point. The team might start out with a macro-flowchart and then add in detail later or only where it is needed.

2. **Determine the steps in the process**
   - Brainstorm a list of all major activities, inputs, outputs, and decisions on a flipchart sheet from the beginning of the process to the end.

3. **Sequence the steps**
   - Arrange the steps in the order they are carried out. Use Post-it™ notes so you can move them around. Don't draw in the arrows yet.

   Tip Unless you are flowcharting a new process, sequence what *is*, not what *should be* or the ideal. This may be difficult at first but is necessary to see where the probable causes of the problems are in the process.

4. **Draw the Flowchart using the appropriate symbols**

   An oval is used to show the materials, information or action (inputs) to start the process or to show the results at the end (output) of the process.

   A box or rectangle is used to show a task or activity performed in the process. Although multiple arrows may come into each box, usually only one output or arrow leaves each activity box.

   A diamond shows those points in the process where a yes/no question is being asked or a decision is required.

   A circle with either a letter or a number identifies a break in the Flowchart and is continued elsewhere on the same page or another page.

   Arrows show the direction or flow of the process.

   - Keep the Flowchart simple using the basic symbols listed above. As your experience grows, use other, more graphic symbols to represent the steps. Other symbols sometimes used include:
     - A half or torn sheet of paper for a report completed and/or filed
     - A can or computer tape wheel for data entry into a computer database
     - A large "D" or half circle to identify places in the process where there is a delay or wait for further action
   - Be consistent in the level of detail shown.
     - A macro-level flowchart will show key action steps but no decision boxes.
     - An intermediate-level flowchart will show action and decision points.
     - A micro-level flowchart will show minute detail.
   - Label each process step using words that are understandable to everyone.
   - Add arrows to show the direction of the flow of steps in the process. Although not a rule, if you show all "yes" choices branching down and "no" choices branching to the left, it is easier to follow the process. Preferences and space will later dictate direction.
   - Don't forget to identify your work. Include the title of your process, the date the diagram was made, and the names of the team members.

5. **Test the Flowchart for completeness**
   - Are the symbols used correctly?
   - Are the process steps (inputs, outputs, actions, decisions, waits/delays) identified clearly?
   - Make sure every feedback loop is closed, i.e., every path takes you either back to or ahead to another step.
   - Check that every continuation point has a corresponding point elsewhere in the Flowchart or on another page of the Flowchart.
   - There is usually only one output arrow out of an activity box. If there is more than one arrow, you may need a decision diamond.
   - Validate the Flowchart with people who are not on the team and who carry out the process actions. Highlight additions or deletions they recommend. Bring these back to the team to discuss and incorporate into the final Flowchart.

6. **Finalize the Flowchart**
   - Is this process being run the way it should be?
   - Are people following the process as charted?
   - Are there obvious complexities or redundancies that can be reduced or eliminated?
   - How different is the current process from an ideal one? Draw an ideal Flowchart. Compare the two (current versus ideal) to identify discrepancies and opportunities for improvements.

5

Variations

The type of Flowchart just described is sometimes referred to as a "detailed" flowchart because it includes, in detail, the inputs, activities, decision points, and outputs of any process. Four other forms, described below, are also useful.

Macro Flowchart

Refer to the third bulleted item in Step 1 of this section for a description. For a graphic example, see Step 2 of the Improvement Storyboard in the Problem-Solving/Process Improvement Model section.

Top-down Flowchart

This chart is a picture of the major steps in a work process. It minimizes the detail to focus only on those steps essential to the process. It usually does not include inspection, rework, and other steps that result in quality problems. Teams sometimes study the top-down flowchart to look for ways to simplify or reduce the number of steps to make the process more efficient and effective.

Planning a Party

1.0 Determine party size → 2.0 Find location → 3.0 Invite guests → • • •

1.1 Decide on budget
1.2 Decide on guest list

2.1 Decide theme
2.2 Select location

3.1 Complete invitations
3.2 Send invitations

6

Deployment Flowchart

This chart shows the people or departments responsible and the flow of the process steps or tasks they are assigned. It is useful to clarify roles and track accountability as well as to indicate dependencies in the sequence of events.

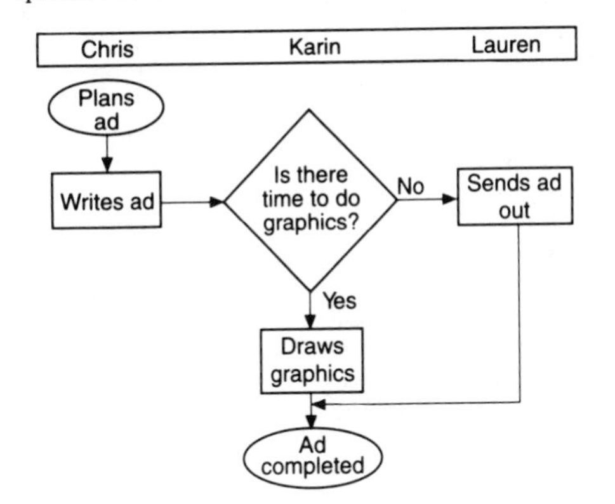

Workflow Flowchart

This type of chart is used to show the flow of people, materials, paperwork, etc., within a work setting. When redundancies, duplications, and unnecessary complexities are identified in a path, people can take action to reduce or eliminate these problems.

7

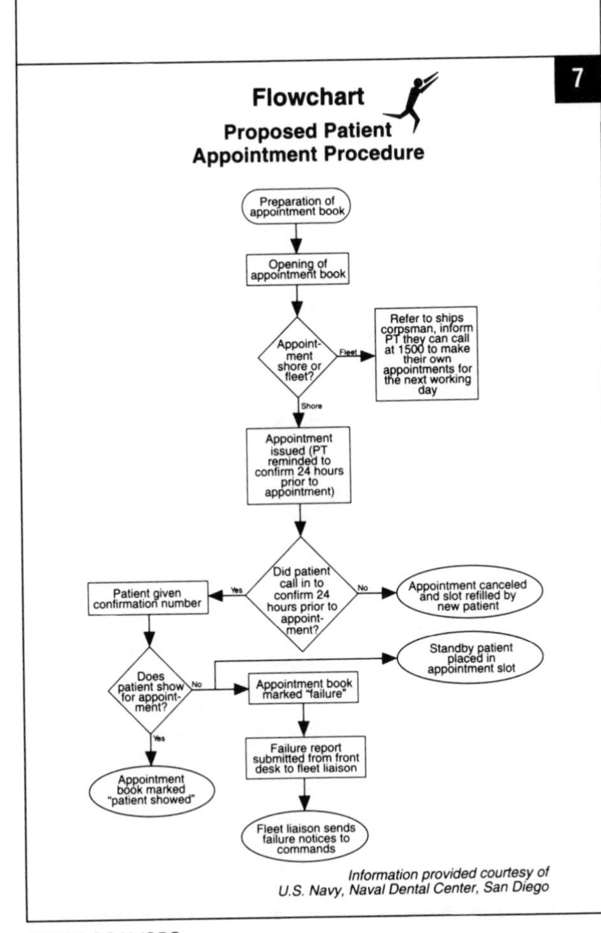

Information provided courtesy of U.S. Navy, Naval Dental Center, San Diego

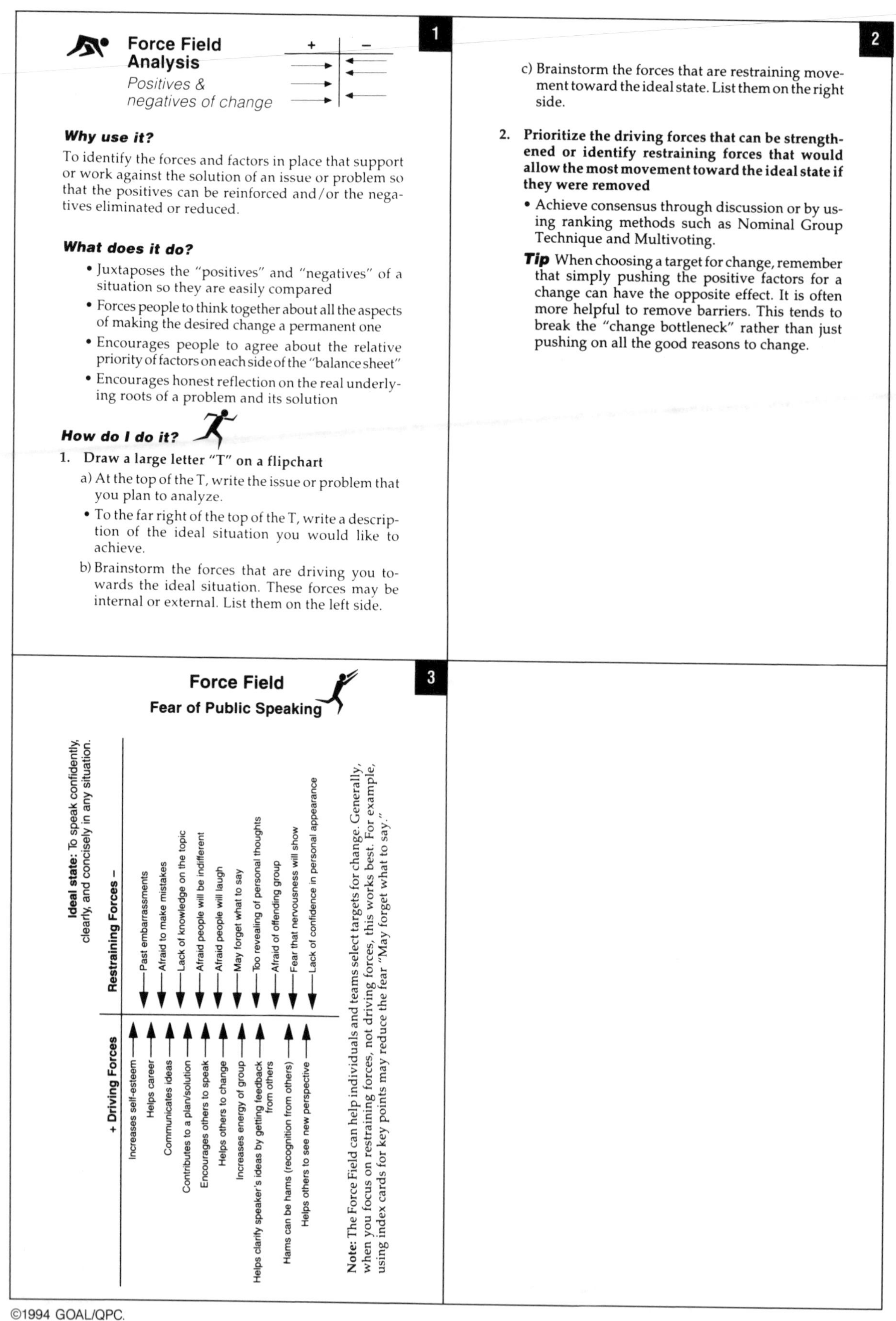

1

Force Field Analysis

Positives & negatives of change

Why use it?

To identify the forces and factors in place that support or work against the solution of an issue or problem so that the positives can be reinforced and/or the negatives eliminated or reduced.

What does it do?

- Juxtaposes the "positives" and "negatives" of a situation so they are easily compared
- Forces people to think together about all the aspects of making the desired change a permanent one
- Encourages people to agree about the relative priority of factors on each side of the "balance sheet"
- Encourages honest reflection on the real underlying roots of a problem and its solution

How do I do it?

1. **Draw a large letter "T" on a flipchart**

   a) At the top of the T, write the issue or problem that you plan to analyze.

   - To the far right of the top of the T, write a description of the ideal situation you would like to achieve.

   b) Brainstorm the forces that are driving you towards the ideal situation. These forces may be internal or external. List them on the left side.

2

   c) Brainstorm the forces that are restraining movement toward the ideal state. List them on the right side.

2. **Prioritize the driving forces that can be strengthened or identify restraining forces that would allow the most movement toward the ideal state if they were removed**

   - Achieve consensus through discussion or by using ranking methods such as Nominal Group Technique and Multivoting.

   Tip When choosing a target for change, remember that simply pushing the positive factors for a change can have the opposite effect. It is often more helpful to remove barriers. This tends to break the "change bottleneck" rather than just pushing on all the good reasons to change.

3

Force Field

Fear of Public Speaking

Ideal state: To speak confidently, clearly, and concisely in any situation.

+ Driving Forces	Restraining Forces –
Increases self-esteem	Past embarrassments
Helps career	Afraid to make mistakes
Communicates ideas	Lack of knowledge on the topic
Contributes to a plan/solution	Afraid people will be indifferent
Encourages others to speak	Afraid people will laugh
Helps others to change	May forget what to say
Increases energy of group	Too revealing of personal thoughts
Helps clarify speaker's ideas by getting feedback from others	Afraid of offending group
Hams can be hams (recognition from others)	Fear that nervousness will show
Helps others to see new perspective	Lack of confidence in personal appearance

Note: The Force Field can help individuals and teams select targets for change. Generally, when you focus on restraining forces, not driving forces, this works best. For example, using index cards for key points may reduce the fear "May forget what to say."

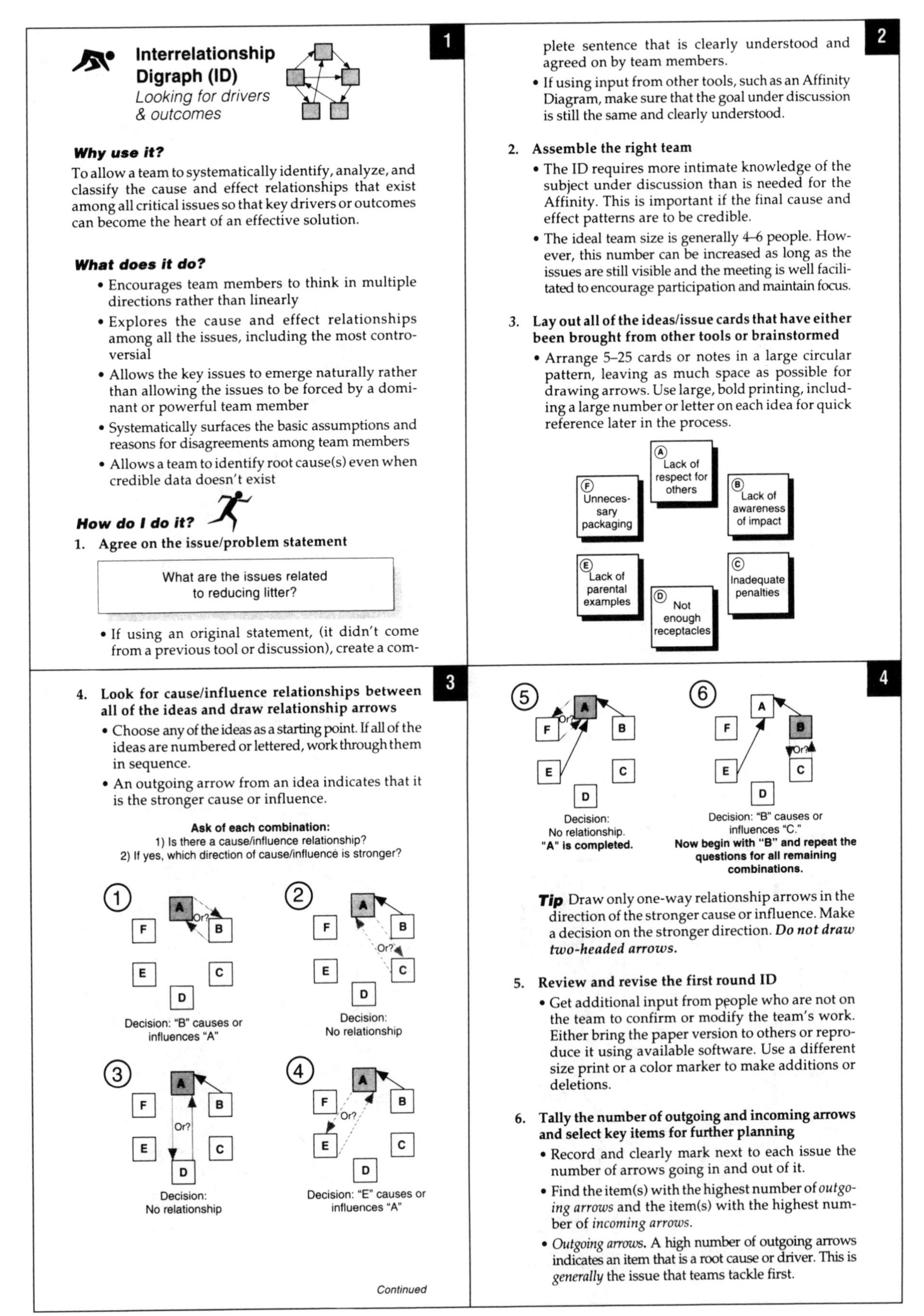

1

Interrelationship Digraph (ID)

Looking for drivers & outcomes

Why use it?

To allow a team to systematically identify, analyze, and classify the cause and effect relationships that exist among all critical issues so that key drivers or outcomes can become the heart of an effective solution.

What does it do?

- Encourages team members to think in multiple directions rather than linearly
- Explores the cause and effect relationships among all the issues, including the most controversial
- Allows the key issues to emerge naturally rather than allowing the issues to be forced by a dominant or powerful team member
- Systematically surfaces the basic assumptions and reasons for disagreements among team members
- Allows a team to identify root cause(s) even when credible data doesn't exist

How do I do it?

1. **Agree on the issue/problem statement**

What are the issues related to reducing litter?

- If using an original statement, (it didn't come from a previous tool or discussion), create a complete sentence that is clearly understood and agreed on by team members.
- If using input from other tools, such as an Affinity Diagram, make sure that the goal under discussion is still the same and clearly understood.

2

2. **Assemble the right team**
   - The ID requires more intimate knowledge of the subject under discussion than is needed for the Affinity. This is important if the final cause and effect patterns are to be credible.
   - The ideal team size is generally 4–6 people. However, this number can be increased as long as the issues are still visible and the meeting is well facilitated to encourage participation and maintain focus.

3. **Lay out all of the ideas/issue cards that have either been brought from other tools or brainstormed**
   - Arrange 5–25 cards or notes in a large circular pattern, leaving as much space as possible for drawing arrows. Use large, bold printing, including a large number or letter on each idea for quick reference later in the process.

3

4. **Look for cause/influence relationships between all of the ideas and draw relationship arrows**
   - Choose any of the ideas as a starting point. If all of the ideas are numbered or lettered, work through them in sequence.
   - An outgoing arrow from an idea indicates that it is the stronger cause or influence.

Ask of each combination:
1) Is there a cause/influence relationship?
2) If yes, which direction of cause/influence is stronger?

Continued

4

Tip Draw only one-way relationship arrows in the direction of the stronger cause or influence. Make a decision on the stronger direction. ***Do not draw two-headed arrows.***

5. **Review and revise the first round ID**
   - Get additional input from people who are not on the team to confirm or modify the team's work. Either bring the paper version to others or reproduce it using available software. Use a different size print or a color marker to make additions or deletions.

6. **Tally the number of outgoing and incoming arrows and select key items for further planning**
   - Record and clearly mark next to each issue the number of arrows going in and out of it.
   - Find the item(s) with the highest number of *outgoing arrows* and the item(s) with the highest number of *incoming arrows.*
   - *Outgoing arrows.* A high number of outgoing arrows indicates an item that is a root cause or driver. This is *generally* the issue that teams tackle first.

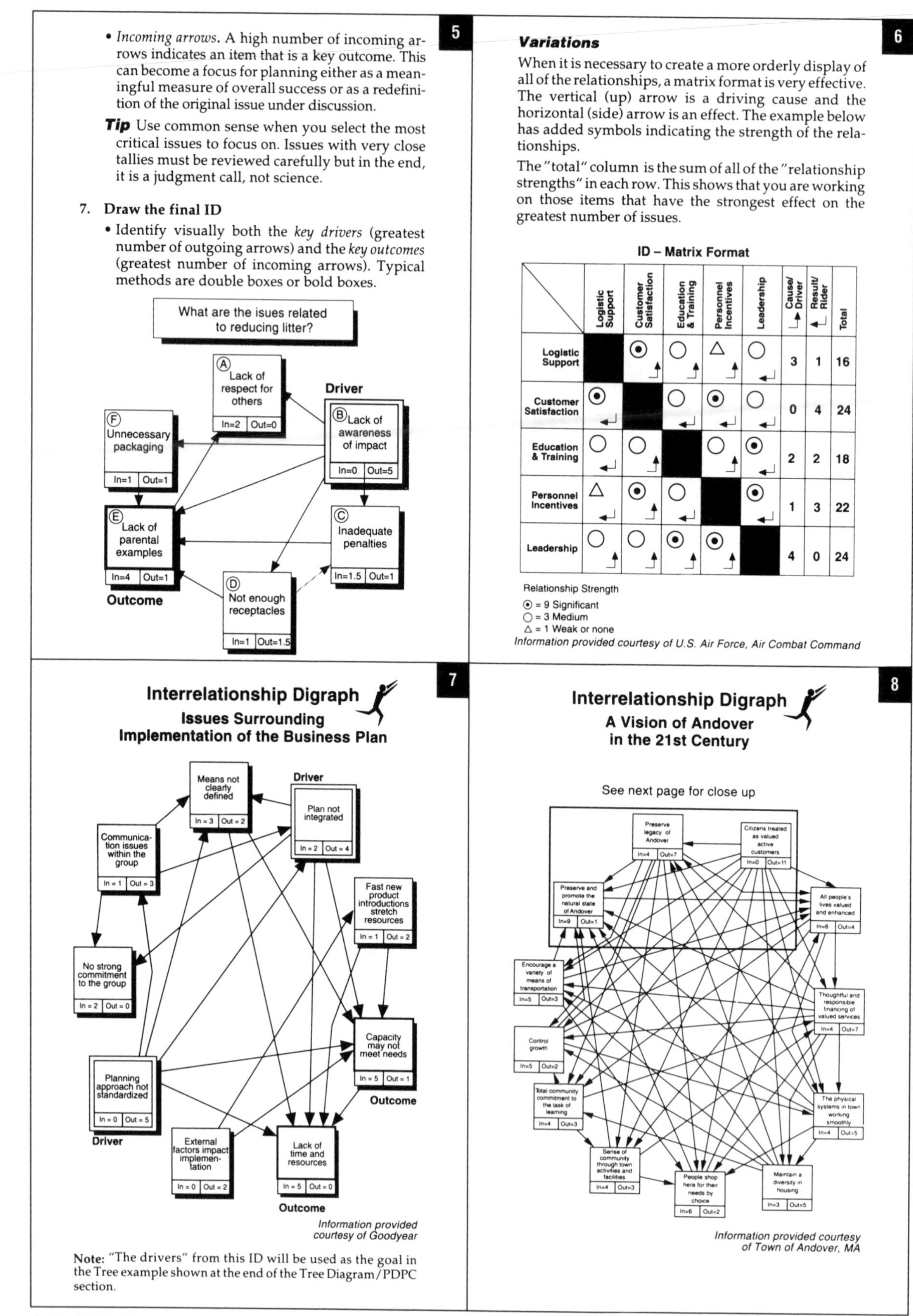

5

- *Incoming arrows.* A high number of incoming arrows indicates an item that is a key outcome. This can become a focus for planning either as a meaningful measure of overall success or as a redefinition of the original issue under discussion.

Tip Use common sense when you select the most critical issues to focus on. Issues with very close tallies must be reviewed carefully but in the end, it is a judgment call, not science.

7. **Draw the final ID**
   - Identify visually both the *key drivers* (greatest number of outgoing arrows) and the *key outcomes* (greatest number of incoming arrows). Typical methods are double boxes or bold boxes.

6

Variations

When it is necessary to create a more orderly display of all of the relationships, a matrix format is very effective. The vertical (up) arrow is a driving cause and the horizontal (side) arrow is an effect. The example below has added symbols indicating the strength of the relationships.

The "total" column is the sum of all of the "relationship strengths" in each row. This shows that you are working on those items that have the strongest effect on the greatest number of issues.

ID – Matrix Format

	Logistic Support	Customer Satisfaction	Education & Training	Personnel Incentives	Leadership	Cause/ Driver ↑	Result/ Rider ←	Total
Logistic Support	■	⊙ ↑	○ ↑	△ ↑	○ ←	3	1	16
Customer Satisfaction	⊙ ←	■	○ ←	⊙ ←	○ ←	0	4	24
Education & Training	○ ←	○ ↑	■	○ ↑	⊙ ←	2	2	18
Personnel Incentives	△ ←	⊙ ↑	○ ←	■	⊙ ←	1	3	22
Leadership	○ ↑	○ ↑	⊙ ↑	⊙ ↑	■	4	0	24

Relationship Strength
⊙ = 9 Significant
○ = 3 Medium
△ = 1 Weak or none

Information provided courtesy of U.S. Air Force, Air Combat Command

7

Interrelationship Digraph
Issues Surrounding Implementation of the Business Plan

Information provided courtesy of Goodyear

Note: "The drivers" from this ID will be used as the goal in the Tree example shown at the end of the Tree Diagram/PDPC section.

8

Interrelationship Digraph
A Vision of Andover in the 21st Century

See next page for close up

Information provided courtesy of Town of Andover, MA

9

Interrelationship Digraph

A Vision of Andover in the 21st Century

Close up

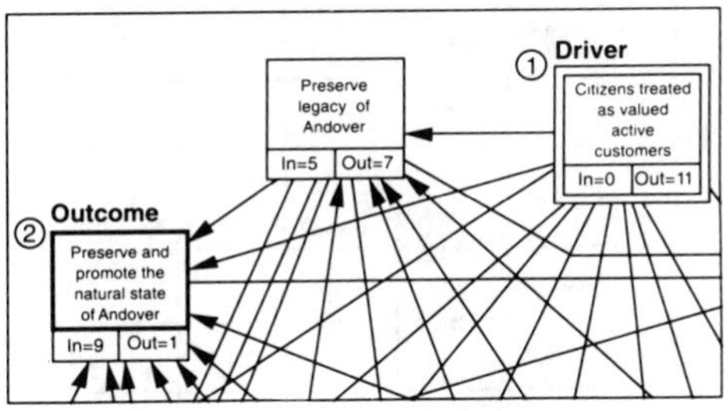

Information provided courtesy of Town of Andover, MA

① This is the driver. If the focus on the citizen as a customer becomes the core of the town's vision then everything else will be advanced.

② This is the primary outcome. It puts the preservation of nature in the town as a key indicator of the vision working.

1

Matrix Diagram
Finding relationships

Why use it?

To allow a team or individual to systematically identify, analyze, and rate the presence and strength of relationships between two or more sets of information.

What does it do?

- Makes patterns of responsibilities visible and clear so that there is an even and appropriate distribution of tasks
- Helps a team get consensus on small decisions, enhancing the quality and support for the final decision
- Improves a team's discipline in systematically taking a hard look at a large number of important decision factors

Types of Matrices

Most Common

- *L-shaped matrix*. Two sets of items directly compared to each other or a single set compared to itself.

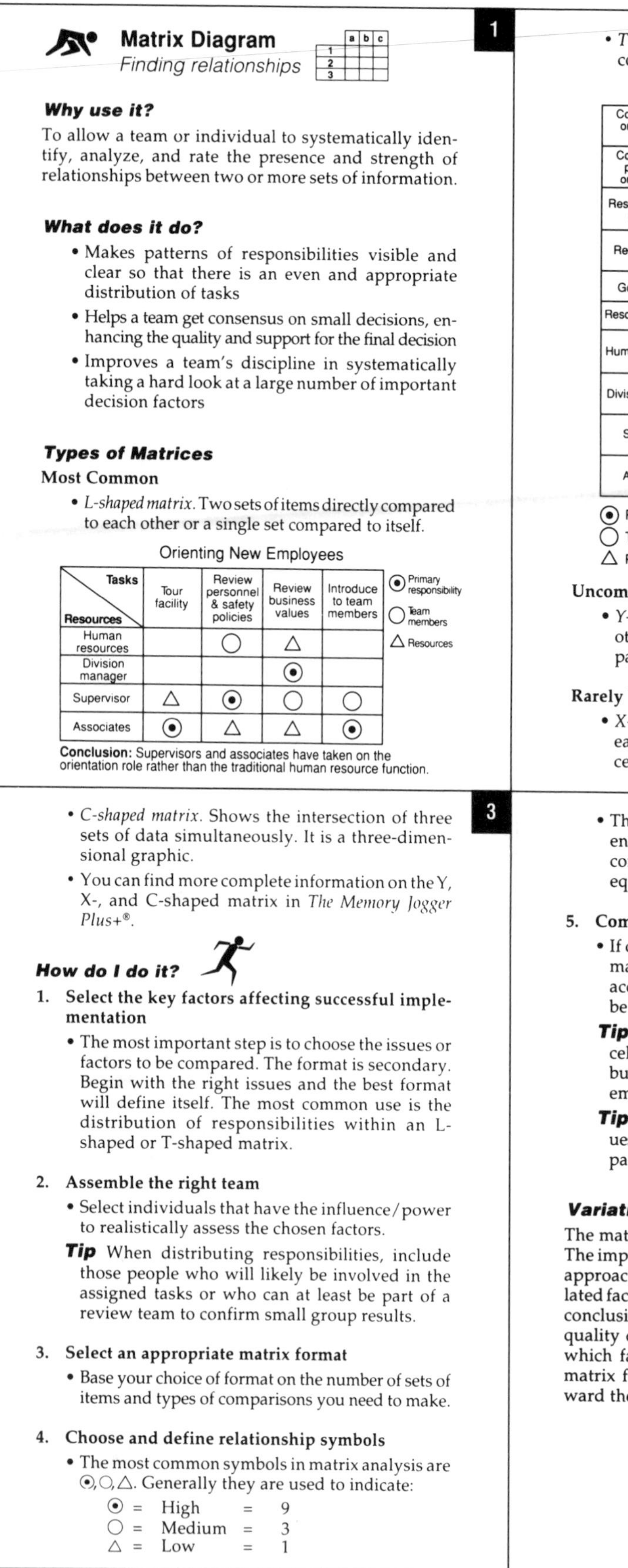

Orienting New Employees

Tasks / Resources	Tour facility	Review personnel & safety policies	Review business values	Introduce to team members
Human resources		○	△	
Division manager			⊙	
Supervisor	△	⊙	○	○
Associates	⊙	△	△	⊙

⊙ Primary responsibility
○ Team members
△ Resources

Conclusion: Supervisors and associates have taken on the orientation role rather than the traditional human resource function.

2

- *T-shaped matrix*. Two sets of items compared to a common third set.

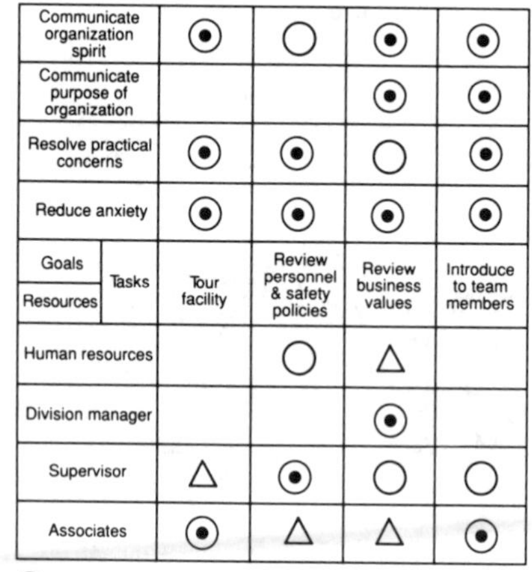

Orienting New Employees

Goals / Resources	Tour facility	Review personnel & safety policies	Review business values	Introduce to team members
Communicate organization spirit	⊙	○	⊙	⊙
Communicate purpose of organization			⊙	⊙
Resolve practical concerns	⊙	⊙	○	⊙
Reduce anxiety	⊙	⊙	⊙	⊙
Human resources		○	△	
Division manager			⊙	
Supervisor	△	⊙	○	○
Associates	⊙	△	△	⊙

⊙ Primary responsibility
○ Team members
△ Resources

Conclusion: The most important purpose of orientation is to reduce anxiety, and the most effective tasks focus on the personal issues.

Uncommon

- *Y-shaped matrix*. Three sets of items compared to each other. It "bends" a T-shaped matrix to allow comparisons between items that are on the vertical axes.

Rarely Used

- *X-shaped matrix*. Four sets of items compared to each other. It is essentially two T-shaped matrices placed back to back.

3

- *C-shaped matrix*. Shows the intersection of three sets of data simultaneously. It is a three-dimensional graphic.
- You can find more complete information on the Y, X-, and C-shaped matrix in *The Memory Jogger Plus+®*.

How do I do it?

1. **Select the key factors affecting successful implementation**
   - The most important step is to choose the issues or factors to be compared. The format is secondary. Begin with the right issues and the best format will define itself. The most common use is the distribution of responsibilities within an L-shaped or T-shaped matrix.
2. **Assemble the right team**
   - Select individuals that have the influence/power to realistically assess the chosen factors.

   Tip When distributing responsibilities, include those people who will likely be involved in the assigned tasks or who can at least be part of a review team to confirm small group results.
3. **Select an appropriate matrix format**
   - Base your choice of format on the number of sets of items and types of comparisons you need to make.
4. **Choose and define relationship symbols**
   - The most common symbols in matrix analysis are ⊙, ○, △. Generally they are used to indicate:

     ⊙ = High = 9
     ○ = Medium = 3
     △ = Low = 1

4

- The possible meanings of the symbols are almost endless. The only requirement is that the team comes to a clear understanding and creates an equally clear legend with the matrix.

5. **Complete the matrix**
   - If distributing responsibilities, use only one "primary responsibility" symbol to show ultimate accountability. All other core team members can be given secondary responsibilities.

   Tip Focus the quality of the decision in each matrix cell. Do not try to "stack the deck" by consciously building a pattern of decisions. Let these patterns emerge naturally.

   Tip Interpret the matrix using total numerical values only when it adds value. Often the visual pattern is sufficient to interpret the overall results.

Variations

The matrix is one of the most versatile tools available. The important skill to master is "matrix thinking." This approach allows a team to focus its discussion on related factors that are explored thoroughly. The separate conclusions are then brought together to create high-quality decisions. Use your creativity in determining which factors affect each other, and in choosing the matrix format that will help focus the discussion toward the ultimate decision.

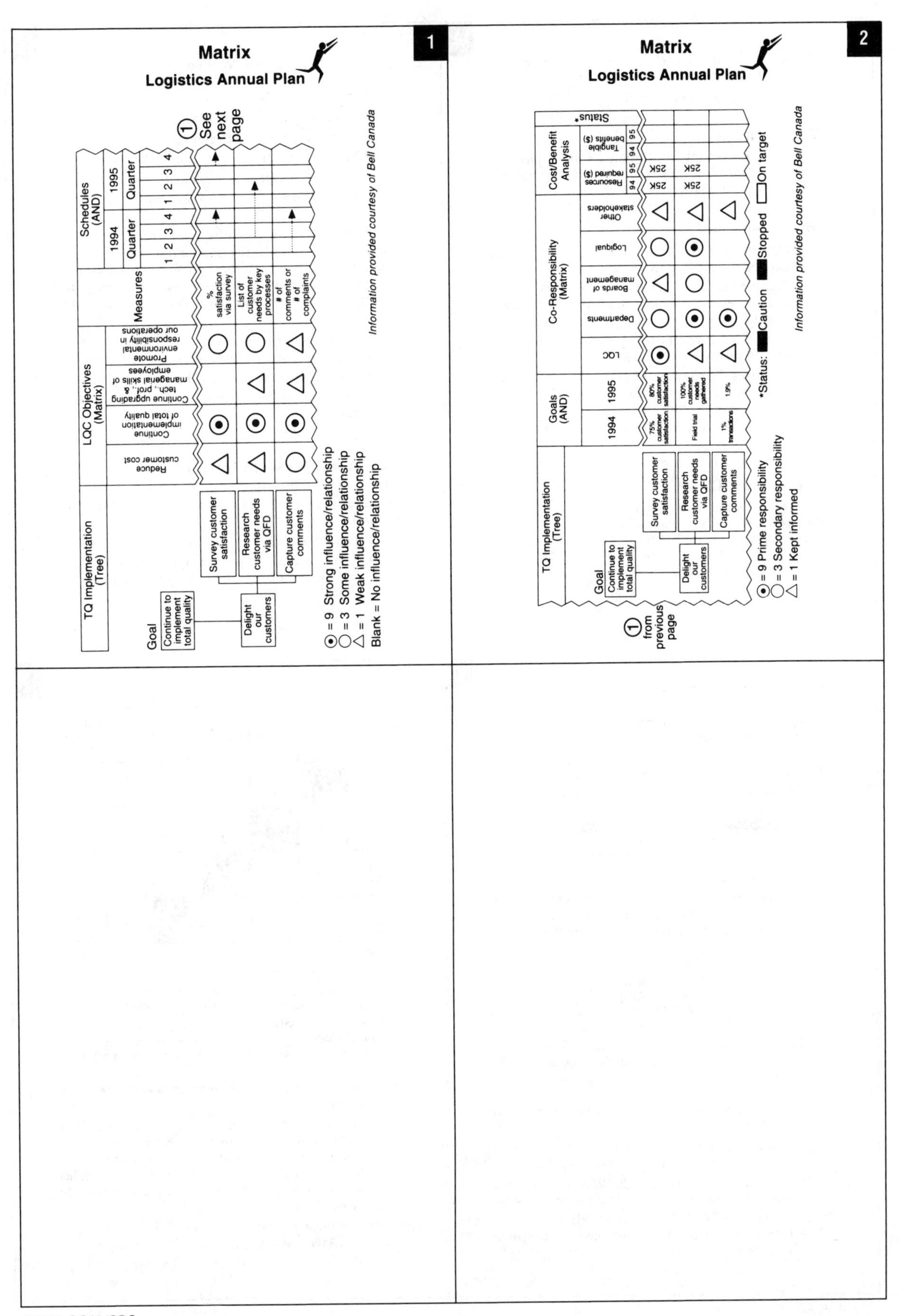
1
Matrix
Logistics Annual Plan
TQ Implementation (Tree)
LQC Objectives (Matrix)
Measures
Schedules (AND)
Goal
Continue to implement total quality
Delight our customers
Survey customer satisfaction
Research customer needs via QFD
Capture customer comments
See next page
◉ = 9 Strong influence/relationship
○ = 3 Some influence/relationship
△ = 1 Weak influence/relationship
Blank = No influence/relationship
Information provided courtesy of Bell Canada
2
Matrix
Logistics Annual Plan
TQ Implementation (Tree)
Goals (AND)
Co-Responsibility (Matrix)
Cost/Benefit Analysis
from previous page
◉ = 9 Prime responsibility
○ = 3 Secondary responsibility
△ = 1 Kept informed
*Status: Caution Stopped On target
Information provided courtesy of Bell Canada

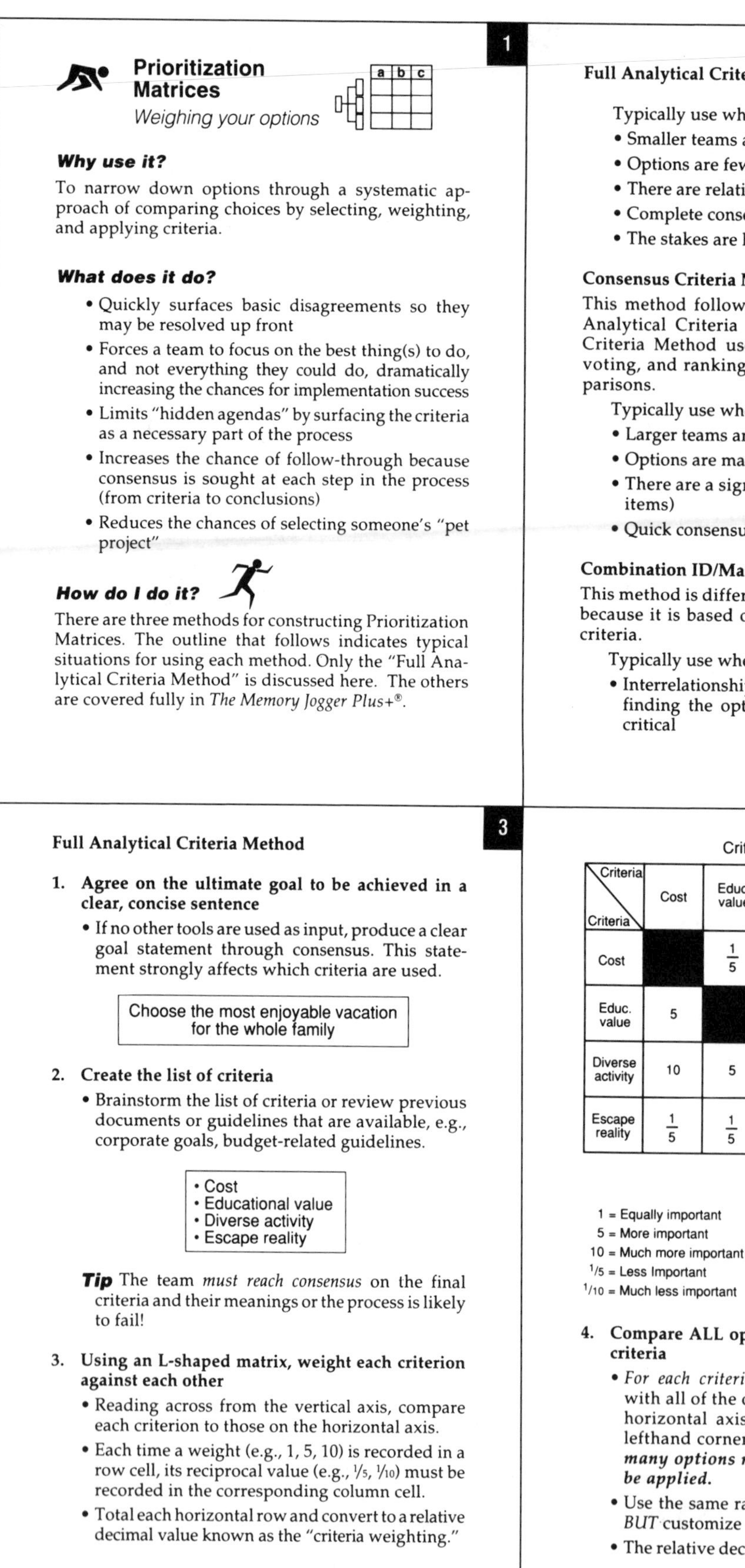

1

Prioritization Matrices

Weighing your options

Why use it?

To narrow down options through a systematic approach of comparing choices by selecting, weighting, and applying criteria.

What does it do?

- Quickly surfaces basic disagreements so they may be resolved up front
- Forces a team to focus on the best thing(s) to do, and not everything they could do, dramatically increasing the chances for implementation success
- Limits "hidden agendas" by surfacing the criteria as a necessary part of the process
- Increases the chance of follow-through because consensus is sought at each step in the process (from criteria to conclusions)
- Reduces the chances of selecting someone's "pet project"

How do I do it?

There are three methods for constructing Prioritization Matrices. The outline that follows indicates typical situations for using each method. Only the "Full Analytical Criteria Method" is discussed here. The others are covered fully in *The Memory Jogger Plus+®*.

2

Full Analytical Criteria Method

Typically use when:

- Smaller teams are involved (3–8 people)
- Options are few (5–10 choices)
- There are relatively few criteria (3–6 items)
- Complete consensus is needed
- The stakes are high if the plan fails

Consensus Criteria Method

This method follows the same steps as in the Full Analytical Criteria Method except the Consensus Criteria Method uses a combination of weighted voting, and ranking is used instead of paired comparisons.

Typically use when:

- Larger teams are involved (8 or more people)
- Options are many (10–20 choices)
- There are a significant number of criteria (6–15 items)
- Quick consensus is needed to proceed

Combination ID/Matrix Method

This method is different from the other two methods because it is based on cause and effect, rather than criteria.

Typically use when:

- Interrelationships among options are high and finding the option with the greatest impact is critical

3

Full Analytical Criteria Method

1. Agree on the ultimate goal to be achieved in a clear, concise sentence

- If no other tools are used as input, produce a clear goal statement through consensus. This statement strongly affects which criteria are used.

> Choose the most enjoyable vacation for the whole family

2. Create the list of criteria

- Brainstorm the list of criteria or review previous documents or guidelines that are available, e.g., corporate goals, budget-related guidelines.

> • Cost
> • Educational value
> • Diverse activity
> • Escape reality

Tip The team *must reach consensus* on the final criteria and their meanings or the process is likely to fail!

3. Using an L-shaped matrix, weight each criterion against each other

- Reading across from the vertical axis, compare each criterion to those on the horizontal axis.
- Each time a weight (e.g., 1, 5, 10) is recorded in a row cell, its reciprocal value (e.g., 1/5, 1/10) must be recorded in the corresponding column cell.
- Total each horizontal row and convert to a relative decimal value known as the "criteria weighting."

4

Criterion vs. Criterion

Criteria \ Criteria	Cost	Educ. value	Diverse activity	Escape reality	Row Total	Relative Decimal Value
Cost		1/5	1/10	5	5.3	.15
Educ. value	5		1/5	5	10.2	.28
Diverse activity	10	5		5	20	.55
Escape reality	1/5	1/5	1/5		.60	.02
				Grand Total	36.1	

1 = Equally important
5 = More important
10 = Much more important
1/5 = Less Important
1/10 = Much less important

Row Total
Rating scores added
Grand Total
Row totals added
Relative Decimal Value
Each row total ÷ by the grand total

4. Compare ALL options relative to each weighted criteria

- *For each criterion,* create an L-shaped matrix with all of the options on both the vertical and horizontal axis and the criteria listed in the lefthand corner of the matrix. ***There will be as many options matrices as there are criteria to be applied.***
- Use the same rating scale (1, 5, 10) as in Step 3, *BUT* customize the wording for each criterion.
- The relative decimal value is the "option rating."

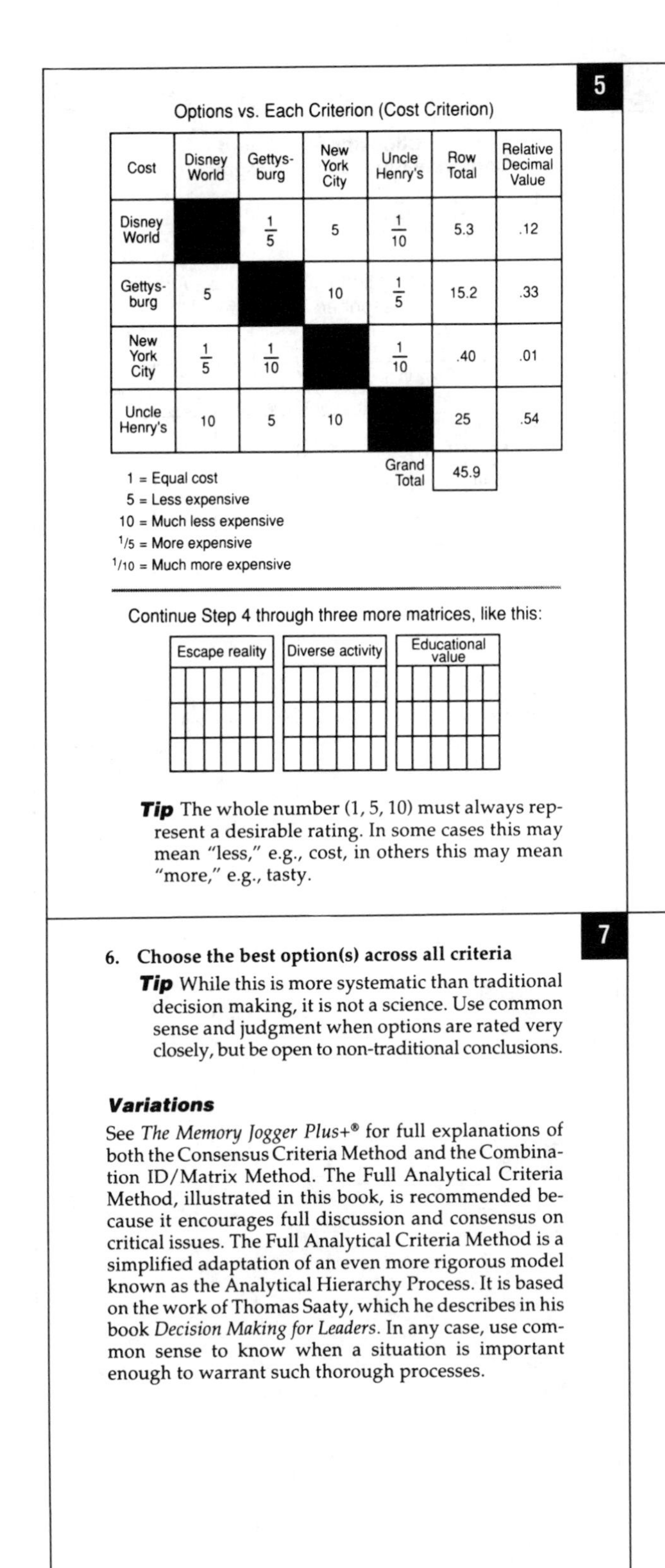

5

Options vs. Each Criterion (Cost Criterion)

Cost	Disney World	Gettys-burg	New York City	Uncle Henry's	Row Total	Relative Decimal Value
Disney World		1/5	5	1/10	5.3	.12
Gettys-burg	5		10	1/5	15.2	.33
New York City	1/5	1/10		1/10	.40	.01
Uncle Henry's	10	5	10		25	.54
				Grand Total	45.9	

1 = Equal cost
5 = Less expensive
10 = Much less expensive
1/5 = More expensive
1/10 = Much more expensive

Continue Step 4 through three more matrices, like this:

Tip The whole number (1, 5, 10) must always represent a desirable rating. In some cases this may mean "less," e.g., cost, in others this may mean "more," e.g., tasty.

6

5. Using an L-shaped summary matrix, compare each option based on all criteria combined

- List all criteria on the horizontal axis and all options on the vertical axis.
- In each matrix cell multiply the "criteria weighting" of each criterion (decimal value from Step 3) by the "option rating" (decimal value from Step 4). This creates an "option score."
- Add each option score across all criteria for a row total. Divide each row total by the grand total and convert to the final decimal value. Compare these decimal values to help you decide which option to pursue.

Summary Matrix
Options vs. All Criteria

Criteria / Options	Cost (.15)	Educa-tional value (.28)	Diverse activity (.55)	Escape reality (.02)	Row Total	Relative Decimal Value
Disney World	.12 x .15 (.02)	.24 x .28 (.07)	.40 x .55 (.22)	.65 x .02 (.01)	.32	.32
Gettys-burg	.33 x .15 (.05)	.37 x .28 (.10)	.10 x .55 (.06)	.22 x .02 (0)	.22	.22
New York City	.01 x .15 (0)	.37 x .28 (.10)	.49 x .55 (.27)	.12 x .02 (.01)	.38	.38
Uncle Henry's	.55 x .15 (.08)	.01 x .28 (0)	.01 x .55 (.01)	.01 x .02 (0)	.09	.09
				Grand Total	1.01	

7

6. Choose the best option(s) across all criteria

Tip While this is more systematic than traditional decision making, it is not a science. Use common sense and judgment when options are rated very closely, but be open to non-traditional conclusions.

Variations

See *The Memory Jogger Plus+®* for full explanations of both the Consensus Criteria Method and the Combination ID/Matrix Method. The Full Analytical Criteria Method, illustrated in this book, is recommended because it encourages full discussion and consensus on critical issues. The Full Analytical Criteria Method is a simplified adaptation of an even more rigorous model known as the Analytical Hierarchy Process. It is based on the work of Thomas Saaty, which he describes in his book *Decision Making for Leaders*. In any case, use common sense to know when a situation is important enough to warrant such thorough processes.

8

Prioritization

Choosing a Standard Corporate Spreadsheet Program

① Weighting criteria (described in Step 3)

This is a portion of a full matrix with 14 criteria in total.

Criteria	Best use of hardware	Ease of use	Maximum functionality	Best performance	Total (14 criteria)	Relative Decimal Value
Best use of hardware		.20	.10	.20	3.7	.01
Ease of use	5.0		.20	.20	35.4	.08
Maximum functionality	10.0	5.0		5.0	69.0	.17
Best performance	5.0	5.0	.20		45.2	.11
				Grand Total (14 criteria)	418.1	

Information provided courtesy of Novacor Chemicals

Note: This constructed example, illustrated on three pages, represents only a portion of the prioritization process and only a portion of Novacor's spreadsheet evaluation process. Novacor Chemicals assembled a 16-person team, comprised mainly of system users and some information systems staff. The team developed and weighted 14 standard criteria and then applied them to choices in word processing, spreadsheet, and presentation graphics programs.

This example continued next page

9

Prioritization

Choosing a Standard Corporate Spreadsheet Program (cont.)

② Comparing options (described in Step 4)

These are just 2 of 14 matrices.

Best integration –internal	Program A	Program B	Program C	Total	Relative Decimal Value
Program A		1.00	1.00	2.00	.33
Program B	1.00		1.00	2.00	.33
Program C	1.00	1.00		2.00	.33
			Grand Total	6.00	

Lowest ongoing cost	Program A	Program B	Program C	Total	Relative Decimal Value
Program A		.10	.20	.30	.02
Program B	10.00		5.00	15.00	.73
Program C	5.00	.20		5.20	.25
			Grand Total	20.50	

Information provided courtesy of Novacor Chemicals

This example continued next page

10

Prioritization

Choosing a Standard Corporate Spreadsheet Program (cont.)

③ Summarize Option Ratings Across All Criteria (described in Step 5)

This is a portion of a full matrix with 14 criteria in total.

Criteria / Options	Easy to use (.08)	Best integration int. (.09)	Lowest ongoing cost (.08)	Total (across 14 criteria)	Relative Decimal Value
Program A	.03 (.01)	.33 (.03)	.02 (0)	.16	.18
Program B	.48 (.04)	.33 (.03)	.73 (.06)	.30	.33
Program C	.48 (.04)	.33 (.03)	.25 (.02)	.44	.49
			Grand Total	.90	

Information provided courtesy of Novacor Chemicals

Result: Program C was chosen. Even though 14 out of the 16 team members were not currently using this program, the prioritization process changed their minds, and prevented them from biasing the final decision.

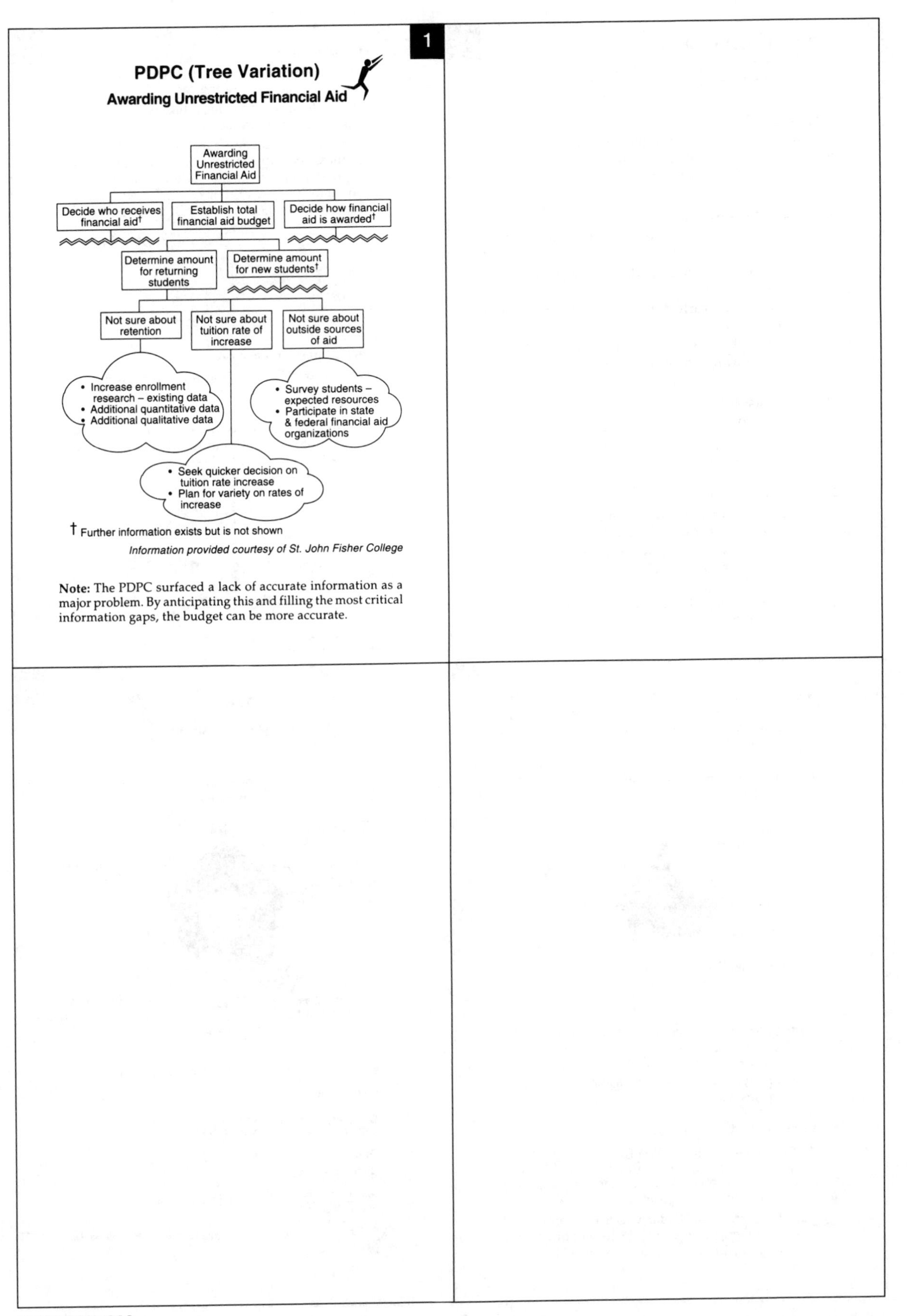

Note: The PDPC surfaced a lack of accurate information as a major problem. By anticipating this and filling the most critical information gaps, the budget can be more accurate.

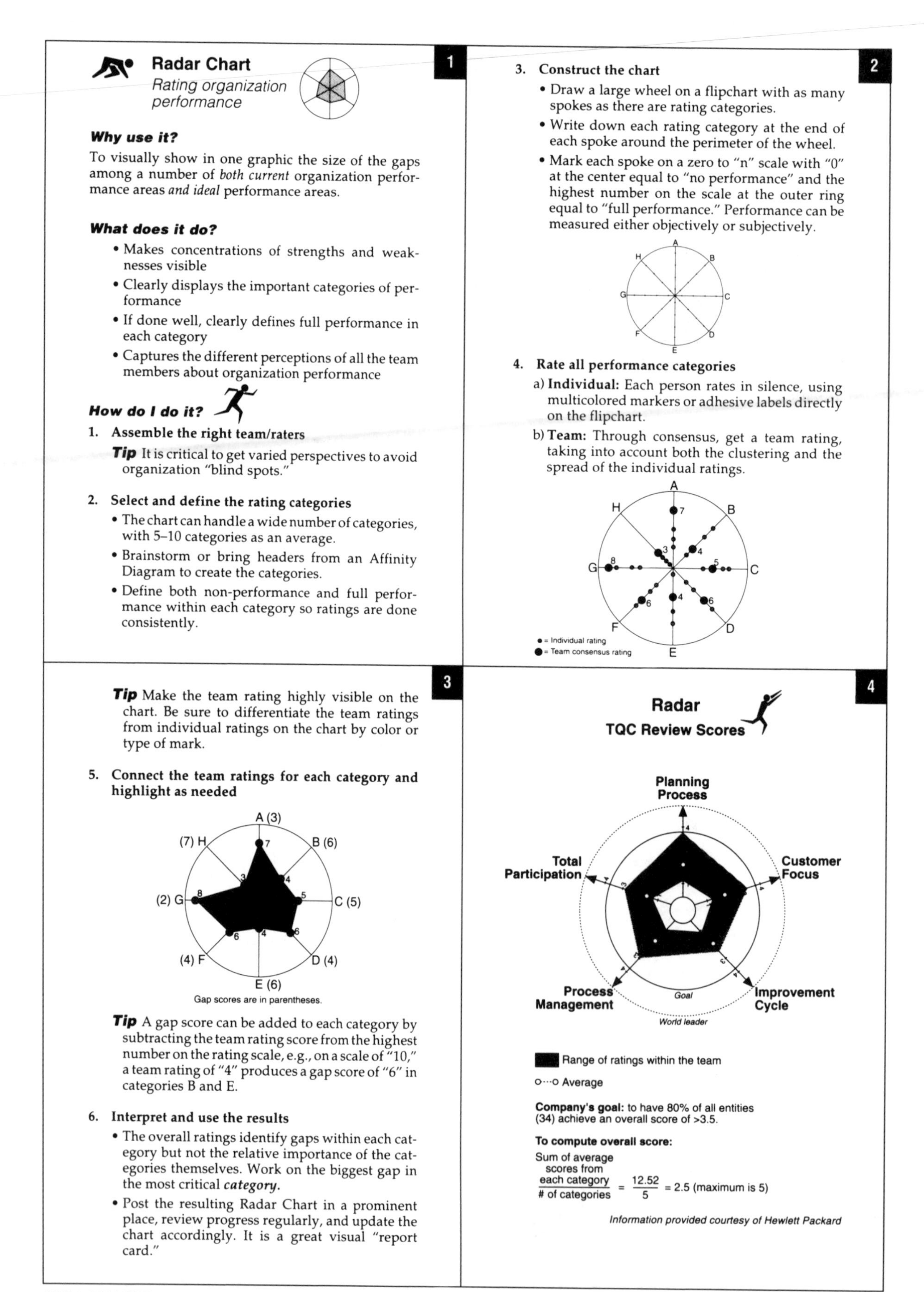

Radar Chart

Rating organization performance

Why use it?

To visually show in one graphic the size of the gaps among a number of *both current* organization performance areas *and ideal* performance areas.

What does it do?

- Makes concentrations of strengths and weaknesses visible
- Clearly displays the important categories of performance
- If done well, clearly defines full performance in each category
- Captures the different perceptions of all the team members about organization performance

How do I do it?

1. **Assemble the right team/raters**

   Tip It is critical to get varied perspectives to avoid organization "blind spots."

2. **Select and define the rating categories**
   - The chart can handle a wide number of categories, with 5–10 categories as an average.
   - Brainstorm or bring headers from an Affinity Diagram to create the categories.
   - Define both non-performance and full performance within each category so ratings are done consistently.

3. **Construct the chart**
   - Draw a large wheel on a flipchart with as many spokes as there are rating categories.
   - Write down each rating category at the end of each spoke around the perimeter of the wheel.
   - Mark each spoke on a zero to "n" scale with "0" at the center equal to "no performance" and the highest number on the scale at the outer ring equal to "full performance." Performance can be measured either objectively or subjectively.

4. **Rate all performance categories**

   a) **Individual:** Each person rates in silence, using multicolored markers or adhesive labels directly on the flipchart.

   b) **Team:** Through consensus, get a team rating, taking into account both the clustering and the spread of the individual ratings.

Tip Make the team rating highly visible on the chart. Be sure to differentiate the team ratings from individual ratings on the chart by color or type of mark.

5. **Connect the team ratings for each category and highlight as needed**

Gap scores are in parentheses.

Tip A gap score can be added to each category by subtracting the team rating score from the highest number on the rating scale, e.g., on a scale of "10," a team rating of "4" produces a gap score of "6" in categories B and E.

6. **Interpret and use the results**
   - The overall ratings identify gaps within each category but not the relative importance of the categories themselves. Work on the biggest gap in the most critical *category*.
   - Post the resulting Radar Chart in a prominent place, review progress regularly, and update the chart accordingly. It is a great visual "report card."

Radar
TQC Review Scores

Company's goal: to have 80% of all entities (34) achieve an overall score of >3.5.

To compute overall score:

$$\frac{\text{Sum of average scores from each category}}{\text{\# of categories}} = \frac{12.52}{5} = 2.5 \text{ (maximum is 5)}$$

Information provided courtesy of Hewlett Packard

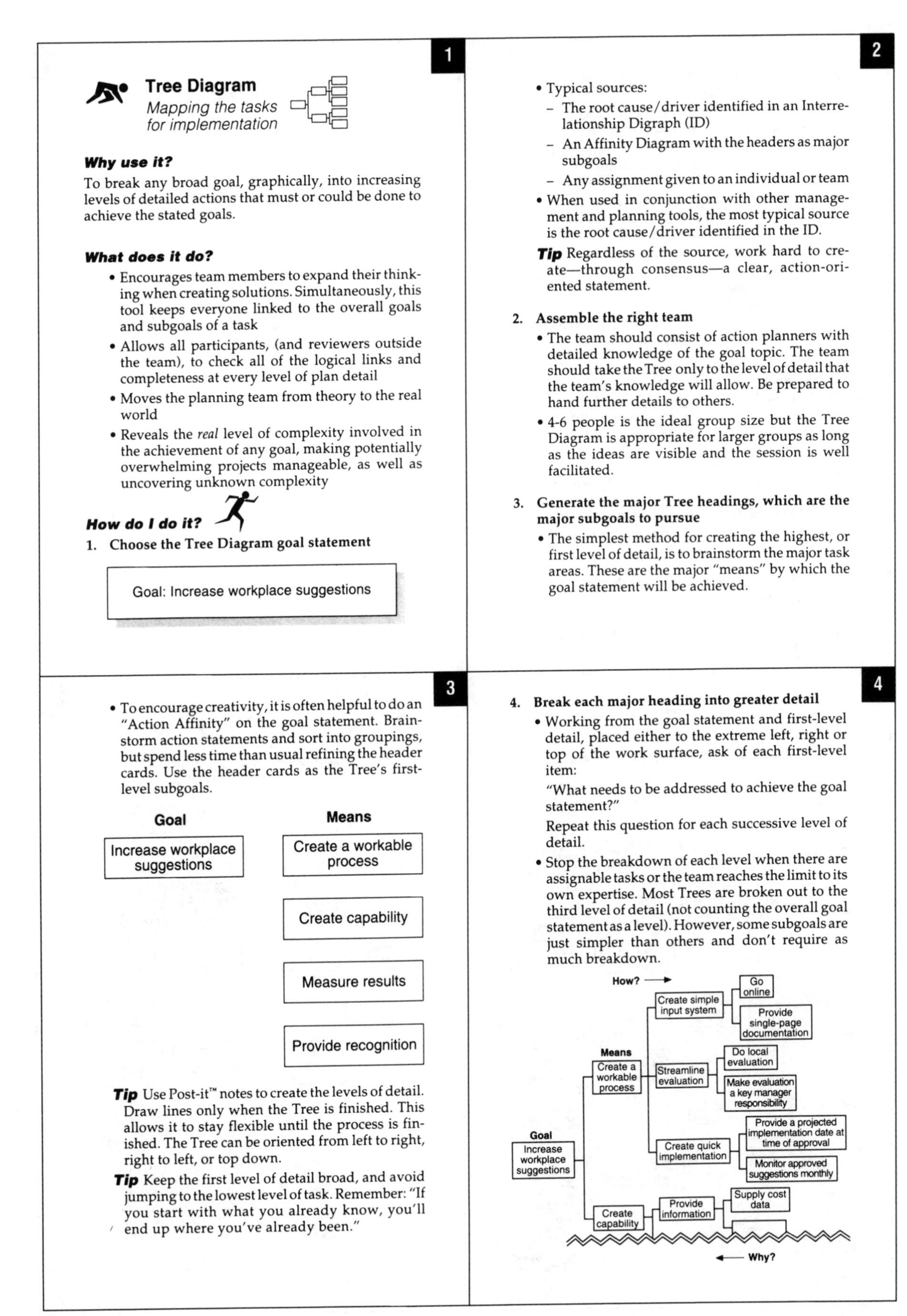

1

Tree Diagram

Mapping the tasks for implementation

Why use it?

To break any broad goal, graphically, into increasing levels of detailed actions that must or could be done to achieve the stated goals.

What does it do?

- Encourages team members to expand their thinking when creating solutions. Simultaneously, this tool keeps everyone linked to the overall goals and subgoals of a task
- Allows all participants, (and reviewers outside the team), to check all of the logical links and completeness at every level of plan detail
- Moves the planning team from theory to the real world
- Reveals the *real* level of complexity involved in the achievement of any goal, making potentially overwhelming projects manageable, as well as uncovering unknown complexity

How do I do it?

1. **Choose the Tree Diagram goal statement**

2

- Typical sources:
  - The root cause/driver identified in an Interrelationship Digraph (ID)
  - An Affinity Diagram with the headers as major subgoals
  - Any assignment given to an individual or team
- When used in conjunction with other management and planning tools, the most typical source is the root cause/driver identified in the ID.

Tip Regardless of the source, work hard to create—through consensus—a clear, action-oriented statement.

2. **Assemble the right team**
   - The team should consist of action planners with detailed knowledge of the goal topic. The team should take the Tree only to the level of detail that the team's knowledge will allow. Be prepared to hand further details to others.
   - 4-6 people is the ideal group size but the Tree Diagram is appropriate for larger groups as long as the ideas are visible and the session is well facilitated.

3. **Generate the major Tree headings, which are the major subgoals to pursue**
   - The simplest method for creating the highest, or first level of detail, is to brainstorm the major task areas. These are the major "means" by which the goal statement will be achieved.

3

- To encourage creativity, it is often helpful to do an "Action Affinity" on the goal statement. Brainstorm action statements and sort into groupings, but spend less time than usual refining the header cards. Use the header cards as the Tree's first-level subgoals.

Tip Use Post-it™ notes to create the levels of detail. Draw lines only when the Tree is finished. This allows it to stay flexible until the process is finished. The Tree can be oriented from left to right, right to left, or top down.

Tip Keep the first level of detail broad, and avoid jumping to the lowest level of task. Remember: "If you start with what you already know, you'll end up where you've already been."

4

4. **Break each major heading into greater detail**
   - Working from the goal statement and first-level detail, placed either to the extreme left, right or top of the work surface, ask of each first-level item:

     "What needs to be addressed to achieve the goal statement?"

     Repeat this question for each successive level of detail.
   - Stop the breakdown of each level when there are assignable tasks or the team reaches the limit to its own expertise. Most Trees are broken out to the third level of detail (not counting the overall goal statement as a level). However, some subgoals are just simpler than others and don't require as much breakdown.

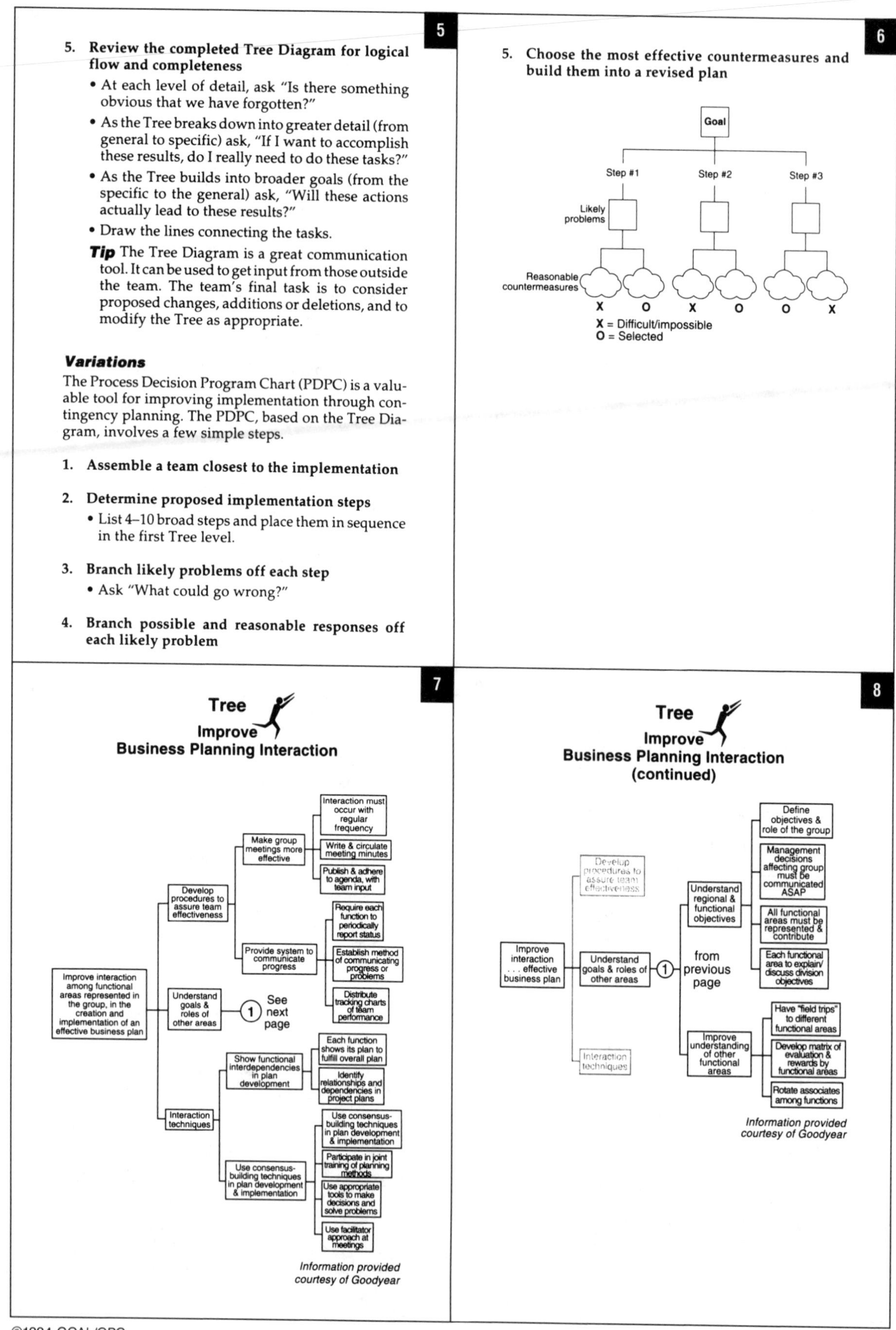

5

5. Review the completed Tree Diagram for logical flow and completeness

- At each level of detail, ask "Is there something obvious that we have forgotten?"
- As the Tree breaks down into greater detail (from general to specific) ask, "If I want to accomplish these results, do I really need to do these tasks?"
- As the Tree builds into broader goals (from the specific to the general) ask, "Will these actions actually lead to these results?"
- Draw the lines connecting the tasks.

Tip The Tree Diagram is a great communication tool. It can be used to get input from those outside the team. The team's final task is to consider proposed changes, additions or deletions, and to modify the Tree as appropriate.

Variations

The Process Decision Program Chart (PDPC) is a valuable tool for improving implementation through contingency planning. The PDPC, based on the Tree Diagram, involves a few simple steps.

1. Assemble a team closest to the implementation

2. Determine proposed implementation steps

- List 4–10 broad steps and place them in sequence in the first Tree level.

3. Branch likely problems off each step

- Ask "What could go wrong?"

4. Branch possible and reasonable responses off each likely problem

6

5. Choose the most effective countermeasures and build them into a revised plan

7

Tree
Improve Business Planning Interaction

Information provided courtesy of Goodyear

8

Tree
Improve Business Planning Interaction (continued)

Information provided courtesy of Goodyear

APPENDIX C

Sample Hoshin Plans (Excerpts)

This appendix contains samples of three hoshin plans. These excerpts have been provided by Fletcher Allen Health Care and The Miriam Hospital and include target/means matrixes; a diagram of annual objectives, targets, and means; and a hospital-wide summary means and objectives matrix.

Target/Means Matrixes

Level 1 (President)
Target: Align medical manpower

Activity	President	Chief Medical Officer	Director of Clinical Systems	VP Planning	1993 Q1	1993 Q2	1993 Q3	1993 Q4
1. Approve policy through VMC board	⊙			▲	—			
2. Open window to transition		⊙	●			—	—	—
3. Charter manpower plan		⊙					—	
4. Complete plan			●	⊙				—

Level 2 (VP Planning)
Target: Manpower plan completed

Activity	VP Planning	Director of Development Market	Director of Clinical Systems	Director of VMC	1993 Q1	1993 Q2	1993 Q3	1993 Q4
1. Inventory physicians	⊙	●			—			
2. Calculate population base	⊙	●				—		
3. Research planning ratios	⊙	●	▲			—	—	
4. Calculate requirements	⊙	●	▲	▲				—

Level 3 (Director of VMC)
Target: Regulate Panel Size

Activity	Director of VMC	Clinical Chiefs	Director of Clinical Systems	1994 Q1	1994 Q2	1994 Q3	1994 Q4
1. Manpower plan communicated	⊙	▲	▲	—			
2. Recruitment plans adjusted		⊙		—	—		
3. Board training and development	●		⊙		—		
4. Appeals strategy developed	⊙	▲	●			—	

Level 4 (Director of Clinical Systems)
Target: Ratio of needed to actual in balance

Activity	Director of Clinical Systems	Director of VMC	VMC Board	VP Planning	1994 Q1	1994 Q2	1994 Q3	1994 Q4
1. Application process developed	⊙	●			—			
2. Board decisions re: applications			⊙	▲		—		
3. Appeals considered			⊙	▲		—	—	—
4. Inventory updated	▲	▲	▲	⊙		—	—	—

⊙ Primary responsibility ● Secondary responsibility ▲ Needs to know

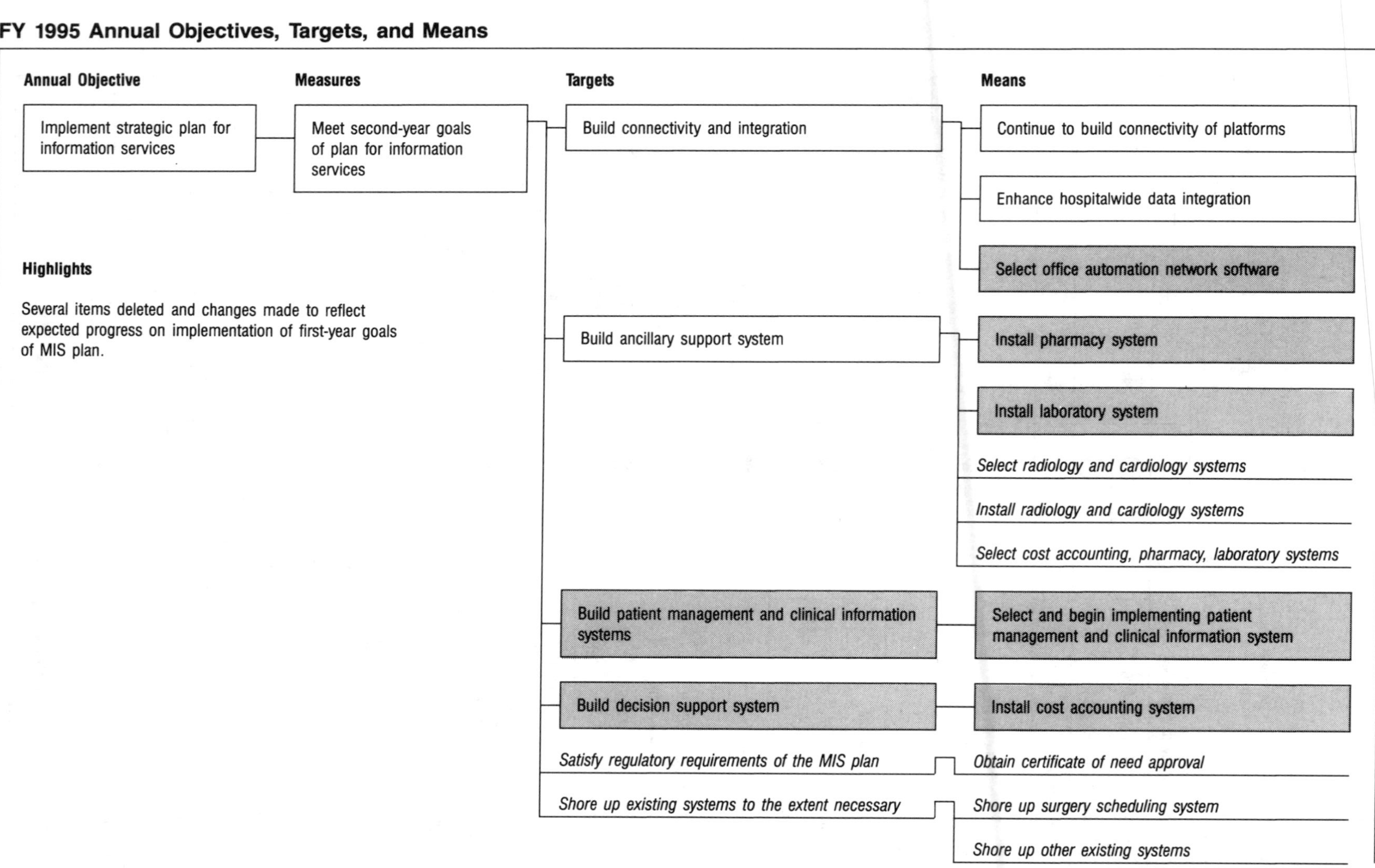
FY 1995 Annual Objectives, Targets, and Means
Annual Objective
Measures
Targets
Means
Implement strategic plan for information services
Meet second-year goals of plan for information services
Build connectivity and integration
Continue to build connectivity of platforms
Enhance hospitalwide data integration
Select office automation network software
Highlights
Several items deleted and changes made to reflect expected progress on implementation of first-year goals of MIS plan.
Build ancillary support system
Install pharmacy system
Install laboratory system
Select radiology and cardiology systems
Install radiology and cardiology systems
Select cost accounting, pharmacy, laboratory systems
Build patient management and clinical information systems
Select and begin implementing patient management and clinical information system
Build decision support system
Install cost accounting system
Satisfy regulatory requirements of the MIS plan
Obtain certificate of need approval
Shore up existing systems to the extent necessary
Shore up surgery scheduling system
Shore up other existing systems

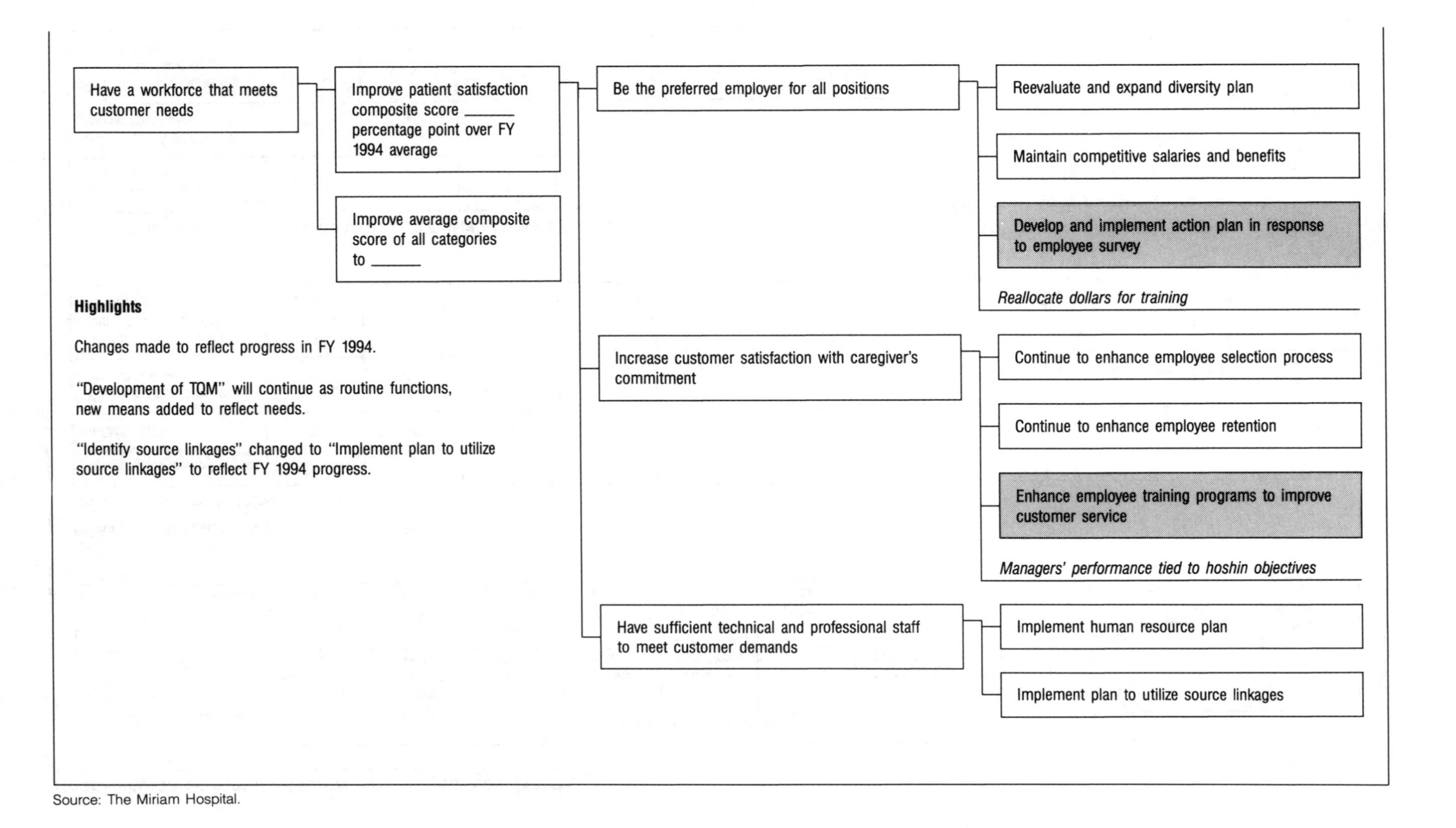

Source: The Miriam Hospital.

Hospitalwide Summary Means and Objectives Matrix

Annual Objective:	Limit Incr. in Cost/Adj. Dis.	Particip. Mgd Care Vent.	Improve Quality Meas.	Finalize Brown Agrmt.	Svs. & Cap. Meet Needs	MDs See TMH as Partner	Inf. Services Strat. Plan	Workforce Meets Needs	Count of Relationship Types			Admin. Resp.		Means Completion Date
Measure:	No Incr. in Cost/Adj. Dis.	Addtl Mgd Care Lives	Impr. Identified Qual. Meas.	3 Centers of Excel.	Impr. Inpt. Satisf.	Improve MD Satisf.	MIS Strat. Plan	Impr. Inpt. & Empl. Satisf.	X	O	—	Prim.	Sec.	

(Columns "Limit Incr. in Cost/Adj. Dis." through "Workforce Meets Needs": Annual Objectives & Measures)

OBJECTIVE: LIMIT INCREASE IN COST/ADJUSTED DISCHARGE

Target: Have Cost Accounting System with Cost/Case by Payor

Means	Limit Incr. in Cost/Adj. Dis.	Particip. Mgd Care Vent.	Improve Quality Meas.	Finalize Brown Agrmt.	Svs. & Cap. Meet Needs	MDs See TMH as Partner	Inf. Services Strat. Plan	Workforce Meets Needs	X	O	—	Prim.	Sec.	Means Completion Date
Obtain Cost/Case by Payor from Curr. System (CQMS, SMS)	X	X	—	—	O	X	—	—	3	1	4	SC	ES	Sep 94
Review & Utilize Insurance Plan Capabilities	O	X	—	—	O	O	—	—	1	3	4	SC	ES	Jan 94
Develop Plan to Provide Comp. Cost Accounting Information	X	X	—	—	X	X	X	—	5	0	3	SC	ES	May 94

Target: Allow No Increase in Supply Costs/Adjusted Discharge (Case Mix Adjusted) from FY 1993

Means	Limit Incr. in Cost/Adj. Dis.	Particip. Mgd Care Vent.	Improve Quality Meas.	Finalize Brown Agrmt.	Svs. & Cap. Meet Needs	MDs See TMH as Partner	Inf. Services Strat. Plan	Workforce Meets Needs	X	O	—	Prim.	Sec.	Means Completion Date
Apply Value Analysis to All New Purchases	X	X	0	—	X	0	0	0	3	4	1	RB	JM CM	Jan 94
Develop L/T Action Plan for Further Cost Savings	X	X	0	—	X	0	0	0	3	4	1	ES	SC CM	Oct 93
Prep. Budgets w/No Incr. in Supply Cost/Case (Case Mix Adj.)	X	X	0	—	X	0	0	0	3	4	1	SC	ALL	Oct 93

Target: Have Lowest Price for Selected Product Lines (CVD, Orthopedics, Oncology)

Make Orthopedics Profitable	X	X	X	—	X	X	—	X	6	0	2	RB	JM CM	Sep 94
Realign Charge Structure	—	X	—	—	—	X	—	0	2	1	5	SC	—	Sep 94
Achieve Overall LOS below FY 1993	X	X	X	—	X	X	0	X	6	1	1	JM	ES CM	Sep 94
Dev. & Impl. Action Plan for Crit. Path Var (High Vol/Cost DRGs)	X	X	X	—	X	X	0	X	6	1	1	JM	ES CM	Mar 94
Identify Nonessential, Nonprofitable Services	X	X	—	—	X	0	—	—	3	1	4	SC	JL CM	Sep 94

Target: Reduce FTEs/Adjusted Occupied Bed (Excluding Research) from FY 1993 Levels

Apply Updated Prod. Stds. in All Appropriate Departments	X	X	X	—	X	0	0	X	5	2	1	ES	SC	Sep 94
Utilize QI Process @ All Levels	X	X	X	—	X	0	—	X	5	1	2	ALL	—	Sep 94
Implement Improved Staffing Flexibility Plan	0	0	—	—	X	0	—	X	2	3	3	DB	ALL	Jun 94

Source: The Miriam Hospital.

Resources for Additional Information

Akao, Y., ed. *Hoshin Kanri: Policy Deployment for Successful TQM.* Cambridge, MA: Productivity Press, 1991.

AT&T Quality Steering Committee. *Policy Deployment: Setting the Direction for Change.* Indianapolis: AT&T Customer Information Center, 1992, Select Code 500-453.

Barker, J. *Discovering the Future: The Business of Paradigms.* St. Paul, MN: I.L.I. Press, 1985.

Block, P. *Stewardship: Choosing Service Over Self-Interest.* San Francisco: Berrett-Koehler Publishers, 1993.

Brassard, M. *Memory Jogger Plus+™.* Methuen, MA: GOAL/QPC, 1989.

Colletti, J. *Hoshin Kanri.* GOAL/QPC course notebook. Methuen, MA: GOAL/QPC, 1994.

Collins, B., and Huge, E. *Management by Policy: How Companies Focus Their Total Quality Efforts to Achieve Competitive Advantage.* Milwaukee, WI: ASQC Quality Press, 1993.

Covey, S. *The Seven Habits of Highly Effective People®.* New York City: Simon & Schuster, 1989.

Demers, D. Tutorial: Implementing hoshin planning at the Vermont Academic Medical Center. *Quality Management in Health Care* 1(4):64–72, Summer 1993.

Deming, W. E. *Out of the Crisis.* Cambridge, MA: MIT Center for Advanced Engineering Study, 1986.

Drucker, P. *The Effective Executive.* New York City: Harper Colophon, 1967.

Durbin, S., Haglund, C., and Dowling, W. Integrating strategic planning and quality management in a multi-institutional system. *Quality Management in Health Care* 1(4):24–34, Summer 1993.

Ernst & Young Quality Improvement Consulting Group. *Total Quality: An Executive's Guide for the 1990s.* Homewood, IL: Dow Jones-Irwin, 1990.

GOAL/QPC. *The Memory Jogger.* Methuen, MA: GOAL/QPC, 1988.

GOAL/QPC Research Committee. *Cross-Functional Management.* Methuen, MA, GOAL/QPC, 1991.

GOAL/QPC Research Committee. *Hoshin Planning: A Planning System for Implementing Total Quality Management (TQM).* Research Report No. 89-10-03. Methuen, MA: GOAL/QPC, 1989.

GOAL/QPC Research Committee. *Integrated Planning Model.* Research Report No. 92-01R. Methuen, MA: GOAL/QPC, 1992.

Hamel and Prahalad. Core competence of the corporation. *Harvard Business Review,* Nov.–Dec. 1990, pp. 111–19.

Hamel and Prahalad. Strategic intent. *Harvard Business Review,* May–June 1990, pp. 63–76.

Hayden, G. TQC starts with policy deployment. *TQC World* [Texas Instruments], June 1989, pp. 12–13.

Health Care Advisory Board. *Total Quality Management.* Vol. 2. *TQM-14 Tactics for Improving the Quality Process.* Washington, DC: The Advisory Board, 1992.

Henderson, B. *Henderson on Corporate Strategy.* Cambridge, MA: Abt Books, 1979.

Ishikawa, K. *What Is Total Quality Control? The Japanese Way.* Englewood Cliffs, NJ: Prentice Hall, 1985.

Juran, J. M. *Juran on Leadership for Quality.* New York City: Free Press, 1992.

Juran, J. *Managerial Breakthrough: A New Concept of the Manager's Job.* New York City: McGraw-Hill Book Co., 1964.

Kano, N. A perspective on quality activities in American firms. *California Management Review,* Spring 1993, pp. 12–31.

Kanter, R. M. *The Change Masters: Innovation for Productivity in the American Corporation.* New York City: Simon & Schuster, 1983.

King, B. *Hoshin Planning: The Developmental Approach.* Methuen, MA: GOAL/QPC, 1989.

Melum, M. M. *CAPD: Check-Analyze-Plan-Do Quick Reference.* St. Paul, MN: Mara Melum & Associates, 1993.

Melum, M. M., and Sinioris, M. K. *Total Quality Management: The Health Care Pioneers.* Chicago: American Hospital Publishing, 1992.

Monteforte, L., and Seemer, R. Winning more than the Malcolm Baldrige National Quality Award at AT&T Transmission Systems. *National Productivity Review,* Spring 1993, pp. 143–65.

Moran, J. W., Collett, C., and Cote, C. *Daily Management: A System for Individual and Organizational Optimization.* Methuen, MA: GOAL/QPC, 1991.

Porter, M. *Competitive Advantage: Creating and Sustaining Superior Performance.* New York City: The Free Press, 1985.

Rieley, J. Closing the loop: an effective planning process in higher education. Unpublished paper. The Center for Continuous Quality Improvement at Milwaukee Area Technical College.

Sahney, V., and Warden, G. The role of CQI in the strategic planning process. *Quality Management in Health Care* 1(4):1–11, Summer 1993.

Scholtes, P. R. *The Team Handbook.* Madison, WI: Joiner Associates, 1988.

Senge, P. M. *The Fifth Discipline: The Art and Practice of the Learning Organization.* New York City: Doubleday, 1990.

Sheridan, B. *Policy Deployment: The TQM Approach to Long-Range Planning.* Milwaukee, WI: ASQC Quality Press, 1993.

Tersteeg, D. Hoshin planning at Zytec. In GOAL/QPC Conference Notes. Methuen, MA: GOAL/QPC, 1991.

Voehl, F. W. Hoshin kanri, American style. *Quality Digest,* Oct. 1991, pp. 31–36.

Walton, M. *The Deming Management Method.* New York City: Dodd, Mead & Co., 1986.

Glossary

activity network diagram: One of the seven management and planning tools. Plots the sequence of steps in a plan. Shows where steps can be done simultaneously; also shows the longest (critical) path of steps. These are two forms of the activity network diagram—activity on node and activity on arrow (sometimes referred to as an arrow diagram). See *management and planning (MP) tools.*

affinity diagram: One of the seven management and planning tools. A method to organize ideas into natural groupings or themes, this tool stimulates the creative thinking that is an essential first step in breakthrough planning. Also known as KJ method.

alignment: The bringing together of parts of an organization (for example, departments or individuals) or multiple organizations into agreement or cooperation. The coordination of efforts and resources to develop and implement a plan. Such coordination may occur vertically (within a given work unit) or horizontally (across work units).

benchmarking: A process of measuring current products, services, and critical processes (business, clinical, technical) against those of the best in the world for the purpose of improving them.

breakthrough: Dramatic improvement in an organization's capabilities to provide products or services. Requires fundamental changes in organizational systems and/or structures.

CAPD cycle: See *check-analyze-plan-do (CAPD) cycle.*

catchball: An iterative, participative approach to develop, communicate, and finalize plans. As targets (or objectives) are developed, they are communicated to those involved in implementing them. Implementers give input to the development of means to achieve the targets. Dialogue about targets and means proceeds within and across departments until the plan is developed in sufficient detail. Then the process reverses itself: As the plan is finalized, it is rolled back up the organization and checked for gaps, overlaps, and feasibility.

cause-and-effect diagram: One of the seven basic process improvement tools. To identify all possible causes of a given effect or problem, the tool can be used to identify "root" causes so that problems are solved at a fundamental rather than a symptomatic or surface level. Also known as an Ishikawa or fishbone diagram.

check-analyze-plan-do (CAPD) cycle: A four-step approach that applies problem solving and management and planning tools to process improvement. The CAPD cycle involves the following steps:

1. *Check:* Develop a general understanding of the process to be improved.
2. *Analyze:* Measure customer expectations and identify root causes of problems.
3. *Plan:* Develop improvements that will solve the problems and exceed customer expectations.
4. *Do:* Implement the improvement plan, measure the results, and hold the gains.

check sheet: One of the seven basic process improvement tools. A form used to systematically record and compile data from historical sources or ongoing observations so that patterns and trends can be detected. In process improvement, check sheets help teams convert opinion hypotheses into fact.

continuous quality improvement (CQI): Management philosophy and methods that lead to ongoing efforts to do work better for the benefit of the customer. This improvement is usually accomplished by reducing variation or by improving the mean (average) performance of work processes.

control chart: One of the seven basic process improvement tools. A graph of process measurement data with statistically defined upper and lower control limits. Used to tell if a process is behaving as expected.

countermeasure: A means to solve a problem. A backup or contingency plan.

critical processes: The vital few business and/or technical procedures that, when performed successfully, allow an organization to fulfill its mission and to satisfy its customers. These processes form the infrastructure of the daily management system. Performance data from these processes are a source of input in selecting the organization's focus in hoshin planning.

cross-functional: Involving two or more departments or work units.

daily management system: The system that allows each work unit to identify, measure, control, and improve the work processes that are vital to achieving customer satisfaction and fulfilling the organization's mission. The daily management system works in concert with the hoshin planning system in two ways:

1. Process data from the daily management system reflect the health of critical organizational processes. These data are a vital input during step 1 of the hoshin planning process (choose the organization's focus).
2. The daily management system becomes important once again during development of the hoshin annual plan (step 2: align the organization with the focus). The means to achieve a part of the hoshin plan may require that certain critical processes be improved – incrementally or radically. Those improvements are monitored (step 3: implement the plan and monitor progress) and documented (step 4: review and improve) as a part of the hoshin planning process. Once institutionalized, they are sustained systematically as a part of the improved daily management system.

deploy/deployment: The act of converting the plan from strategic targets to action items, from general to specific. Deploying a hoshin plan involves cascading high-level targets down and across an organization, developing increasing detail and specificity. Deployment is a vehicle both for development and communication. While a plan is being deployed, those who will be involved in implementing the plan are given the opportunity to discuss and refine the meaning of the plan – before it goes into effect.

empowerment: The commitment to give people the vision, authority, capability, opportunity, and trust to make decisions and correct problems, improve processes, and satisfy customers.

fishbone diagram: See *cause-and-effect diagram.*

flag system: A method to display progress and contribution of departments toward an organizational target. The charts resemble flags on staffs.

flowchart: Sometimes included in lists of the seven basic process improvement tools. Used to show activities or sequential steps in a process – to make a process visible.

focus: Out of all the items of strategic importance to an organization, the focus is selected systematically and consciously as the area most vital to customer satisfaction and organizational success. Through the hoshin planning process, the focus is developed into a detailed plan designed to bring about a breakthrough level of improvement.

gap analysis: A method to display visually the difference between current and expected (or ideal) performance. The radar chart is a tool for conducting a gap analysis on a variety of factors. Also called spider diagram.

Golden Thread: A term used at AT&T to describe organizational alignment. Refers to the plan, made up of interconnected targets and means, the thread that aligns everyone around the same organizational focus. The "thread" is tied from each customer satisfier, to the company's leaders, to managers, and to all workers.

histogram: One of the seven basic process improvement tools. The chart displays variation in measurement data – for example, temperature or dimensions, which vary naturally over time if enough repeated measurements are taken. A histogram looks like a bar graph of data arranged in categories, ranging from low to high numbers. The height of the bar over each category of data represents how many data points fall into that category. The overall appearance of the histogram shows how widely the data points vary (from low to high) and in which categories most of the data points are concentrated.

hoshin: A Japanese term that refers to shiny metal, pointing or setting direction (like a compass).

hoshin kanri: A Japanes phrase that embodies two concepts: *hoshin* ("shining metal" or "pointing direction," like a compass) and *kanri* ("management" or "control"). Taken together, *hoshin kanri* means a systematic approach to setting and achieving strategic targets.

hoshin planning: A strategic planning and management system that focuses and aligns the organization to achieve breakthroughs for customers.

indicator: Sometimes called "a measure." A concept or progress of a piece of a plan (target or means) or status of a process.

integration: Coordinated, often cross-functional efforts to develop or carry out a plan.

interrelationship digraph: One of the seven management and planning tools. Displays the relationships among all the factors in a complex system or situation.

Ishikawa diagram: See *cause-and-effect diagram.*

KJ method: See *affinity diagram.*

Malcolm Baldrige National Quality Award: An award designed to recognize and share best practices in quality management systems within U.S. organizations. The award is managed by the National Institute of Standards and Technology, an agency of the United States Department of Commerce.

management and planning (MP) tools: A body of seven tools, also known as the seven new tools, used to gather, sort, and organize idea data during a planning process. They include the affinity diagram and interrelationship digraph (used in selecting the organization's focus); the tree diagram, prioritization matrix, and matrix diagram (used to develop means to achieve the focus); and the process decision program chart and activity network diagram (used to troubleshoot the detailed plan and chart out the final sequence of planning steps).

management by objectives (MBO): An approach whereby management specifies targets or objectives and holds work units and individuals accountable for obtaining results.

management by policy (MBP): Another name for hoshin planning.

matrix diagram: One of the seven management and planning tools. Used to show the existence and strength of relationships between two or more sets of factors.

MBO: See *management by objectives.*

MBP: See *management by policy.*

means: A way to accomplish a target.

mission: The purpose or charter statement of an organization. The reason for the organization's existence.

monthly or bimonthly review: Self-evaluation of performance against targets. An examination of things that helped or hindered performance and the corrective actions taken. Reviews emphasize both the progress made (outcomes/results) *and* the methods by which progress was achieved (process). Results and supporting data are summarized and documented for use in quarterly and annual reviews.

organizational culture: The pattern of shared beliefs, values, and behaviors acquired over time by members of an organization.

Pareto chart: One of the seven basic process improvement tools. A vertical bar chart that arranges causes by frequency of occurrence in descending order from left to right. Designed to identify which causes contribute most significantly to an observed effect.

PDPC: See *process decision program chart.*

plan-do-check-act (PDCA) cycle: Originally developed by Walter Shewhart, popularized by W. Edwards Deming. Scientific method by which improvements are planned, tried, and checked to see if they should be implemented, adapted, or abandoned.

policy deployment: One English translation for *hoshin kanri.*

prioritization matrix: One of the seven management and planning tools. Used to determine priorities among a variety of options, often based on multiple, weighted criteria.

problem-solving tools: The basic process improvement tools, which may include: cause-and-effect (fishbone) diagram, check sheet, run chart, Pareto chart, flowchart, histogram, control chart, and scatter diagram. In Japan, they are often collected in groups of seven, based on which tools are most used in an organization. Called the "seven quality control (7QC) tools," they are designed to analyze and display data and ideas.

process: A series of steps leading to a defined result. Processes transform inputs into outputs. In a collective sense, all people, machines, materials, and methods required to accomplish a task.

process capability: A measure that determines whether a process can deliver products and/or services that will satisfy customers by comparing the statistically derived limits of the process (what the process is capable of delivering) to the specification limits the customers place on the process (what the customers want).

process decision program chart (PDPC): One of the seven management and planning tools. Identifies what can go wrong in a plan, along with appropriate countermeasures – both preventive and contingency plans.

process improvement tools: See *problem-solving tools.*

process management: The activity that focuses on monitoring and improving processes to produce good results. Involves use of the seven basic process improvement tools.

quality function deployment (QFD): A process applied to understand customer expectations (the voice of the customer); to translate that voice into the language of the organization (technical terminology and measurements); and to carry the voice all the way through the design, development, and production of customer-pleasing products and services.

radar chart: A graphic display of how well several (5 to 15) elements in a system perform compared to a desired standard. Also known as a "spider diagram," the radar chart is a gap analysis tool. It gives a visual "report card" to the elements being assessed and identifies the biggest gaps between current and desired performance. In hoshin planning, the radar chart is useful as a focusing technique. See also *gap analysis.*

run chart: One of the seven basic process improvement tools. Displays process measurement data over time to see if the long-range average is changing. Also known as a time series graph.

scatter diagram: One of the seven basic process improvement tools. Used to test for the existence and strength of a relationship between two variables. Shows graphically what happens to one variable as the other variable changes.

seven new tools: See *management and planning (MP) tools.*

SDCA cycle: See *standardize-do-check-act cycle.*

7MP tools: See *management and planning tools.*

Shewhart cycle: See *plan-do-check-act (PDCA) cycle.*

SPC: See *statistical process control.*

spider diagram: See *gap analysis* and *radar chart.*

standardization maintenance: The method that ensures that everyone follows the current best practice for a process. Includes documenting and institutionalizing process improvements to ensure that gains are sustained.

standardize-do-check-act (SDCA) cycle: A variation of the PDCA cycle, wherein the first step involves planning to establish and maintain a process standard throughout the organization.

statistical process control (SPC): The act of using control charts to monitor process variation. Based on the nature of variation, a decision is made to allow the process to operate in its current state or to intervene and improve it.

strategic planning: A method by which an organization develops a dream of what it wants to be, develops plans to achieve that desired future state, and evaluates the implementation of those plans.

stratification: The act of breaking down the whole into smaller related parts, especially when the parts represent significantly different data sources.

system: A group of parts or processes that work together to accomplish a specific purpose.

target: A specific end result.

target/means matrix: Developed by Yoji Akao to show the relationship between the desired results of a plan and the methods used to achieve those results. The coupling of targets and means is a distinguishing feature of hoshin planning.

total quality management (TQM): A strategy to integrate quality philosophy and methods into the management of all aspects of an organization. Involves commitment to meeting and exceeding customer needs through continuous improvement of the work processes of everyone in the organization.

tree diagram: One of the seven management and planning tools. Assists in intermediate planning by breaking down plans into component parts. Systematically maps out the tasks and subtasks required to accomplish a plan.

values: Shared beliefs and attitudes, borne out by consistent behaviors that determine the character of an organization.

vision: An organization's dream of what it wants to be in the future. Based on a careful assessment of the most important directions for the organization, a vision provides direction for the hoshin planning process.

Note: Some definitions were adapted from glossaries in the following sources:

AT&T Quality Steering Committee. *Policy Deployment.* Indianapolis: AT&T, 1992.

Collins, B., and Huge, E. *Management by Policy.* Milwaukee, WI: ASQC Quality Press, 1993.

King, B. *Hoshin Planning: A Developmental Approach.* Methuen, MA: GOAL/QPC, 1989.

Index